NMS Q & A Family Medicine

2nd EDITION

NMS Q&A Family Medicine

2nd EDITION

David R. Rudy, MD, MPH

Professor, Former Chairman
Department of Family and Preventive Medicine
The Chicago Medical School
North Chicago, IL

Wolters Kluwer | Lippincott Williams & Wilkins
Health
Philadelphia · Baltimore · New York · London
Buenos Aires · Hong Kong · Sydney · Tokyo

Acquisitions Editor: Donna Balado
Managing Editors: Liz Stalnaker, Cheryl Stringfellow
Marketing Manager: Jennifer Kuklinski
Associate Production Manager: Kevin P. Johnson
Designer: Holly Mclaughlin
Compositor: Aptara

351 West Camden Street
Baltimore, MD 21201

530 Walnut Street
Philadelphia, PA 19106

The publisher is not responsible (as a matter of product liability, negligence, or otherwise) for any
injury resulting from any material contained herein. This publication contains information relating
to general principles of medical care that should not be construed as specific instructions for individual patients. Manufacturers' product information and package inserts should be reviewed for
current information, including contraindications, dosages, and precautions.

Printed in the United States of America

Library of Congress Cataloging-in-Publication Data

Rudy, David R.
    Family medicine / David R. Rudy. — 2nd ed.
        p. ; cm. — (NMS Q&A)
    ISBN–13: 978–0–7817–9188–5
    1. Family medicine—Examinations, questions, etc. I. Title. II. Series.
    [DNLM: 1. Family Practice—Examination Questions. WB 18.2 R917f 2008]
    RC58. R83 2008
    616—dc22

                                                                                    2007021018

*The publishers have made every effort to trace the copyright holders for borrowed material. If they have
inadvertently overlooked any, they will be pleased to make the necessary arrangements at the first
opportunity.*

To purchase additional copies of this book, call our customer service department at **(800) 638-3030**
or fax orders to **(301) 223-2320.** International customers should call **(301) 223-2300.**

Visit Lippincott Williams & Wilkins on the Internet: http://www.LWW.com. Lippincott Williams &
Wilkins customer service representatives are available from 8:30 am to 6:00 pm, EST.

06 07 08 09 10
1 2 3 4 5 6 7 8 9 10

This work is dedicated to my wife, Rose Mary S. Rudy, MA; our children Douglas David Rudy, Steven William Rudy, Katharine Rudy Hoffer, and Hunter Ashley Elam; and to our five grandchildren in descending order of age: Elizabeth Lynn Rudy, Michael Robert Rudy, Steven Douglas Rudy, Jacob Rudy Hoffer, and Molly Nicole Hoffer. Finally, I dedicate this work to the memory of my parents, Robert Sale Rudy, CPA, late retired CFO of the White Castle Corporation and Lois May Arthur Rudy.

Contents

SECTION XIII ALLERGIES

SECTION XIV PREVENTIVE CARE AND HEALTH

SECTION XV BEHAVIOR AND PSYCHOLOGY IN PRIMARY CARE

SECTION XVI MISCELLANEOUS AREAS OF CLINICAL PRACTICE

Foreword to the First Edition

Family medicine was the first specialty to require recertification to ensure that family physicians remain current in advances in medicine. We are continually challenging ourselves with questions of the type presented in this book. These questions help us remain abreast of new information and prepare for written examinations, whether they be the in-training exams given in the medical clerkships, to family practice residents, or the certification and recertification exams taken by physicians in practice.

The questions in this book focus on practical issues also presented in *Family Medicine: The House Officer Series*. The answers not only give the preferred course of action, but also discuss why other options are incorrect. New information is added, supplementing that provided in *Family Medicine: The House Officer Series*. These questions and the discussions of the answers give the reader insight into the problem-solving process in primary care, which often differs from that in the consulting specialties.

Dr. Rudy has, through *Family Medicine: The House Officer Series* and *NMS Q&A Family Medicine*, provided the reader with an excellent overview of our discipline by reflecting the variety of problems encountered in practice. It is this variety that keeps us perpetually challenged. These books let us keep pace with modern advances and help us sustain the excitement and satisfaction of primary care.

Robert E. Rakel, MD

Preface

The second edition of *Family Medicine Q&A*, in the respected NMS series, is again intended to provide study material for students in preparation for USMLE Steps 2 and 3 and Family Medicine clerkships. Every item from the first edition was revisited; obsolete material was deleted and material still relevant was presented anew from different pedagogical angles. Obviously there is new material presented on the basis of being well enough processed by the medical establishment that it enters into approved clinical practice. Only a few pithy questions that bear repetition were included in unchanged form from the first edition. As with the first edition, the exacting standards of Lippincott Williams & Wilkins ensure that the work remains worthy of the NMS. And once again, the project itself has been engrossing and fulfilling. I hope that the student and resident will benefit significantly.

David R. Rudy, MD, MPH

Acknowledgments

For the contributions to medical education I hope will be conveyed through book, I wish to acknowledge a great debt owed to Dean Arthur Ross and the faculty of the Chicago Medical School. They allowed me to devote a sabbatical year to the bulk of this work as I retired from the Chair of Family and Preventive Medicine. Further, I greatly appreciate the professionalism of Cheryl Stringfellow and Liz Stalnaker, managing editors with Lippincott Williams & Wilkins, with whom I worked throughout the project. Finally, I wish the best for Charley Mitchell, my first contact at Williams & Wilkins.

SECTION **I**

Problems of the Head, Eyes, Ears, Nose, and Throat

chapter **1**

Problems of the Ears, Throat, and Sinuses

Examination questions: *Unless instructed otherwise, choose the ONE lettered answer or completion that is BEST in each case.*

1 A 25-year-old, cigarette-smoking male sales manager makes an appointment for complaint of a prolonged course of a cold. He noted the onset of coryza 2.5 weeks ago; his rhinorrhea has persisted, producing a tenacious discharge, sometimes blood streaked, from the right naris. He gets bouts like this at least once every winter but has not sought treatment for the last 3 years until now. He admits to frequent "summer colds." When he leans forward, he feels a pain in his right facial region and sometimes a sense of shifting fluid in the right cheek. On examination he manifests tenderness of the right nasal rim of the orbit. Which of the following would be a logical therapeutic plan?

(A) Refer for allergy evaluation

(B) Obtain an otolaryngology consultation

(C) Prescribe a course of levofloxacin

(D) Administer a 500-mg injection of ceftriaxone

(E) Prescribe 500 mg of amoxicillin three times per day

2 The patient in Question 1, immediately after filling his prescription, joined friends on a canoeing trip into the wilds of the great north woods of Canada. On the third day he accidentally drops his pill bottle overboard. After the group reaches a distance equivalent to 5 days' travel from motorized transportation, the 25-year-old man, with known ethmoid and maxillary sinusitis, notes the onset of diplopia and the inability to direct his right eye gaze within the normal range. His friends notice the right eye has become chemotic (shows excessive edema of the conjunctivae). In addition, the man complains of blurred vision in his right eye. Which of the following is his likely complication?

(A) Brain abscess

(B) Osteomyelitis of the frontal bone

(C) Mucocele of the ethmoid

(D) Cavernous sinus thrombosis

(E) Orbital cellulitis

3 A 4-year-old girl has had five middle ear infections in each of the last 3 years; now, on March 15, she comes to you with an acute attack of earache on the right side, with a Weber test lateralizing to the left ear and a red, immobile eardrum with pus-fluid level on the right. The previous September you administered both influenza and pneumococcal vaccines, and you prescribed a regimen of daily amoxicillin between December 1 and March 1. What should be your next therapeutic move?

(A) Prescribe inhaled glucocorticoids

(B) Prescribe ventilation tubes

(C) Consult an otolaryngologist for possible adenoidectomy

(D) Consult an otolaryngologist for possible tonsillectomy

(E) Perform a skin test for desensitization

4 A 24-year-old man is in the examining room to complain of stuffy nose in the aftermath of a viral cold of 5 days' duration. He relates that he has taken a proprietary nasal spray for self-treatment of this symptom for the last 3 days, and he notes that the stuffiness has become bilateral and now interferes seriously with his sleep. Which of the following is an accepted rational approach to the treatment of this condition?

(A) Breathe through warm moist towels to open the nasal passages or mist for nasal inhalation combined with inhaled glucocorticoids for a brief period of time while the topical medication is withdrawn

(B) Prescribe more potent vasoconstrictors in a topical preparation

(C) Prescribe longer-acting nasal decongestants

(D) Perform skin testing and desensitization to treat atopic allergies

(E) Use a topical application of a basophile-stabilizing agent such as cromolyn

5 An African American mother brings to you her 4-year-old son, who is also African American. The child has an earache with onset the previous night and an associated fever with a temperature of 38.3°C (101°F). The mother is concerned because her son has had five bouts of middle-ear infection over the last year, three of which have occurred in the last 6 months. It is the month of February. The most likely underlying risk factor in the recurrence of the child's condition is

(A) Atopic constitution

(B) African American ancestry

(C) Exposure to cold winds

(D) Tonsillar hypertrophy, tonsillitis, or both

(E) Anterior attached frenulum

6 A 2-year-old child is brought to you for apparent dyspnea 4 days following coryza and fever (temperature, 39.5°C, 103.1°F). The fever has abated over the last 24 hours but the child is now coughing. The child's respiratory rate is 50 breaths per minute. The lung fields manifest a prolonged expiratory phase as well as diffuse wheezes and crackles during the expiratory phase. Which of the following statements is true regarding this condition?

(A) It is caused by influenza A/B.

(B) The chances of follicular tonsillitis are increased.

(C) There is a scant chance of future respiratory sequelae.

(D) The possibility of coincident otitis media is higher than that with other upper respiratory infections.

(E) It is caused by an adenovirus.

7 His mother brings to you a 4-year-old child for 12 hours of right-sided earache following 3 days of coryza, giving way to cough over the last 2 days. Neither the external ear nor the temperomandibular

joint is tender. The eardrum is retracted, fiery red, and slightly bulging, and it reveals a pus-fluid level. What are the three top-ranking bacterial organisms in the causation of this condition, in descending order of frequency?

(A) *Streptococcus pyogenes, Staphylococcus aureus, Klebsiella pneumoniae*

(B) *Moroxella catarrhalis, S. pyogenes, S. aureus*

(C) *M. catarrhalis, Pseudomonas sp, Haemophilus influenzae*

(D) *H. influenzae, S. pyogenes, S. aureus*

(E) *S. pneumoniae, H. influenzae, M. catarrhalis*

8 In the preceding vignette, which of the following ranges approximates the proportion of organisms involved in otitis media that would be expected to be resistant to penicillin and ampicillin?

(A) 10% to 20%

(B) 20% to 30%

(C) 30% to 40%

(D) 40% to 50%

(E) 50% to 75%

9 A 26-year-old woman complains of gradually developing hearing loss on the left side. Her left tympanic membrane appears to be discolored red as compared with the right. Which of the following must be present in order to make the diagnosis of otitis media?

(A) Pain located in the ear area without external tenderness

(B) Temperature >101°F

(C) Fiery red tympanic membrane

(D) Local tenderness of the tragus

(E) Conductive hearing loss in the involved ear

10 A 5-year-old girl is brought in by her mother for a routine physical examination to meet health standards requirements before entry into the first grade in school. During the examination you are reminded that you treated the girl for otitis media 5 weeks ago, her third attack since birth, and you note a fluid level behind the tympanic membrane that manifests a purplish color. When you mention this to the mother, she expresses concern and asks whether further treatment is required. Which of the following is your most appropriate answer?

(A) Yes. Otitis media should be entirely cleared by 10 days after treatment.

(B) Yes. Otitis media should be entirely cleared by 3 weeks after treatment.

(C) No. Treatment failure of otitis media is not established until 6 weeks have passed.

(D) No. Treatment failure of otitis media is not established until 16 weeks have passed.

(E) No. Treatment failure of otitis media is not established until 24 weeks have passed.

11 A 24-year-old man with type I diabetes mellitus comes to you with complaint of severe pain in the right ear with onset over the previous 24 hours. On examination you find the ear to be extremely tender upon light touch of the tragus and slight manipulation of the auricle. You diagnose external otitis and consider the possibility of malignant otitis externa. Which of the following defines that condition?

(A) Conductive hearing loss

(B) *Pseudomonas* sp

(C) Associated diabetes mellitus

(D) Osteomyelitis of the bony canal or mastoid

(E) Requirement of intravenous antibiotics

12 A 35-year-old woman who works on a noisy assembly line received a routine audiogram at her place of employment that showed a conductive hearing loss on the left. She was vaguely aware of increasingly turning her right ear toward conversation and using it for talking on the telephone. She denies pain, recent upper respiratory infection, and atopic constitution or allergic symptoms. Both eardrums move briskly when the patient performs a modified Valsalva maneuver (forced expiration against a closed nasopharyngeal cavity). The tympanic membrane exhibits a color more erythematous than the right eardrum does. Which of the following is the most likely diagnosis?

(A) Mild otitis media of the left ear

(B) Otosclerosis

(C) Noise-induced sensorineural hearing loss

(D) Ménière disease

(E) Labyrinthitis

13 An 18-year-old male patient complains of a sore throat, which began 5 days ago. There has been neither preceding or accompanying coryza nor cough, and the pain becomes worse toward the day's end. On examination you see a diffusely red posterior palate, and the anterior lymph nodes are enlarged and tender. Assuming a bacterial cause, which of the following is the most likely causation?

(A) *Neisseria meningitidis*

(B) *S. aureus*

(C) *M. catarrhalis*

(D) Beta-hemolytic *S. pyogenes*

(E) *K. pneumoniae*

14 A 45-year-old man, a right-handed, devout game hunter, complains that his wife notes he often turns his left ear to her in order to understand her in conversation. Which of the following is the most likely pattern to be found on a multiple-frequency audiogram?

(A) Flat audiogram across multiple frequencies in both ears

(B) Low-frequency hearing loss in the right ear

(C) Early complaint of difficulty hearing at a conversational level

(D) Deep involvement of the 4,000-Hz frequency in the right ear

(E) Crisp response to a hearing aid

15 A 45-year-old female patient is sent to you for follow-up from your junior partner's care 2 days ago with a diagnosis of left otitis media for which she was prescribed amoxicillin and told to see you, her personal physician, within a few days. You ask for what symptom she sought treatment, and she answers that she complained of hearing loss, which gradually increased over several months before she felt it necessary to seek a medical opinion. She denies previous coryza and vertigo. She does not shoot guns and works in an office as a public accountant. She feels tinnitus has gradually become prominent on the left. You examine her and find that her tympanic membrane is mobile but the color of the left eardrum is red streaked as compared with the right. The Weber test indicates sensorineural loss on the left (i.e., lateralizes to the right). Which of the following is the most likely cause of this woman's symptoms?

(A) Ménière disease

(B) Mild otitis media of the left ear

(C) Acoustic neuroma

(D) Impacted cerumen in the left ear

(E) Acoustic trauma to the left ear

16 Your 38-year-old patient, a Mexican-American man who runs his own landscaping business, comes to you for a routine physical examination, interested in knowing the status of his lipids and blood sugar. On routine otoscopy you notice that the anatomy of the left ear in the region of the tympanic membrane is unrecognizable. The patient then says that he has had a perforated eardrum for several years. Weber and Rinne tests indicate conductive hearing loss on the left side. Which of the following is the diagnosis?

(A) Otosclerosis

(B) Malignant external otitis

(C) Cholesteatoma

(D) Ménière disease

(E) Bullous myringitis

17 A 55-year-old woman comes to you for vertigo of recent and violent onset. She denies hearing loss and tinnitus. Which of the following characteristics reveals this as of peripheral origin (labyrinth) as opposed to central origin?

(A) Immediate onset of nystagmus and vertigo with the Hallpike maneuver

(B) Violent symptoms after a latent period upon motion of the head affecting the semicircular canals

(C) The causes include basilar artery insufficiency

(D) Associated nystagmus exhibiting a pendular motion

(E) It is associated with a conductive hearing loss

18 A 3-year-old girl presents with foul-smelling post-nasal drip, a temperature of 102°F, and perceptible swelling of the face. Which of the following is the most important reason to diagnose and treat this condition in a timely fashion?

(A) The patient presents with a malodorous discharge.

(B) Ethmoiditis may occur within the first 12 months of life.

(C) It may be caused by lactamase-producing organisms.

(D) Orbital cellulitis is a feared complication.

(E) Treatment must be carried out for 3 weeks.

19 A 55-year-old man complains of gradually increasing tinnitus over the last 2 years as well as two bouts of sudden drop in his hearing acuity noted on the right side, lasting 2 days in the first instance and for 12 hours in the second. With the first attack he noted vertigo and was treated with a meclizine-containing prescription drug by another physician. A Weber test lateralizes to the left ear. You suspect Ménière disease. Which of the following is an acceptable characterization of the pathophysiology of Ménière disease?

(A) This disease is caused by recurrent otitis media in childhood.

(B) The pathophysiology may involve an increased permeability of the Reissner membrane.

(C) The condition is autoimmune based and responds in many cases to glucocorticoid administration.

(D) Vertigo attacks are present in virtually all cases.

(E) The ossicles become adherent to one another.

20 A 23-year-old graduate student complains of sore throat for 3 days and requests an antibiotic to "head off strep," which he states he has been treated for frequently. He says he began having nasal discharge yesterday and has a slight cough. Although his throat was quite sore when he woke up this morning and when he called to make the appointment, the soreness abated by 11 AM. Which of the following is most likely the cause of his illness?

(A) Viral infections

(B) *Neisseria gonorrheae*

(C) *H. influenzae*

(D) *Corynebacterium diphtheriae*

(E) Beta-hemolytic *S. pyogenes*

21 You have diagnosed streptococcal pharyngitis in a child. What is the age range of susceptibility to the first attack of rheumatic fever in untreated streptococcal pharyngitis?

(A) 1 to 5 years

(B) 3 to 10 years

(C) 5 to 15 years

(D) 10 to 20 years

(E) 5 to 30 years

22 The patient in Question 21 is 12 years old. In order to prevent rheumatic fever in this child, how soon must treatment begin to eradicate the streptococcus (days or hours after onset)?

(A) 48 hours

(B) 5 days

(C) 9 days

(D) 15 days

(E) 20 days

23 A 22-year-old male medical student complains of severe sore throat for 3 days and says that he has been unable to ingest solid foods for the last 3 days. He appears moderately ill and in pain, with his head held in a "sniffing" type position; his lips are slightly parted, and he grimaces while swallowing saliva. The patient has muffled speech and sounds as though he is trying to talk with a hot potato in his mouth. There is no stridor. His temperature is 101°F (38.3°C). His cervical lymph nodes are visibly and palpably enlarged; tonsils are present and show an exudate whose color is a mixture of white and yellowish against an erythematous and edematous background. There are palatal petechiae. The rim of the epiglottis is visible above the base of the tongue and appears normal in color and size. Survey for other adenopathy yields nothing of note and an abdominal examination is negative for masses and organomegaly. A rapid streptococcal screen is negative. Therefore, you order a stat spot test for infectious mononucleosis, which is also negative. Despite the latter findings, because of the patient's state of illness, you elect to treat him with 250 mg of penicillin VK qid for 10 days. He returns in 4 days complaining that he is not improved and in fact is "miserable"; he appears just as uncomfortable as during the last visit and the cervical adenopathy has not abated discernibly. Which of the following is the most logical measure you should take at this time?

(A) Change the antibiotic to 500 mg of ampicillin tid for the balance of 10 days and instruct the patient to return in 48 to 72 hours

(B) Repeat the stat spot test for infectious mononucleosis

(C) Change the antibiotic to a newer macrolide (e.g., azithramycin) for the balance of 10 days

(D) Check HIV status and assume cytomegalovirus (CMV) is the cause of the patient's seronegative mononucleosis

(E) Hospitalize and consult an infectious disease specialist

24 A 35-year-old woman complains of cough that has become debilitating, though not very productive. The onset of her illness was 2 days before and was gradual, with low-grade fever, malaise, headache, and cough, which was at first mild. On inspection she does not appear seriously ill; she manifests tender red nodules on her anterior lower legs. Otologic examination reveals an abnormality of the left eardrum. The patient denies hearing loss and the eardrum moves when the patient performs a modified Valsalva maneuver, but the Weber test subtly lateralizes to the left side. Which of the following is the most logical empiric therapeutic approach to this patient?

(A) Prescribe 250 mg of penicillin VK four times per day for 10 days

(B) Prescribe a codeine-containing antitussive medication

(C) Prescribe 500 mg of extended release clarithramycin, two tablets daily for 3 weeks

(D) Prescribe 875 mg of amoxicillin three times a day for 10 days

(E) Prescribe an expectorant and reassure the patient

Examination Answers

1. The answer is E. Prescribe 500 mg of amoxicillin three times per day. This patient has typical right ethmoid sinusitis (by examination) as well as right maxillary sinusitis (by the history of shifting fluid in the cheek area). Ethmoiditis seldom occurs without concurrent maxillary sinusitis. Levofloxacin and ceftriaxone are too radical for this sinusitis, which has not been treated for at least 3 years and hence is not expected to involve exotic or resistant organisms. These drugs should be held in reserve. The sinusitis is likely a complication of allergic rhinitis, for which summer "cold" is a code word. Uncomplicated, it responds to antihistamines throughout the season of allergic symptoms, unlike viral colds, in which antihistamines remediate symptoms for no more than 3 to 4 days. Allergists seldom have anything to offer during the acute phase of complications. An ear, nose, and throat (ENT) consultation would be grossly premature.

2. The answer is D. This complication of ethmoid sinusitis is cavernous sinus thrombosis. At first glance it may be easily confused with orbital cellulitis, also a complication of ethmoid sinusitis. The difference in clinical presentation is that the latter manifests as proptosis of the involved eye and edema of the eyelids, as opposed to chemosis and ophthalmoplegia. Both conditions are medical emergencies and require rapid intervention with intravenous antibiotics (the outdoorsman in the vignette must phone in for life flight out of the bush). Mucocele is relatively benign by comparison and requires only aspiration and evacuation by an otolaryngologist. Brain abscess can be a complication of sinusitis and would present with neurologic symptoms and signs. Osteomyelitis of the frontal bone is a complication of frontal sinusitis and presents with swelling of the frontal bone.

3. The answer is A. Prescribe inhaled glucocorticoids to attempt to prevent recurrences of otitis media. Choices B and C, ventilation tubes and referral for adenoidectomy, would be the second and third choices, in that order.

4. The answer is A. Use warm moist towels to open the nasal passages or mist for nasal inhalation combined with inhaled glucocorticoids for a brief period following momentary withdrawal is an accepted rational approach to the treatment of *rhinitis medicamentosa*. Another approach is to use short-term systemic glucocorticoids. Prescription of longer-lasting topical decongestants is not a solution to this problem, which has been brought on by the overuse of such medications. When prescribed, topical decongestants should be used only intermittently, most likely on one side of the nose only and at the time of sleep onset. Although this condition may be more prevalent in atopic individuals, allergy is not the proximate cause and the condition is not served by skin testing at this point in the course.

5. The answer is A. Atopic constitution is an underlying factor in the recurrence of otitis media; in fact, it is probably the most prevalent one in this disorder. Native American but not African American race is a factor. Contrary to earlier teaching, tonsillar hypertrophy or tonsillitis is not a factor, though adenoidal hypertrophy is the second most prevalent underlying risk factor. Congenital palatal deformity renders one susceptible to recurrent otitis media. Anterior attached frenulum, or "tongue tied" state, is not a risk factor for recurrent otitis media. Because the most common precipitating insult is viral upper respiratory infection, superimposed on one of the foregoing risks, exposure to a population with increased incidence of viral upper respiratory infection is also an underlying risk factor.

6. The answer is D. The child has a respiratory infection and bronchiolitis caused by a respiratory syncytial virus (RSV), a member of the family Paromyxiviridae, sp *pneumovirus*. RSV carries a 30% to 60% risk of otitis media as a sequela, as compared with about 10% of cases of respiratory infections caused by the plurality of common colds, rhinoviruses (about 25% of common colds). Expiratory rales or "crackles" are unique to bronchiolitis in children. It is felt that children who have had bronchiolitis caused by RSV are at increased risk for asthma in their future.

7. The answer is E. *S. pneumoniae, H. influenzae,* and *M. catarrhalis* are the three most frequent bacterial causes of otitis media. *S. pyogenes,* the cause of "strep" pharyngitis and tonsillitis, is the agent of otitis media in just 5% of the cases, according to a typical study finding by Del Baccaro et al.

8. The answer is B. The range of 20% to 30% approximates the proportion of organisms involved in otitis media that would be expected to be resistant to penicillin and ampicillin. One-third of the 19% of otidides mediae caused by *H. influenzae* (some 6% of the total) are highly lactamase producing, whereas 80% to 90% of the 22% of cases caused by *M. catarrhalis* (some 20% of the total) are "low grade" producers.

9. The answer is E. Hearing loss in the involved ear that is conductive in character is a sine qua non for otitis media (assuming it is a hearing ear). A common mistake is to overinterpret perceived color change in the eardrum without checking to find whether there is a conductive hearing loss before making the diagnosis. Color changes attendant to otitis media vary from fiery red through purple and the creamy hue of pus, and apparent color change may be the stable state of an eardrum that is overlain with vascular ectasia.

10. The answer is D. Although most children will show nearly normal middle-ear findings by 3 to 4 weeks after treatment is instituted (or often even without treatment), otolaryngologists will not define a case as failure to respond on the basis of persistent effusion until 16 weeks have passed.

11. The answer is D. Osteomyelitis of the bony canal or mastoid is present by definition in malignant otitis externa. The characteristics listed in the distracters are all true, except that conductive hearing loss, though often present in external otitis secondary to debris that is blocking the canal, is not necessary for the diagnosis and not necessarily present in either uncomplicated or malignant external otitis. *Pseudomonas* sp remains the most common pathogen. Associated diabetes mellitus is the most common underlying condition rendering the patient susceptible, and there is virtually always a requirement of intravenous antibiotics.

12. The answer is B. In otosclerosis a conductive loss occurs in the face of completely normal physical examination, including mobile tympanic membrane. The perceived color change of the eardrum on the affected side is a "red herring." Otitis media cannot exist without a conductive hearing loss. In all other forms of conductive hearing loss, either the external canal is occluded on examination or the tympanic membrane is immobile or nearly so, as a result of exudate (purulent or serous), or nonfunctional as a result of perforation. A noise-induced hearing loss is a sensorineural loss, not a conductive loss. Ménière disease also causes a sensorineural loss, and classically it is associated with prominent tinnitus and vertigo. Labyrinthitis causes vertigo without hearing loss. In otosclerosis a conductive loss is the first clinical manifestation. It is a cause of hearing loss that is curable through surgery to free the adhesive new bone formation that prevents vibration of the stapes footplate within the oval window. Otosclerosis is inherited as an incompletely penetrant Mendelian-dominant trait that affects whites more than other racial groups. Its progress is accelerated by pregnancy.

13. The answer is D. Beta-hemolytic *S. pyogenes* is virtually the only cause of bacterial pharyngitis. Other bacterial causes are relatively rare. *Corynebacterium diphtheriae* and *Neisseria gonorrheae* make up about 5% of the cases of bacterial pharyngitis. Epiglottitis is caused by *H. influenzae*. Although it is often said that no one historical or physical finding can differentiate streptococcal from viral pharyngitis, the constellation shown in this vignette is significant and helpful: The first and continuing dominant symptom is sore throat; symptoms are worse toward the end of the day (whereas viral sore throat is more often worst in the morning); coryza and cough are absent.

14. The answer is D. The patient has hearing loss caused by chronic exposure to noise, affecting the right ear selectively in a right-handed rifle shooter. On an audiogram the vertical axis represents decibels of hearing *loss* ranging from "minus 10" (10 db better than "normal" at the top) to up to a 60-db loss going downward on the chart. The horizontal axis shows the sound frequencies in the hearing range in cycles per second or Hertz moving upward in frequency from left to right (connecting the points of hearing threshold, one would see that normal hearing would be a flat line across the top of the graph). The 4,000-Hz frequency is the first and most severely affected frequency (deepest loss on a tonal audiogram) involved in noise-induced hearing loss. As the 4,000-Hz frequency is more deeply affected, the adjacent frequencies become involved (e.g., 3,000 and 5,000 Hz), producing on the audiogram the noise-induced "V" (see Table 1–1). A flat audiogram showing depression of the threshold uniformly across the frequencies is more characteristic of a conductive hearing loss than of a sensorineural loss. Early involvement of conversational frequencies is not a strong characteristic of noise-induced loss, as most conversation occurs at lower frequencies. However, when conversational frequencies are affected, it involves higher voices, such as those of women and girls, for which the patient first notes a problem. As a sensorineural hearing loss, noise-induced loss is not as amenable to a hearing aid as are conductive losses. Table 1–1 is a depiction of an audiogram showing a noise-induced hearing loss; the dip is earliest and deepest at 4,000 Hz or 4 KHz.

TABLE 1–1   Audiogram Showing the Noise-Induced V Shape

db 500 Hz	1 KHz	2 KHz	3 KHz	4 KHz	5 KHz	6 KHz	7 KHz	8 KHz
0								
10	X	X				X	X	X
20			X		X			
30								
40				X				

15. The answer is C. An acoustic neuroma is a slowly growing benign growth, the most common of cerebellopontine angle tumors, comprising 78% of that category. Gradual expansion may involve other cranial nerves as well; for example, trigeminal and visual dysfunction can result through space occupation. Acoustic neuromas present with hearing loss, sensorineural to be sure, in little more than 50% of cases, with the remainder presenting with tinnitus, vertigo (9%), or unsteadiness. Female individuals are involved more than male individuals, at a ratio of 3:2. When bilateral, acoustic neuroma may be a manifestation of Von Recklinghausen disease. Both otitis media and cerumen impaction cause conductive hearing loss. Acoustic trauma causes sensory hearing loss but comes on more slowly and is associated with clearly identified causes by history. Although Ménière disease may present as isolated hearing loss without vertigo (and acoustic neuroma with vertigo and tinnitus, much like Ménière disease), the course of Ménière disease is always episodic rather than steadily progressive. The perceived color change does not fit with other findings in this case and thus must be attributed to an unrelated cause, such as a vascular variation on the tympanic membrane.

16. The answer is C. Caused by chronic otitis media, this complication is nearly always the result of a nonhealing perforated tympanic membrane. The interaction of the ectodermal and entodermal elements of the eardrum combine to form an expanding "benign" mass that occupies space and may destroy the ossicular chain, impinge on the facial nerve, and lead to such complications as meningitis. Treatment is usually surgical. Neither otosclerosis nor Ménière disease manifests any visible abnormalities on examination. Although this condition may resemble chronic external otitis in that the latter would show debris in the canal, gentle lavage would reveal the deeper-lying findings as middle-ear elements. Bullous myringitis is easily seen as a deformity of the recognized eardrum.

17. The answer is B. Vertigo of peripheral origin is characterized by violent symptoms after a latent period of 15 to 60 seconds, after motion of the head affecting the semicircular canals, such as the Hallpike maneuver. Having symptoms immediately upon motion of the head affecting the semicircular canals is characteristic of centrally based vertigo. This syndrome may be caused by vestibular neuronitis, benign positional vertigo, and Ménière disease, among others, though Ménière disease is usually associated with hearing loss and tinnitus (and would be expected to recur). Nystagmus that is due to a peripheral cause manifests fast and slow phases and tends to be relieved by fixation of gaze upon a fixed point.

18. The answer is D. The patient has ethmoid sinusitis (ethmoiditis). The most important reason to diagnose and treat this condition within a day or two is the feared complication of orbital cellulitis. The other statements are all true as well, except that in cases diagnosed early, treatment may be completed within 10 days instead of a mandatory 3 weeks.

19. The answer is B. The pathophysiology may involve an increased permeability of the Reissner membrane (in Ménière disease). None of the other statements is true regarding Ménière disease. It is a condition that can cause a sensorineural hearing loss, tinnitus, and vertigo. Although severe vertigo is the trademark of Ménière disease, it does not occur at all in some cases. The condition responds in many cases to dietary salt restriction and to judicious use of diuretics. Ablative surgery may be required.

20. The answer is A. Viral infections account for between 62% and 90% of cases of pharyngitis, depending on the time of year and geographic locale; a plurality of 25% are due to rhinoviruses. All other choices are possible bacterial causes, of which beta-hemolytic *S. pyogenes* comprises >95%. In this case the early addition of coryza and cough to the patient's symptoms and the increased soreness when he awakens in the morning underscore the great likelihood of a viral basis.

21. The answer is C. The first attack of rheumatic fever occurs in untreated Group A beta-hemolytic streptococcal infections in persons between the ages of 5 and 15 years.

Subsequent attacks, however, may occur up to the age of 30. Prevention is most effective through monthly injections of 1.2 million units of benzathine penicillin G.

22. The answer is C. Beta strep must be treated within 7 to 9 days in order to be certain of the prevention of rheumatic fever in children infected with Group A beta-hemolytic *S. pyogenes.*

23. The answer is B. Repeat the stat spot test for infectious mononucleosis. The clinical picture is classic for infectious mononucleosis, given the description and severity of symptoms in the absence of tenderness. The immunologic screens and certainly the heterophile agglutination test are known to require 5 to 7 days of illness, and in some cases as long as 4 weeks, before they become positive. Nevertheless, the decision to treat as streptococcal disease was justified, given the degree of illness, even though the streptococcal screen was negative. Rapid screening tests are only 80% to 87% sensitive. Not mentioned is that this patient, if he has infectious mononucleosis, would have >90% chance of developing a maculopapular or sometimes a petechial rash if ampicillin were instituted, compared with 15% in patients with infectious mononucleosis who are not treated with ampicillin. Generalized adenopathy, though expected logically, given the pathophysiology of infectious mononucleosis, is often not appreciable. The cervical adenopathy is frequently notable posteriorly rather than anteriorly as is found in streptococcal disease, but this is not a dependable distinction in this patient. With infectious mononucleosis there is a 50% chance of splenomegaly. For that reason patients must be cautioned to avoid contact sports for at least 6 weeks. CMV infection is the most common cause of seronegative mononucleosis (wherein the heterophile antibodies, the basis of the stat spot test for infectious mononucleosis, never rise). Both CMV and toxoplasmosis may present in a similar manner to infectious mononucleosis but are less likely to manifest exudative pharyngitis. CMV can be cultured, but if it is strongly suspected and the culture is negative, then HIV should be tested for as the possible underlying basis for susceptibility to CMV.

24. The answer is C. Given the subacute onset of febrile disease (in influenza, fever is present from the first hours), the hacking, troubling cough, the headache, and the bullous myringitis, a good clinical empiric approach is expectant treatment for mycoplasmal disease. This is the classic cause of the definitive atypical pneumonia (although mycoplasma disease causes pneumonia in only 5% to 10% of patients who have the infection). Mycoplasma responds to tetracyclines and to the macrolides, including clarithramycin—not to the penicillins. Expectorants and antitussives are needed as supportive therapy but are not truly therapeutic. Bullous myringitis comprises a bleb on the eardrum, with fluid dissecting the ectodermal and entodermal elements of the tympanic membrane, without eustachian tube dysfunction necessarily being present. Because of the awkwardness of eardrum mobility, it might be expected for there to be a mild conductive hearing loss.

References

Del Baccaro MA, Mendelman PM, Inglis AF, et al. Bacteriology of acute otitis media: A new perspective. *J Pediatr.* 1992; 120: 81–84.

Handzel O, Halperin D. Necrotizing (malignant) external otitis. *Am Fam Physician.* 2003; 68:309–312.

Neff M. AAP, AAFP, AAO-HNS release guideline on diagnosis and management of otitis media with effusion. *Am Fam Physician.* 2004; 69:2929–2931.

Rudy DR. Problems of the ears, throat and sinuses. In: Rudy DR, Kurowski K, eds. *Family Medicine: House Officers Series.* Baltimore: Williams & Wilkins; 1997:1–26.

chapter 2

Problems of the Oral Cavity

Examination questions: Unless instructed otherwise, choose the ONE lettered answer or completion that is BEST in each case.

1 A new mother brings in her 2-month-old daughter for routine well baby care. She was born vaginally at 40 weeks of gestation and has had an uneventful course to date. The mother asks about dental care. Which of the following statements is true regarding routine pediatric dental care and prevention of caries?

(A) Dental care need not be initiated until the secondary teeth have all erupted.

(B) Because the family lives in a community that has fluoridation of the water system, caries will not be a problem.

(C) As long as the child is trained to avoid sugars, caries can be evaded.

(D) Starting between 6 and 12 months of age, the child is at risk of developing caries.

(E) Prevention of caries is a moot point in dealing with deciduous teeth.

2 The mother of the child in Question 1 asks which of the following food substances is the most likely to cause cavities for her child's teeth. Your answer is

(A) Cow's milk

(B) Enfamil

(C) Soy formula with sucrose

(D) Similac

(E) On-demand mother's milk

3 The mother of the child in Question 1 asks also when (at what age of the child) to expect the eruption of the last of the deciduous dentition. Your answer is

(A) 18 months

(B) 2.5 years

(C) 3.5 years

(D) 4 years

(E) 6 years

4 A few years later, the mother of the child in Question 1 brings in her daughter, now 6 years old. She has a neighbor with a child of the same age who has "sprouted" her front teeth, and she is concerned because her daughter has not shown eruption of any of her adult teeth. You reassure her with the statement that the first permanent teeth should erupt at which of the following ages:

(A) 4 to 6 years

(B) 6 to 7 years

(C) 9 to 10 years

(D) 12 to 13 years

(E) 17 to 22 years

5 The mother of an 18-month-old male child notes that there is no fluoridation of the water in her community. She asks if there are any side effects to fluoride treatments for children at that age. Your answer is

(A) No. The child can only *benefit* from fluoride treatments because of prevention of caries.

(B) Yes. Fluorosis may result but only if oral fluoride is the mode of administration.

(C) Yes. Fluorosis may result but only if the fluoride is applied topically.

(D) Yes. Fluorosis may result whether topical or systemic (oral) fluoride is the mode of treatment.

(E) No. Fluoride is a harmless substance.

6 Apropos the previous question, what is the standard concentration of fluoride in the treated public water supply?

(A) 0.6 parts per million (ppm)

(B) 1 ppm

(C) 2 ppm

(D) 2 mg/kg/day

(E) 5 mg/kg/day

7 The foregoing notwithstanding, at what age should a child be started on fluoride treatments?

(A) Birth

(B) 3 months

(C) 6 months

(D) 1 year

(E) 2 years

8 You warn the mother in Question 5 that children may acutely overdose on fluoride; they are at risk for each of the following toxic sequelae *except*

(A) Hypocalcemia

(B) Diastolic myocardial dysfunction

(C) Convulsions

(D) Ventricular dysrhythmias

(E) Tetany

9 Which of the following statements about *home* dental care of children is true?

(A) The parents should take the child to the dentist for the first time by the age of 26 months, about the age of eruption of the last of the deciduous teeth.

(B) If a child under the age of 18 months is irritable and teething, the child may have a low-grade fever.

(C) Bottle propping is acceptable as long as the bottle does not contain sugary liquids.

(D) Dental caries in parents may lead to dental caries in their children.

(E) The earliest sign of caries in children is a brown or black concavity in a tooth.

10 A 75-year-old man complains for 3 weeks of irritation of the tongue. An examination shows fiery redness of the entire dorsum of the tongue. The causes of this condition include all but *which* of the following?

(A) Pernicious anemia

(B) Riboflavin deficiency

(C) Iron deficiency

(D) Excessive smoking

(E) Rubeola

11 Regarding the man featured in Question 10, which of the following would tend to support a diagnosis of riboflavin deficiency?

(A) The patient has a history of melena.

(B) The patient has a chronic cough and sits with lips pursed and shoulders hunched.

(C) The patient has spider angiomata scattered over the anterior chest.

(D) There are Koplik spots in the buccal mucosa.

(E) The patient is unable to perform the finger-to-nose test with his eyes closed.

12 A 22-year-old woman complains of an increasingly severe sore throat over the last 4 days, worse in the evening, without evolution to coryza or cough. The appearance of the throat is that of diffuse redness; anterior cervical lymph nodes are tender. Which of the following organisms is virtually the sole possible bacterial cause of this condition?

(A) *Streptococcus pneumoniae*

(B) *Streptococcus pyogenes*

(C) *Staphylococcus aureus*

(D) *Moraxella catarrhalis*

(E) *Haemophilus influenzae*

13 A 35-year-old male patient comes to you for a second opinion, having been to his dentist by whom he was advised to undergo extraction of his remaining three unerupted third molars ("wisdom teeth"). One month ago he had undergone incision and drainage of an abscess formed around his left lower third molar, which had been only partially erupted, showing two cusps above the gum line. In your response, which of the following do you indicate is the most significant sequela of failure of eruption and consequent impaction of third molars?

(A) Malocclusion

(B) Cosmetic implications

(C) Inability to masticate with the molars

(D) Formation of dentigerous cysts

(E) Abscess formation

14 A 17-year-old girl is brought to you for the complaint of sore throat. You note the presence of petechiae of the mucosa overlying the hard palate. Cervical lymph nodes are notably enlarged and palpable but not tender. Which of the following *nonbacterial* diseases could explain the foregoing?

(A) Herpes simplex I

(B) Infectious mononucleosis

(C) Herpes simplex II

(D) Influenza A virus

(E) Rhinovirus

15 A male teenager and his family complain of his having severe mouth soreness for the last 10 days. Examination discloses a fetid odor and fibrous pseudomembranes on many gingival crests. Which of the following diagnoses best fits this situation?

(A) Acute necrotizing gingivitis

(B) Periodontal abscess

(C) Dentigerous cyst

(D) Herpes labialis

(E) Molar impaction

16 A 55-year-old man was found sleeping in an alley and smelling of alcohol. He complained of swelling of the anterior neck and is brought to the emergency department of your hospital. Physical examination shows edema and erythema of the area of the anterior neck as it merges with the floor of the mouth. Percussion of the teeth reveals a tender area surrounding a lower partially erupted third molar. What is this form of oral cavity infection called?

(A) Caseous scrofula

(B) Cavity formation with secondary lymph nodes

(C) Coronary insufficiency

(D) Ludwig angina

(E) Mucosal epidermolysis

Examination Answers

1. The answer is D. Children are at risk of development of caries from the age of their first (primary) dentition. The central maxillary incisors erupt when the child is between the ages of 6 and 12 months. At about 1 year, the first molars erupt; at 2 years, the second or posterior molars erupt. Fluoridation of water or systemic fluoridation by medication reduces the chances of caries formation by 50%. Avoidance of sugar is important but not a guarantor against tooth decay. Soy-based formulas have a tendency to contain sucrose, which is an obvious risk factor for caries formation.

2. The answer is C. Cow's milk (which is also the basis of Enfamil and Similac) and mother's milk are the least likely among baby foods to predispose babies to caries formation. The lactose of cow's milk may actually be protective. Indigenously present sugars, such as fructose, are less cariogenic than introduced sugars such as sucrose. Premature birth (low birth weight) and low socioeconomic status are strong risk factors for caries formation. Bottle propping, especially when the feed contains sweetening, predisposes to cavities. Propping, a substitute for attention, presumably results in unnecessarily prolonged exposure to the cariogenic substance. Having carious deciduous teeth constitutes a risk factor for having caries in permanent dentition.

3. The answer is B. The last teeth should have erupted by the time the child reaches the age of 30 months. The peak times of eruption for the individual teeth are as follows (note that they erupt in mesiolateral order, front to back): Maxillary and mandibular incisors, 6 to 12 months; mandibular and maxillary lateral incisors, 11 to 13.2 months; mandibular and maxillary cuspids ("canines"), 15.6 to 16 months; mandibular and maxillary first molars, 19.5 to 19.6 months; and mandibular and maxillary second molars, 26.5 to 28 months.

4. The answer is B. The peak times for eruptions of the various permanent dentition are as follows: First premolars, 6 to 6.3 years; central and lateral mandibular incisors, 7.2 years; maxillary incisors, 8.5 years; mandibular cuspids or canines, 9.7 years; maxillary cuspids, 11.6 years; maxillary premolars, 10 to 10.7 years; mandibular premolars, 10.7 to 11.5 years; first molars, 6 to 7 years; second molars, 10.7 to 11.5 years; and third molars or wisdom teeth, 20 to 20.5 years.

5. The answer is D. Administering fluoride topically (e.g., by using fluoride-containing toothpastes) or orally before the age of 2 years appears to carry an increased risk of fluorosis, which is mottling of the teeth. Fluorosis in these children is mild when dosing has been reasonable.

6. The answer is B. The standard for fluoride supplementation in public water supplies is 1 ppm; 0.6 ppm is the point below which prescriptive supplementation should be initiated. A major overdosage would be 2.2 mg /kg/day; however, 2.2 mg of sodium fluoride daily is the recommended dosage to obtain 1 mg of fluoride in communities without supplementation in their water supply, at or above 0.03 ppm for children in the age range of 6 to 16 years. In a single dose, 5 mg/kg constitutes a critical toxic dose (see Question 8).

7. The answer is C. Children should start receiving fluoride at 6 months of age. This would be in the form of a supplement if the well water or household water is not fluoridated commercially or publicly at a concentration of more than 6 ppm. Supplement should be topical, oral, or both. The child should not receive fluoride supplementation if he or she is breastfeeding, and in any event not until the age of 6 months.

8. The answer is B. Acute toxicity from fluoride may cause each of the listed sequelae except for diastolic myocardial dysfunction. In fact, all of the other listed effects emanate from the hypocalcemia that ensues from an acute overdose of fluoride: tetany, convulsions, and ventricular dysrhythmias. Myocardial contractility in fact is decreased, the opposite of what occurs in diastolic dysfunction. Acute fluoride overdose at doses less than 5 mg/kg can cause nausea and vomiting. For an average-sized 5-year-old child, this amounts to half of a 95-mL tube of fluoridated toothpaste. Prescriptions for fluoride supplement should not exceed a total of 120 mg.

9. The answer is D. Bacteria that cause dental caries (i.e., mutans streptococci in the great majority) can be transferred among members of a household, including from

[handwritten margin notes: "Decidous Teeth Eruption" and "Permanent Teeth Eruption"]

mother to newborn child. Children should be taken to the dentist by the age of 1 year. Teething is not a cause of fever in infants. Bottle propping is unacceptable according to dental opinion, for many reasons: First, because of the temptation to overfeed improper foods; second, there may eventually be mechanical effects on the dentition. The typical yellow to brown to black discoloration is not the first appearance of caries. They are preceded by white spots or lines.

10. The answer is E. Rubeola or "hard measles," although classically producing the buccal Koplik spot, does not cause glossitis. All the other listed conditions may be associated with glossitis.

11. The answer is C. Most vitamin deficiencies in the United States occur in multiples and are associated with alcoholism, malabsorption, or iatrogenic causes such as medications, renal dialysis, and total parenteral nutrition. Alcoholism looms high on the list, and a classic sign thereof is the existence of spider angiomata and other forms of telangiectasia. Melena is a sign of gastrointestinal blood loss, a chief cause of iron deficiency. The hunched, dyspneic patient is likely a smoker with chronic obstructive lung disease who is not necessarily malnourished. Inability to perform finger-to-nose testing is a sign of poor proprioception and hence can be associated with pernicious anemia (subacute combined degeneration).

12. The answer is B. Beta-hemolytic streptococcus is virtually the only bacterial cause of bacterial pharyngitis. Streptococcal pharyngitis causes increasingly severe symptoms throughout the day, whereas viral pharyngitis, as the harbinger of a viral upper respiratory infection, is worst in the morning upon awakening. Although there is no single reliable symptom or sign of streptococcal infection in the throat, the combination of the chronicity and progression of symptoms in this case, along with tenderness of the anterior cervical nodes and the cellulitic appearance of the throat, point to such an infection. *S. pneumoniae*, the most common cause of bacterial pneumonia, is not an oral pathogen; nor are Staphylococci (except in unusual circumstances), *M. catarrhalis*, or *H. influenzae*.

13. The answer is D. The third molars are commonly only partially erupted in the adult. For this reason, they are the foci of frequent abscesses that are due, of course, to the beta-hemolytic *S. pyogenes*. Further, when third molars or wisdom teeth remain totally unerupted, they

may form dentigerous cysts (expansions of the original cocoon of the molar roots); these may grow slowly over time, taking on the characteristics of benign tumors, dislodging other teeth, and eroding the maxillary or mandibular arch. Malocclusion is not a significant occurrence in this condition. There are no cosmetic implications with unerupted third molars. Chewing is seldom a problem except in the partially erupted molar that has abscess formation.

14. The answer is B. Infectious mononucleosis and streptococcal pharyngitis each may cause petechiae over the hard palate, though the question regards nonbacterial cause only. In children, herpangina (not mentioned among the choices) causes palatal petechiae and occurs mostly in preschool-age children, generally up to 4 years of age. It may occur, however, as late in childhood as 16 years. In the present case, the existence of impressive lymphadenopathy without tenderness is typical of mononucleosis.

15. The answer is A. Periodontitis progresses to gingivitis, which, if untreated and severe, leads to acute necrotizing gingivitis or trench mouth. Periodontal abscess consists of a focal lesion under pressure, which is quite painful. Dentigerous cysts are not visible on oral examination. Molar impaction is the primary lesion from which dentigerous cysts form, nearly always involving a third molar that has not erupted and that impinges on surrounding structures, especially after cyst formation (see the discussion of Question 13).

16. The answer is D. Ludwig angina is cellulitis of the submandibular space by extension from the sublingual area. It usually results from an infection of a dental site, such as that from an infected extraction site, root canal therapy, or abscessed third molar. Scrofula is tuberculous involvement of cervical nodes and as such consists of obvious adenopathy. Coronary insufficiency may cause anginal pains that radiate into the neck, but nearly always this occurs unilaterally and is not associated with local findings. Mucosal epidermolysis occurs on the mucosa, not the skin.

References

Tryon AF, Stechfus CF. Problems of the oral cavity. In: Rudy DR, Kurowski K, eds. *Family Medicine: House Officer Series*. Baltimore: Williams & Wilkins; 1997:27–42.

U.S. Preventive Services Task Force. Prevention of dental caries in preschool children: Recommendations and rationale. *Am Fam Physician*. 2004; 70:1529–1532.

chapter **3**

Headache and Neuralgic Pain Management

1 A patient enters your practice with complaint of recent onset of acute headache. Which of the following would be the least indicative of serious pathology underlying the cause of the headache?

(A) Occipitonuchal distribution

(B) Age 50 years

(C) Headache waking the patient from sleep

(D) History of taking ibuprofen daily for arthritis

(E) Increasing frequency of the headaches over time

2 A 35-year-old woman complains of headaches that are throbbing and frontal or occipital in distribution. These have been occurring for most of her adult life but have become more severe over the last several days, lasting the whole day, several times per week. They require her to take over-the-counter ibuprofen once or twice weekly and usually respond thereto. Although the headaches remit during sleep, they recur during the day. Neurological history (including inquiry regarding visual and other neurological symptoms accompanying the headaches) and examination are negative. Funduscopy is negative for hemorrhages, exudates, and papilledema. Blood pressure is 116/75. Which of the following is most likely as the diagnosis of the headaches?

(A) Tension headache

(B) Cluster headache

(C) Migraine headache

(D) Intracranial hemorrhage

(E) Sinusitis

3 The patient in Question 2 was treated successfully 2 years ago and did well until the last 3 months, during which time the headaches have increased in frequency. For the last 4 weeks her headaches have occurred daily. She is now taking ibuprofen three times per week and also complains of fatigue despite her increased sleep requirements. The headaches may be unilateral or retro-orbital in distribution. The examination is otherwise unchanged from that of 2 years ago. Which of the following most likely explains the new pattern of her headaches?

(A) Cluster headache

(B) Migraine headache

(C) Carotid artery dissection

(D) Sinusitis

(E) Tension headache

4 A 45-year-old man complains of daily unilateral headaches associated with rhinorrhea and tearing for the past several weeks. Vascular examination is normal. There are no visual or musculoskeletal symptoms. Which of the following is the most likely diagnosis?

(A) Migraine headache

(B) Temporal arteritis

(C) Cluster headache

(D) Hemicrania continua

(E) Sinusitis

5 A 42-year-old woman complains of recent onset of facial pain in the areas of the left cheek, left jaw, and the ante-auricular area on the left side. There has been no rash and this is the first time the patient has experienced these symptoms. The pain is lancinating, and it is precipitated by touching the skin of the affected areas, by chewing, and sometimes by talking. Which of the following is possibly associated with this syndrome?

(A) Dental abscess

(B) Temporomandibular joint arthritis

(C) Vascular compression of the gasserian ganglion

(D) Maxillary sinusitis

(E) Herpes zoster (HZ)

6 A patient presents exactly as the person in Question 5 except that she complains also of disturbed vision and recent onset of urinary retention. Which of the following is the most likely cause of this patient's symptoms?

(A) Vascular impingement on the gasserian ganglion

(B) Posterior fossa epidermoid cyst

(C) Multiple sclerosis

(D) Sepsis

(E) Amyotrophic lateral sclerosis

7 Your female patient, an elementary school teacher, complains of paroxysms of right occipital pain. Examination is negative except for local tenderness over the right side of the occipital scalp at the ridge, and tapping the area produces a shocklike pain in the area of the headache. What is this pain called?

(A) Tension headache

(B) Occipital neuralgia

(C) Migraine variant

(D) Cluster headache

(E) Giant cell arteritis

8 Which of the following patients with HZ (or shingles) is *least* likely to suffer from post-herpetic neuralgia?

(A) A 25-year-old woman with abdominal zoster, one dermatome involved

(B) A 76-year-old man with abdominal dermatomal involvement

(C) A 25-year-old man with HZ involvement of the ophthalmic branch of the trigeminal nerve

(D) A 45-year-old person with sacral involvement

(E) A 55-year-old person with sciatic branch involvement

9 You are examining a 66-year-old man who was brought to you by a friend; the man states that less than an hour earlier he was walking from his yacht club to

his car and abruptly developed a very severe headache in his occipital area and upper neck. He had never before experienced a headache. There is no reported drug use and he denies taking any prescription medication. Vital signs are normal, except for blood pressure, which is 150/90. The patient's head shows no ecchymosis, and stethoscopy reveals no bruits. For the eyes, the pupils are equal and reactive. Fundi appear normal; extraocular movements are normal. There is resistance to flexing and rotation in the neck. Neurologically, the patient is sleepy but arousable. He can respond to questions, but they must frequently be repeated. He can move all extremities and sensation to touch is intact in all extremities. Deep tendon reflexes are normally reactive and symmetrical. Which of the following would you order first to evaluate this patient?

(A) A computed tomography (CT) scan of head without contrast

(B) A CT scan of head with contrast

(C) A magnetic resonance image (MRI) of the brain

(D) A cerebrospinal fluid examination

(E) An erythrocyte sedimentation rate

10 A 71-year-old man complains of right-sided headache, coming on only within the last several months. Last week he noted that, when he was chewing enthusiastically, his jaw on the right side began to be stiff and painful. Examination reveals tenderness of the right temporal artery. Dental examination is negative. A complete blood count is within normal limits, except that the sedimentation rate is 65 mm/hour. Which of the following is the most likely diagnosis?

(A) Migraine headache

(B) Subarachnoid hemorrhage

(C) Cluster headache

(D) Giant cell arteritis

(E) Dental infection in the right mandibular arch

11 All of the following are associated with the condition diagnosed in Question 10, *except* which one?

(A) Pain in the hip and shoulder girdle

(B) Unilateral vision loss

(C) Pain in the jaw muscles during mastication

(D) A photosensitive, macular rash over the facial cheeks

(E) A fever

12 A 60-year-old man complains of a 1-week history of generalized mild headaches occurring on the right side. He denies any history of trauma. He denies experiencing any chronic headaches in the past. Over the last week he has also noted pain in his jaw muscles with chewing. He denies visual disturbance. On further questioning, he alludes to difficulty putting on his clothes in the morning as a result of stiffness and pain about the shoulder girdle. The temporal artery on the right side is not particularly enlarged or tender. The shoulder girdle stiffness does not particularly remit after he has been up for hours, and the patient denies metacarpophalangeal joint and proximal interphalangeal joint pain and stiffness. Neurologic history and examination are negative. Which of the following is the best first test to order?

(A) A CT scan of the head without contrast

(B) A CT scan of the head with contrast

(C) An MRI of the brain

(D) An erythrocyte sedimentation rate

(E) A temporal artery biopsy

13 A 30-year-old woman complains of headaches that have often occurred during her menstrual periods. Recently she has begun hearing her own pulsation in her right ear. She weighs 120 lb (54.4 kg) and is 5 ft, 4 in. (1.63 m) tall; she has no blood pressure or lipid abnormalities. You place your stethoscope over her optic orbits and hear no abnormal sounds. When you move the scope to the mastoid areas, you hear on the right a bruit timed with her peripheral pulse. What is the most likely explanation of these findings?

(A) Atherosclerotic stenosis of the right external carotid artery

(B) Arteriovenous malformation

(C) Migraine headache

(D) Cluster headache

(E) Temporal arteritis

14 A 25-year-old man riding with his age peers falls off the back of a truck bed and strikes his head on the pavement. He did not lose consciousness, but for several hours he kept asking what day it was and could not remember his phone number. Finally, because of headaches, he visits his family doctor a week later. An office examination of his head showed some tenderness and swelling of the mid frontal scalp. He was alert and oriented to person, place, and time and his ear examination was normal (showed no otorrhea). He had full strength and sensation in all extremities and normal deep tendon reflexes. A CT scan of the head without contrast showed no fracture and no areas of hemorrhage. Plain films of the cervical spine were negative for vertebral fracture or dislocation. Three weeks later he has no residual

scalp or frontal tenderness but he continues to complain of headaches. He denies a past history of headaches. Which of the following is characteristic of a patient with this type of headache?

(A) The patient has headaches that last only for a few days to a week after the injury.

(B) The patient does not report any associated symptoms such as visual changes, vertigo, or light-headedness.

(C) The patient has headaches that are typically very severe.

(D) The patient is more likely to be seen if he or she suffered a concussion with the head trauma.

(E) The patient with this type of headache has areas of contusion, which would usually be visible with an MRI or a CT scan of the head with contrast.

15 A 28-year-old woman complains of a 10-year history of headaches. These headaches are fronto-occipital in location and are noted often at the end of workdays; they are more likely when sleep has been poor or short and they are generally relieved by sleep. They have always been quickly relieved by the use of nonsteroidal anti-inflammatory drugs. She does note an increase in her headaches when she is under stress or *anticipates* stress. Which of the following characteristics is most commonly associated with this type of headache?

(A) There is an aura about 30 minutes before onset of the headache.

(B) There is nausea and emesis.

(C) There is a gradual, often not precisely noticed, start and end to the headaches.

(D) They are more common in men.

(E) They are frequently brought on by oral contraceptive usage.

16 A 45-year-old man began 2 weeks ago to have headaches on a daily basis. They last 1 to 2 hours and are associated with erythema of the face and rhinorrhea. The man says that he had a string of similar headaches about a year ago. He suffered a concussion 2 years ago and had headaches for several months afterward, but he has had none since until the recurrent headaches a year ago. Which of the following does this patient have?

(A) Allergic rhinitis

(B) Classic migraine

(C) Cluster headache

(D) Tension, vascular headache

(E) Post-traumatic headache

17 Which of the following headache patients would be appropriately treated with oral sumatriptan or its analogs?

(A) A 35-year-old man with cluster headaches and no significant past medical history

(B) A 30-year-old woman, pregnant at 10 weeks gestation

(C) A 28-year-old man with basilar migraine

(D) A 32-year-old woman whose migraine did not respond to a sublingual ergotamine tablet taken 4 hours earlier

(E) A 58-year-old man with hypertension, hypercholesterolemia, and type II diabetes mellitus who has no history of angina

Examination Answers

1. The answer is D. Daily use of medication commonly results in rebound headache. Conversely, daily use of analgesics often fails to respond to preventive therapy. All analgesics may result in this phenomenon, including the triptans. Although occipital and nuchal distribution of headache is common in tension-type (sometimes called vascular) headaches, rapid onset may be a sign of an intracranial vascular phenomenon or cervical spine syndromes. Headache that awakens the patient in the night is unlikely to have a benign cause unless there are associated migraine features or in the case of cluster headache. Increasing frequency of headaches, especially when worse in the mornings or associated with nausea, must be evaluated for intracranial pathology.

2. The answer is A. The description is typical of tension headache, albeit changing in intensity over the recent past. In a patient such as this, the first step after the neurologic history and examination is to investigate for increased tension in her life. Sources of such tension might be recent relative sleep deprivation, onset of anxiety or depression, onset of a systemic condition such as a chronic infection, a metabolic abnormality or anemia, or other life changes. Cluster headache is strictly unilateral and occurs daily or several times per day, albeit lasting less than 4 hours. Migraine headaches don't usually occur in the frequency given in this vignette and are classically unilateral. Intracranial hemorrhage is unlikely, given the overall chronicity. Ninety percent of patients who complain of "sinus headache" have identifiable forms of headache.

3. The answer is E. Tension headache is a nonspecific response to a variety of stresses in patients who are susceptible. Carotid artery dissection is unlikely in a 35-year-old normotensive woman. Another cause of chronic daily headaches (CDHs) is migraine transformation, which is a case of typical migraine (i.e., hemicranial, with aura) that is "transformed" to a CDH. See the explanation of Question 4.

4. The answer is D. Hemicrania continua is associated with autonomic symptoms such as rhinorrhea and tearing. So are cluster headaches; however, cluster headaches are not persistent and do not last throughout the day. Temporal arteritis is associated with tenderness of the temporal artery. Migraine is classically hemicranial as well but is not daily in frequency. It appears that all types of CDH are treated with the same battery of medications, with the exception that migraine and cluster headaches are treated specifically with the triptan group in addition.

5. The answer is C. This patient has typical trigeminal neuralgia ("tic douloureux"). Causes have become better understood within the past few years, and in fact a majority of these cases are now thought to be caused by anatomic aberrations, including posterior fossa tumors, meningioma, schwannoma, epidermoid cyst, and basilar artery aneurysm. Another surgically approachable cause is arterial or venous pressure on the gasserian (trigeminal) ganglion. Other invasive approaches include methods of destruction of the ganglion or the root, such as radio frequency, glycerol, or balloon compression, all three of which may result in corneal anesthesia. The surgery is dramatically successful. Regardless, the initial treatment should be conservative, to which 70% of patients will respond. CT scan and MRI are often negative in the foregoing syndromes, so exploration has become more common for making the diagnosis. The first drug of choice is carbamazepine (Tegretol). Other drugs used are phenytoin, baclofen, lamotrigine (Lamictal), gabapentin (Neurontin), topiramate (Topamax), and clonazepam (Klonopin). Neither temporomandibular joint syndrome nor maxillary sinusitis has sensory stimulatory precipitation. HZ acutely causes a typical rash. Postherpetic (zoster) pain is precipitated by sensory stimulation, but this patient had no preceding rash.

6. The answer is C. Multiple sclerosis can be a cause of trigeminal neuralgia. The common pathological pathway of trigeminal neuralgia includes demyelination of the nerve root near the ganglion, which may be on a mechanical basis as described in Question 5 or by the mechanism involved in multiple sclerosis. Sepsis could not explain the symptoms described without having more than one focus. Amyotrophic lateral sclerosis is entirely a motor degenerative neurologic disease. Mechanical causes of compression of the ganglion would not explain the urinary and the ophthalmologic symptoms.

7. The answer is B. Occipital neuralgia is caused by compression of the greater occipital nerve, by such underlying entities as posterior head trauma or compression of the occipital nerves by muscle tension (a possible cause in a "burned out" elementary school teacher). Tapping to stimulate electric shocklike pain is called here the Tinel sign, just as it is in relationship to carpal tunnel syndrome. Such muscle tension can be secondary to osteoarthritis of the cervical spine, and on occasion the cause cannot be found. Tension headache is not characterized by local tenderness or other neuralgic traits, although some patients complain of generalized scalp tenderness; migraine and cluster headaches are not neuralgic in character. Giant cell arteritis does not produce nerve tenderness.

8. The answer is A. Postherpetic neuralgia occurs increasingly with increasing age of the patient, rising from 9% in younger people to as high as 70% in patients older than 75 years. The other significant risk factor is acute HZ involvement of the ophthalmic branch of the trigeminal nerve. Sacral involvement may result in bladder dysfunction but no particular risk for post-herpetic neuralgia. Incidence in all settings is reduced by acute (within 72 hours of onset) treatment with antiviral agents, such as acyclovir and famciclovir.

9. The answer is A. A CT scan of head without contrast should be taken. Sudden severe headache, sometimes called "the worst headache I've ever had," should be assumed to be due to subarachnoid hemorrhage (SAH) until proven otherwise. A CT scan of the head without contrast is 90% sensitive in detecting SAH. Using a contrast agent or MRI confers no greater sensitivity; these procedures also require more time and cost more. Cerebrospinal fluid examination is not necessary if blood is visible in the ventricles on the CT scan. Such procedures should be resorted to in the event of a negative CT study, when SAH is still suspected, to avoid brainstem herniation. Sedimentation rate elevation is sensitive for temporal arteritis, which occurs in the age group of this patient. SAH is a neurosurgical emergency.

form of vasculitis

10. The answer is D. Giant cell arteritis is the cause of temporal arteritis, which this patient has. The disease is a medical urgency because it can be the cause of blindness, based on occlusion of the ophthalmic artery. The jaw pain is the ischemic pain of claudication. The diagnosis is confirmed by biopsy of the temporal artery. Giant cell disease can affect many other parts of the arterial vascularity, which accounts for a variety of presentations other than the headache of temporal arteritis. The disease responds dramatically to systemic glucocorticoids, and these do not have to be continued indefinitely. → *1-2 yrs*

Path Not affected by 35 days of prednisone *+ may have tongue claudication + scalp TTP*

11. The answer is D. A photosensitive, macular rash over the facial cheeks is *not* known to be associated with temporal arteritis. Temporal arteritis may be proceeded by the symptoms of polymyalgia rheumatica (or the symptoms of both may develop simultaneously). Unilateral vision loss is present in only about 7% of patients at the time of presentation, but it will develop in about 44% of patients if they are not treated. Temporal arteritis must be considered as a potential source of fever in those patients who are older than 50 years of age. *constitutional sxs*

12. The answer is D. Erythrocyte sedimentation rate should be determined. The clinical history is consistent with polymyalgia rheumatica, especially given the patient's age (>50) and jaw claudication and lack of symptomatology suggesting rheumatoid arthritis. The patient probably also has temporal arteritis, in which polymyalgia rheumatica is associated in 50% of the cases (see Question 11). In the latter condition the artery often lacks enlargement and tenderness; hence the more invasive, expensive, and specific artery biopsy, though kept in consideration, should not be the first test. A markedly elevated sedimentation rate with this history and examination would be sufficient to begin therapy with prednisone and to make arrangements for a temporal artery biopsy in the near future, in order to prevent possible progression to blindness. A CT scan or MRI of the head would not be justified on an urgent basis because there are no neurologic symptoms or signs. *in elderly may present c proximal limb girdle pain, AM stiffness, constitu. sxs + ↑ ESR*

13. The answer is B. There is an intracranial arteriovenous malformation. Arteriovenous malformation may present with headache, seizures, or focal neurologic symptom or hemorrhage, but the latter is the most common, constituting the clinical presentation in 30% to 60% of cases. Headaches are the presenting complaint in 5% to 25% of the cases, and seizures in 20% to 40%. Bruits may be heard over a mastoid bone or an optical orbit. Carotid atheromatous stenosis causes pulsations audible to the patient on occasion but are not often heard by the stethoscope. Carotid atheromas would most likely occur in people with risk factors such as hypertension, dyslipidemia, or diabetes, and nearly always in individuals in their fifth or sixth decades or older. Migraine headaches often recur during various stages of the menstrual cycle, but the bruit would have to be explained otherwise. The same is said regarding cluster headaches, and these do not recur with such wide ranges of time periods between attacks. See Questions 11 and 12 for the clinical setting of temporal arteritis. Although it might briefly be considered, again the bruit would have to be otherwise explained.

14. The answer is D. This is called a post-traumatic headache, and it is more likely to be seen if the patient suffered a concussion with his head trauma. This patient's brief short-term memory loss showed that he had suffered a concussion (epidural and subdural hemorrhage were ruled out by the CT scan of the head). Patients with post-traumatic headache may have moderately intense headaches for months after their head injuries. There may be brief bouts of vertigo. A CT scan or MRI of the brain is usually negative in these patients, though some concussions may be associated with small intracerebral hemorrhages that may not be indications for surgical intervention.

15. The answer is C. These are prototypical tension or vascular headaches. Onsets are gradual, are often not precisely noted, and subside gradually. The presence of aura, as well as exacerbation perimenstrually, perimenopausally, during pregnancy, and with oral contraceptives, is characteristic of migraine headaches. Migraine headaches are frequently associated with nausea and emesis, unlike tension or cluster headaches. Both migraine and tension headaches are more common in women.

16. The answer is C. The patient has typical cluster headaches. The defining pattern is the daily recurring but short-lived headache, the associated facial flushing and rhinorrhea, and the "remission" of a year between clusters. Retro-orbital headache is also a characteristic of cluster headaches. These headaches traditionally affect men eight times as frequently as women and come on between the ages of 30 and 50 years of age. That said, recent reports indicate the gender gap has been closing markedly in recent years. Allergic rhinitis causes rhinorrhea but is not

well noted for headache. (Many people with self-proclaimed sinus headaches may actually have cluster headaches.) Migraine headaches last longer but do not recur in clusters. The patient's history suggests that he once had traumatic headaches following a concussion, but they would not recur after a year's absence. Tension headaches are known for gradual beginnings and endings rather than the sudden starts and stops depicted in the vignette.

17. The answer is A. This is a 35-year-old man with cluster headaches. Sumatriptan may be used for migraine or cluster headaches, but it is contraindicated in basilar or hemiplegic migraine because of the danger of permanent neurologic damage or stroke caused by the vasoconstriction occurring as part of the pharmacologic therapeutic effect. Extra caution is warranted in prescribing it to the older, predominantly male population with cluster headaches, as they are more prone to have recognized and unrecognized coronary artery disease, also susceptible to aggravation by the vasoconstrictive effects of the triptans. Sumatriptan must not be given within 24 hours of receiving ergot preparations because of the dangers associated with the additive vasoconstrictive effects of the two drugs.

References

Beck E, Sioeber WJ, Frejo R. Management of cluster headaches. *Am Fam Physician.* 2005; 71:717–724, 728.

Kurowski K. Headache. In: Rudy DR, Kurowski K, eds. *Family Medicine: House Officer Series.* Baltimore: Williams & Wilkins; 1997:43–56.

Maitzels M. The patient with daily headaches. *Am Fam Physician.* 2004; 70:2299–2306.

chapter **4**

Problems of the Eyes and Vision

Examination questions: Unless instructed otherwise, choose the ONE lettered answer or completion that is BEST in each case.

1 A 71-year-old white woman complains of a visual disturbance over the last 2 days. She read in a family health journal about retinal detachment and fears she may have that problem. Which of the following symptoms would lead you to have her evaluated for that condition?

(A) Sudden loss of central vision in one eye

(B) Homonymous right-side visual field loss

(C) Peripheral visual loss in one eye with progression toward the central visual field over several hours

(D) Diplopia after a head contusion

(E) Irritation and tearing of the right eye over a period of 24 hours

2 A 55-year-old African American man complains of the sensation of "a curtain" dropping over the peripheral visual field of his left eye. He complains of headache as well but no eye pain or photophobia. The patient has worn glasses for farsightedness. He denies past history of intraocular hemorrhage, inflammatory conditions of the eye, eye infections, or eye surgery. He denies any increased incidence of "floaters" over the past weeks or months. Upon obtaining further history, you find the patient has a known history of hypertension that has been treated in the past; however, treatment lapsed about a year ago when the patient moved to his present location from another city. You examine him and find a blood pressure of 220/110. Pupils are equal, round, and reactive to light and accommodation. His fundi show hemorrhages typical of uncontrolled hypertension but there is no papilledema. Which of the following is the best plan of action for today?

(A) Start aggressive treatment (e.g., labetalol, perhaps combined with a thiazide diuretic) to control blood pressure and call for an ophthalmologic opinion

(B) Perform a slit-lamp examination

(C) Hospitalize and start intravenous mannitol at 1 to 2 g/kg

(D) Obtain a magnetic resonance image of the head with and without contrast medium

(E) Obtain a carotid artery duplex Doppler study

3 A 25-year-old mother of two children complains of pain in the right eye immediately after the fifth fingernail of her 6-month-old baby swiped across her eye during bottle feeding 4 hours ago. On physical examination she exhibits striking photophobia. Which of the following is the key aspect of diagnosis of this condition?

(A) Disturbance in visual acuity

(B) Presence of diplopia

(C) Presence of limbal flush

(D) Matting of the eyelids

(E) Presence of green color upon examination of the cornea when a cobalt blue light is shone after application of fluorescein

4 You have diagnosed an 18-year-old man who plays on the high school varsity basketball team and incurred an injury to the left eye when another player poked his finger into the eye an hour ago. Fluorescein staining of the cornea is positive. Which of the following is the mainstay of treatment of this condition?

(A) Topical and oral analgesics with a follow-up in 24 hours

(B) Antibiotic ointment followed by double patching and taping to prevent relative movement of the eye during the healing process

(C) Mydriatic drops followed by patching with follow-up in 24 hours

(D) Meiotic drops followed by patching with follow-up in 24 hours

(E) Immediate referral to an ophthalmologist

5 A 2-year-old boy is brought to your office by his parents for the first time, after a day care attendant expressed concern because the boy's eyes do not appear to be in parallel position. He and the mother are concerned that the child has "cockeyes": One eye falls consistently to the outside of the direction of his gaze. As a permanent condition, this is most often caused by which of the following visual defects?

(A) Myopia

(B) Amblyopia

(C) Hyperopia

(D) Astigmatism

(E) Exotropia

6 A 3-year-old girl exhibits crossed eyes. The parents ask what the implications are to her vision in the future as a result of this problem. You answer that if the condition is not corrected, the child will suffer from which of the following conditions?

(A) Myopia

(B) Amblyopia

(C) Hyperopia

(D) Astigmatism

(E) Exotropia

7 The parents of the patient in Question 6 ask what can be done to avoid complications from this condition. You answer that the defect must be corrected by what age?

(A) 6 to 9 months

(B) 12 to 18 months

(C) 18 to 24 months

(D) 3 to 5 years

(E) 7 years

8 A 3-week-old female infant is brought to you by her mother, who is concerned by the child's left eye; it shows crusting and matting of a conjunctival discharge. The pupils are equal and reactive to light and there appears to be no photophobia. What is the most likely cause of this finding and what must be done, if anything, to remediate the condition?

(A) Bacterial conjunctivitis—use ophthalmic antibiotic drops

(B) Viral conjunctivitis—use ophthalmic antibiotic drops

(C) Iritis—use patching and instill an ophthalmic glucorticoid preparation

(D) Obstructed lacrimal duct—use observation and consider probing the lacrimal duct

(E) Foreign body—perform double eversion of the eyelid and removal of same

9 At what age can the foregoing condition be expected to resolve physiologically?

(A) 3 to 4 weeks

(B) 4 to 5 weeks

(C) 3 to 5 months

(D) 9 to 11 months

(E) 2 to 3 years

10 A 52-year-old white woman calls your office and asks for an appointment today because she has had rapid onset of pain in her right eye. You see her within the hour and notice injection of her right eye and that she is unable to open her eye easily in the bright light of your examining room. She complains of pain that is 8 on a scale of 10, and the pain is felt in the eye as opposed to the anterior aspects of the eye as in foreign body or corneal injury. You have her visual acuity measured while she wears her glasses that correct for myopia. Her right eye, normally correctable to 20/25, is now 20/50 at distance. On examination in the light, the right pupil is dilated as compared with the left. In the dark, however, the right eye pupil dilates no further while the left eye pupil dilates and becomes larger than the right pupil. Which of the following does the patient have until proven otherwise?

(A) Acute iritis

(B) Allergic conjunctivitis

(C) Chronic simple glaucoma

(D) Acute (angle closure) glaucoma

(E) Retinal detachment

11 A 35-year-old white man complains of the onset over 2 days of photophobia and blurred near vision of the left eye. He is not aware of getting a foreign body in his eye and the irritation of which he complains is unlike that of a foreign body sensation. Review of his medical history reveals that he has been diagnosed with psoriasis and has been under treatment for the past 2 years. On examination the pupils are unequal; the left eye is meiotic (constricted) as compared with the right eye. The left eye has been tearing, and the patient has difficulty opening the eye widely when a light is shone into it. His corneae show no fluorescein uptake and no foreign body is found on double upper-lid inversion. Which of the following diagnoses is the most probable explanation of this patient's eye complaints?

(A) Acute angle closure glaucoma

(B) Unseen foreign body in the left eye

(C) Retinal detachment of the left eye

(D) Bacterial conjunctivitis

(E) Anterior uveitis

12 A 58-year-old woman complains of dryness of her eyes for the past several months and that, when she has had occasion to cry, her tear production is sparse. Over the last 2 years she has had a spate of recurrent dental caries. Within the last 2 weeks she has noted soreness of an enlargement behind her left ear and that her mouth is dry most of the time. Which of the following is most likely to be associated with her condition?

(A) Atherosclerosis

(B) Multiple endocrine neoplasia type I

(C) Colorectal cancer

(D) Diabetes type II

(E) Hashimoto thyroiditis

13 You have instituted screening for glaucoma in certain routine preventive complete physical examinations. Which of the following is a risk factor for primary open angle glaucoma?

(A) Age >35 years in the absence of other risk factors

(B) Female sex

(C) Mexican or indigenous American race

(D) Excess exposure to sunlight

(E) African American race

14 A 55-year-old white male patient enters your practice for the first time and has scheduled a complete his-

tory and physical examination. Specifically he asks to be checked for chronic glaucoma, as he works with a person who informs him that he must take drops in his eyes daily for glaucoma. You do a measurement of intraocular tension and find it to be 16 mm Hg OS and 15 mm Hg OD (normal ≤25 mm Hg). However, on completing the general examination you make a finding that tells you that you have not definitely ruled out open angle (chronic) glaucoma in the left eye. Which of the following is that finding?

(A) Optic cup in the left eye is 40% the diameter of the optic disc.

(B) The patient exhibits a change in distant visual acuity with correction from 20/20 to 20/50.

(C) There is erythema of the left eye conjunctiva.

(D) There is papilledema of the left eye.

(E) There is a mydriatic pupil in the left eye.

15 A 20-year-old student is being brought to you directly from the scene of a bar fight in which he received a fist blow to his left eye orbit. He manifests an impressive periorbital hematoma ("black eye"), but no hyphema is seen. The pupils are equal and round and reactive equally to light. He complains of diplopia when he directs his gaze to the right, and you find that his left eye cannot follow your penlight more than 15 degrees past the midline toward the right. Which of the following is the likely cause of this complaint and finding?

(A) Direct blow to the eyeball

(B) Rupture of the eyeball

(C) Fracture of the orbital rim

(D) Traumatic iritis

(E) VI nerve palsy precipitated by trauma in a diabetic patient

16 You have diagnosed chronic (open angle) glaucoma by a Schiotz tonometer and wish to do an in-office check of the patient's peripheral vision in order to make an informed request for consultation of an ophthalmologist. When having the patient count fingers to ascertain visual fields, at what angle from the central visual axis should you hold your fingers?

(A) 15 degrees

(B) 25 degrees

(C) 30 degrees

(D) 45 degrees

(E) 60 degrees

Examination Answers

1. The answer is C. Peripheral loss of vision in a curtain type of blockage, as opposed to central loss, is typical of retinal detachment. Central visual loss occurs in optic neuritis or macular degeneration. Homonymous scotomas are always due to central lesions. Those that involve the right field of both visual fields would occur through a lesion of the left optic radiation or the left visual projection area of the occipital cortex. Diplopia is a result of pathology other than retinal function. Tearing is caused by irritation of anterior structures such as corneae, conjunctivae, or sclerae and also may be a response to pain and irritation associated with iritis and acute glaucoma, among other problems.

2. The answer is A. Given the history, it is likely that the patient has had a serous type of retinal detachment. This is brought about by effusion of serum behind the retina, secondary to uncontrolled disease states such as hypertension or uveitis. Treatment consists of medical control of the underlying disease and usually results in complete recovery of vision. However, most primary care physicians would make early judicious inquiry of an ophthalmologist as they begin to control the hypertension (as in this case). A second type of detachment is tractional retinal detachment and is due to intraocular fibrotic processes caused by previous hemorrhage. Treatment consists of surgical disengagement of the scar tissue from the retina by a trained ophthalmologist. The third type is the most common and is called rhegmatogenous detachment, related to initial detachment of the vitreous from the retina. One-fourth of the population will experience this condition between the ages of 61 and 70 years. At this stage the symptoms are mild, consisting of an increased frequency of vitreous floaters. However, 15% of people with vitreous detachment progress to develop a retinal flap or tear or a hole. Besides the risk factor of age, rhegmatogenous retinal detachment occurs more often in myopic individuals and in those who have undergone cataract removal. The word *rhegmatogenous* is derived from the Greek word for rupture.

Slit-lamp examinations are not normally expected of primary care physicians. Intravenous mannitol is an accepted therapeutic modality for acute angle closure glaucoma. Acute glaucoma is characterized by intraocular pain and ipsilateral midposition fixed pupil. A magnetic resonance image of the head would be indicated for suspicion of vascular accident or neoplastic disease, neither of which is suggested by the findings given. A carotid artery duplex Doppler study would be indicated for suspicion of visual disturbance that is due to carotid artery insufficiency. The latter may cause amaurosis fugax, that is, ipsilateral transient total blindness (or partial visual cuts, such as unilateral quadrantanopsia), caused by embolism of small flakes of coagulum or ruptured plaque from an atherosclerotic site of carotid artery stenosis. This patient did not exhibit that constellation of symptoms.

3. The answer is E. The patient has either a corneal abrasion or corneal laceration. Either lesion shows a green color in the area of abrasion, keratitis, or laceration of the cornea with cobalt blue light after instillation of fluorescein. The shape of the defect will determine whether one is dealing with a laceration or an abrasion. If the injury is associated with an embedded corneal foreign body, the defect will outline the speck. The aforementioned patient might well have a laceration or an abrasion, but it is unlikely that there would be a foreign body. Keratitis, depending on the cause, results in an array of pinpoint fluorescein positive areas, ulceration in patches, or a dendritic pattern. In any event, the course would not be so rapid in onset and would not be associated with trauma. Acute visual disturbance, decreased visual acuity, occurs with many problems of the eye, such as acute glaucoma, marked changes in blood sugar in diabetes, conjunctivitis with profuse exudate, or corneal injury. Limbal flush, which is a thin, red halo surrounding the limbus of the cornea, is reputed to be a hallmark of angle closure glaucoma. Matting of the eyelids, which is crusting of the lids to the point that they tend to stick together upon opening, is a sign of the profusion of exudate. Matting occurs especially in conjunctivitis, more so in bacterial as compared with viral causation.

4. The answer is A. Management of corneal abrasion has been greatly simplified. Essentially, supportive and symptomatic care consisting of topical and oral analgesics is all that is necessary and efficacious. Follow-up in 24 hours by the treating physician is prudent. Healing takes place rapidly and often is virtually complete within 24 hours and certainly so in 3 to 4 days. Patching as management of corneal injury has been eclipsed in light of meta-analyses that show that patching neither promotes more rapid healing nor relieves pain. Antibiotics, whether ointment or drops, are probably irrelevant, although they are often used. Bacterial infection is rare as a complication of corneal abrasion or laceration, as long as the injury is not deforming or ablative. Neither therapeutic mydriasis nor meiosis has a place in the treatment of corneal injury. Mydriasis was once used on the basis of relief of ciliary muscle spasm (there sometimes being ciliary spasm, hence a meiotic pupil as occurs in iritis) and resultant pain. Referral to an ophthalmologist is seldom necessary because of the benign natural course of this condition. However, if healing has not occurred within 4 days, then such referral is warranted and indicated. Many corneal abrasions are secondary to contact lens use. In those cases, if they recur, contact lenses should be discontinued.

5. The answer is A. Myopia is most often the result of a congenitally elongated eyeball. This leads early to unsuccessful attempts to relax accommodation for distance, resulting in relaxation of convergence to a degree that goes beyond parallel and thus is divergent. The resultant divergence is called exotropia. Thus, exotropia is a synonym for divergent gaze, not a cause thereof; the choice of letter E is therefore wrong. Basically the eyeball that is abnormally long in relation to the focal distance capability of the lens and cornea must relax accommodation of the ciliary apparatus even for reading; in the extreme, this is unsuccessful even for reading. Accommodation and convergence are enervated together and act synchronously. In some cases, gaze malalignment occurs only when fusion of gaze is broken up ("lazy eye") and thus shows no visible strabismus under usual circumstances. In such cases the cover–uncover test is performed. The patient is instructed to fix the gaze on a point beyond 20 ft, or 6 m (i.e., "infinity"). Then an obstructing cover is placed over one eye, serving to break up the fusion or point fixation. Upon removal of the cover, in a person with lazy eye, the previously covered eye is seen to return to the original gaze from either a lateral position (exophoria, which is the subclinical phase of exotropia) or medially (esophoria, which is the subclinical phase of esotropia) Eventually the diplopia that occurs is no longer tolerated by the brain and the weaker eye's vision is suppressed. This condition is called suppression amblyopia and such cortical blindness may become permanent. Amblyopia is central blindness as defined herein, but the described case does not illustrate that condition. Hyperopia, farsightedness, is caused by an abnormally shortened eyeball at birth. Astigmatism is a refractory error produced when the cornea, which accounts for 65% to 75% of the refraction of light to the eyes, is set in a less than perfect spherical surface.

6. The answer is B, amblyopia. The child has a strabismus with in-turning nonparallel gaze called esotropia

("cross-eye"). The refractory error that results in the squint is congenitally shortened eyeballs that cause the point of convergence from infinity (distance) to fall in front of the retina (see explanation for Question 5). The relationships among tracking, convergence, and muscle control are the opposite of those for congenital myopia. Thus, attempts to accommodate for near vision and the convergence that goes therewith results in esotropia Attempts to strain for near accommodation even for infinite distance result in inappropriate convergence. In this way, two images are conveyed to the brain instead of a fused single vision (i.e., diplopia).

7. The answer is D. The patient has diplopia caused by uncorrected hyperopia. The relationships among tracking, convergence, and muscle control are the opposite of those for congenital myopia. Thus, attempts to accommodate for near vision and the convergence that goes therewith result in esotropia. If the condition is not corrected by eye exercises during the interval of 3 to 5 years or, if unsuccessful, surgically by the age of 5 years, then the brain will increasingly suppress the image of one of the eyes, favoring instead the "stronger" eye. This timeline applies equally to exotropia, featured in Question 5. The patient becomes blind in the weaker eye and the condition is called suppression amblyopia, which is a permanent condition.

The age range of 3 to 5 years for correction through surgery or eye exercises was chosen so that the child would be mature enough to cooperate in the therapy and the procedure would be early enough for the condition to still be reversible.

8. The answer is D. An obstructed lacrimal duct (physiological) is a common cause of conjunctival discharge after the first month of life. Treatment generally is nonspecific and supportive as the condition is self-limited. Occasionally the lacrimal duct and sac become infected. In either case the pressure on the lacrimal sac expresses fluid from the ipsilateral punctum or through the nose and thereby effects the opening of a congenital obstruction.

9. The answer is D. Congenital impatency of the lacrimal duct should not be expected to be resolved physiologically until 9 months of age. Bacterial conjunctivitis is treated with antibiotic drops, but this diagnosis is much less likely in the described situation. Viral conjunctivitis is more likely to be bilateral and is usually associated with other symptoms of a viral syndrome such as coryza and other symptoms of upper respiratory infection. Congenital impatency is a diagnosis of inference, and although it is usually treated with topical antibiotics, they would not be effective in this case. Iritis does not manifest equal pupillary size. Foreign body would manifest lid spasm, which is not found here. If present, it is diagnosed first by an inspection that usually requires double-lid eversion to be carried out effectively.

10. The answer is D. Angle closure glaucoma is characterized by rapid onset of pain that is in the eye and that exhibits a fixed midpositioned pupil. Intraocular pressure, normally ≤25 mm Hg, is elevated to anywhere from 40 mm Hg to 80 mm Hg. Failure to rapidly lower intraocular pressure will result in chronic uncontrolled intraocular hypertension and permanent loss of vision. Immediate medical therapy includes intravenous mannitol, or oral isosorbide if intravenous equipment is not immediately available, while administering pilocarpine to constrict the pupil and ease the pressure in the Schlemm canals. Ultimately, therapy is surgical, such as laser partial iridectomy.

11. The answer is E. The patient has iritis or anterior uveitis. Posterior uveitis involves the ciliary body (cyclitis), choroid, or both. Iritis is characterized by a meiotic constricted pupil and photophobia. Photophobia is a consequence of the iridospasm and the aggravation thereof by light stimulation. Vision is blurred because of the nonspecific effects of abnormal ciliary body responsiveness but especially so at distance because the spastic ciliary body may disallow relaxation of accommodation for distant vision. Most uveitis is nongranulomatous and associated with and involving autoimmune processes, which can be seen by the presence of psoriasis in this patient. Treatment of anterior uveitis usually consists of topical glucocorticoids after confirmation by an ophthalmologist. Posterior uveitis and panuveitis are often treated by systemic glucocorticoids. Rheumatological consultation would be in order in those situations as well. Infectious causes are unusual and most often associated with immune incompetence; these are treated by appropriate antibiotics. Angle closure glaucoma is characterized by a fixed midpositioned pupil. Foreign bodies are rarely unseen and signaled by the history of instantaneous symptoms. With a corneal embedded foreign body (which would be fluorescein positive) there may be iridospasm that is relieved by removal of the foreign body. Retinal detachment of the left eye would be characterized by a curtainlike loss of vision rather than blurred vision and is usually painless. Bacterial conjunctivitis manifests much purulent exudate, matting of the eyelids, and a fine "sandy" foreign body.

12. The answer is E. The vignette describes Sjögren syndrome. It is an autoimmune disease characterized by dry mouth (carious teeth as a result) and dry eyes, as well as loss of taste and smell, pancreatitis, pleuritis, and chronic obstructive lung disease in the absence of smoking. Among many associated or metachronous conditions are parotid gland enlargement and other autoimmune diseases such as Grave disease, Hashimoto thyroiditis, and vitiligo and rheumatoid arthritis. There is no increased risk of diabetes type II (though there may be an increased risk of type I, an autoimmune disease), atherosclerotic diseases, multiple endocrine neoplasia type II, or colorectal cancers (nor other cancer).

13. The answer is E. Chronic glaucoma (open angle glaucoma), which is increased intraocular pressure that insidiously destroys vision, occurs gradually over a period of years. This occurs without causing pain but eventually causing loss of vision, first in the peripheral fields and then involving central vision. A significant percentage of patients with chronic glaucoma have normal pressure open angle glaucoma. These cases are diagnosed in primary care by funduscopy and visual field testing (see Question 14). Being of African American race confers nearly a fourfold risk of developing primary open angle glaucoma (4.7% prevalence vs. 1.3% for whites). In addition, African Americans are at risk much earlier in life than people of other races, which warrants their screening at an age as young as 20 years. Otherwise, age >50 years is a risk factor (not >35 years). Neither being female nor of Mexican or Indigenous American race is listed as a risk factor for primary open angle glaucoma; nor is exposure to sunlight. However, the latter places one at risk for pterygium (a pinguecula that forms on the sclera and crosses the limbus to extend onto the cornea). Being of Eastern Asian race is a significant risk factor for closed angle or acute glaucoma. Another risk factor for chronic glaucoma is diabetes mellitus. Chronic glaucoma is best prevented by routine intraocular tension measurements, every 2 years after the age of 40 years; abnormal readings are defined as >24 mm Hg on repeated measurement. This measurement may be taken in primary care offices by use of the inexpensive Schiotz tonometer. As mentioned, these cases are diagnosed through more subtle means (see Question 14).

14. The answer is A. A significant proportion of open angle glaucoma occurs without intraocular hypertension. This is a situation analogous to normal pressure hydrocephalus. Diagnosis in most of these cases can be made early by finding a cup/disc ratio >0.3 (30%). The earliest change in vision would be a narrowing of peripheral vision rather than a decrease in central vision (visual acuity). A decrease in distant visual acuity can result from an increase in the index of refraction (refraction density) brought about by hyperglycemia as in new or uncontrolled diabetes, among other causes. Chronic glaucoma exhibits no other physical findings and no symptoms until visual changes are apparent. Therefore, erythema is not a sign of chronic glaucoma. Papilledema does not occur with chronic glaucoma. Acute (angle closure) glaucoma, but not open angle glaucoma, results in pupil change, in the form of relative mydriasis (dilatation).

15. The answer is C. In orbital fracture an extraocular muscle may become entrapped and limit the range of motion of the ipsilateral eye. Although diabetes is a cause of cranial nerve VI (abducens) palsy in diabetics, diabetic VI nerve palsy is not precipitated by trauma. A rupture of the eye would likely result in sluggish gaze movement, but the hallmark of an eyeball contusion is hyphema. The latter may lead to secondary glaucoma. A rupture of the eyeball may cause an irregular pupil, not found here. Iritis could occur after trauma if there were a corneal injury or foreign body, but it would not be found immediately after the trauma.

16. The answer is D, 45 degrees. In this version of confrontational field checking, the acuity of the peripheral field is being testing as well as the range (i.e., discrimination adequate to count fingers). For detection of motion only, the angle from the central axis should be limited only by the anatomic barriers, which are the nose, brow, lateral orbit, and cheek below.

References

Gariano RF, Kim CH. Evaluation and management of suspected retinal detachment. *Am Fam Physician.* 2004; 69:1691–1698.

Savory LM, Krasnow MA, Terry JE. Problems of the eye. In: Rudy DR, Kurowski K, eds. *Family Medicine: House Officer Series.* Baltimore: Williams & Wilkins; 1997:57–70.

Wilson SA, Last A. Management of corneal abrasions. *Am Fam Physician.* 2004; 70:123–130.

SECTION **II**

Cardiovascular Problems

chapter 5

Common Cardiac Problems in Ambulatory Practice

Examination questions: Unless instructed otherwise, choose the ONE lettered answer or completion that is BEST in each case.

1 A 63-year-old white man has had poorly controlled hypertension for at least 8 years. He has a family history of hypertension and type II diabetes. He had been on a calcium channel-blocking agent when he was last seen by you 2.5 years ago. He failed to follow up with you until he became dyspneic with exertion over the last week. Blood pressure (BP) is 160/105, apical heart rate is 110, and the rhythm is irregular. The electrocardiogram shows voltage criteria for left ventricular hypertrophy and the chest x-ray shows a "concentric hypertrophy" pattern in the cardiac silhouette (i.e., hypertrophy without obvious dilatation). Which of the following findings would most certainly apply to this patient?

(A) Distended neck veins

(B) Ejection fraction >50%

(C) Pulmonary venous hypertension

(D) S_3 gallop

(E) Hepatomegaly

2 Regarding the patient in Question 1, what is the most likely type of dysrhythmia?

(A) Multiple premature ventricular contractions

(B) Primary atrial contractions

(C) Sick sinus syndrome

(D) Atrial fibrillation

(E) Second-degree heart block

3 Which of the following is the best therapeutic foundation for managing the patient in Question 1?

(A) BP control and heart-rate reduction

(B) Aggressive diuresis

(C) Angiotensin-converting enzyme inhibitors (ACEIs)

(D) Oxygen therapy

(E) Morphine sulfate injection

4 A 75-year-old man is seeing you for a routine checkup. He has seen few doctors in his lifetime and none in your city since moving there 10 years ago. You hear a diastolic murmur over the apex that radiates to the left axilla. Which of the following is the likely diagnosis?

(A) Aortic stenosis

(B) Mitral stenosis

(C) Dilated cardiomyopathy

(D) Aortic insufficiency

(E) Ventricular septal defect

5 A 17-year-old boy, upon routine preparticipation sports examination, manifests BP of 150/90 in the right arm and 110/90 in the left. Which of the following is the cause of this asymmetry of BP levels in the upper extremities?

(A) Congenital arteriovenous shunt

(B) Congenital abdominal aorta coarctation

(C) Congenital coarctation of the aortic arch

(D) Atherosclerotic blockage of the left subclavian artery

(E) Congenital stenosis of the left subclavian artery

6 In the patient in Question 5, which of the following abnormalities, if any, is most likely to be found upon examination?

(A) Systolic crescendo–decrescendo loudest over the left second interspace near the left sternal border

(B) Low-pitched holosystolic murmur at the apex radiating to the left axilla

(C) Systolic murmur at the lower left sternal border and a hepatojugular reflex

(D) Decrescendo diastolic murmur loudest at the left second interspace on the left sternal border

(E) Machinery murmur loudest along the left sternal border, both systolic and diastolic

7 A 55-year-old woman is scheduled for routine procedures by her private dentist, whose office now calls and inquires as to whether she should undergo endocarditis antibiotic prophylaxis. She has a history of mitral valve prolapse. You consult your record, which confirms mitral valve prolapse (whose evidence is an audible systolic click without a murmur). Which of the following conditions is one of the indications for endocarditis antibiotic prophylaxis before dental procedures?

(A) Previous rheumatic fever without valvulitis

(B) Previous Kawasaki disease without valvular dysfunction

(C) Presence of cardiac pacemaker and implanted defibrillator

(D) Presence of mitral valve prolapse, with click and no murmur

(E) Presence of prosthetic cardiac valves, including bioprosthetic and homograft valves

8 You have followed the patient in Question 7 for another 10 years. Now she has a systolic murmur radiating to the left axilla and in fact manifests fatigue and, three times per week, paroxysmal nocturnal dyspnea. You decide to discuss with her the possibility of referral for mitral valve replacement. Which valvular repair surgery is fraught with the highest perioperative mortality rate?

(A) Aortic valve replacement for aortic regurgitation

(B) Aortic valve replacement for aortic stenosis

(C) Mitral valve replacement

(D) Patent ductus repair

(E) Fracture of mitral valve leaflets for stenosis

9 Which of the following risk factors for coronary artery disease (CAD) is the most potent from the viewpoint of relative risk (rate of coronary disease in the person at risk compared with the rate expected in the population)?

(A) Obesity

(B) Sedentary lifestyle

(C) Hypertension

(D) Smoking

(E) HDL cholesterol <35 mg/dL

10 A 45-year-old man has a family history of CAD in his father, who died of a myocardial infarction (MI) at the age of 52. The patient is a smoker. He comes to your office with chest pain described as pressing, with radiation into the left jaw and medial left arm. The pain has been present for about 45 minutes. The apical rate is 94 and regular. BP is 112/68. Which of the following is the best first action to be taken?

(A) Order the patient to drive to the nearest emergency department

(B) Order and administer subcutaneous morphine sulfate

(C) Administer an aspirin

(D) Start an intravenous line

(E) Call for paramedics plus Choices C and D

11 Regarding the patient in Question 10, what is the earliest one can rule out MI by laboratory tests?

(A) 1 hour

(B) 2 hours

(C) 3 hours

(D) 4 hours

(E) 8 hours

12 Regarding the patient in Questions 10 and 11, in what window of time is it necessary to act to obtain the maximum value of thrombolytic therapy?

(A) 1 hour

(B) 2 hours

(C) 3 hours

(D) 4 hours

(E) 8 hours

13 A 55-year-old type II diabetic male nonsmoker is consulting you electively for the advisability of taking up a controlled exercise program. He has neither history of chest pain or heart disease attacks nor symptoms of heart failure. However, a routine electrocardiogram (EKG) shows a QS configuration in leads II, III, and aVF (deep Q waves; no R wave); there is neither ST elevation nor depression. Each of the following statements is true about this situation except which one?

(A) The patient has had a posterior MI of indeterminate age.

(B) "Silent" MIs carry a worse prognosis than symptomatic MIs.

(C) A silent MI is more likely to occur in people with diabetes.

(D) During the acute phase of this past MI, the patient was likely to exhibit a sinus bradycardia.

(E) During the acute phase of this MI, the patient's symptoms were easily confused with an upper gastrointestinal syndrome.

14 A 55-year-old woman is brought to you by her family because of near-fainting spells. She denies chest pain but admits to shortness of breath upon climbing stairs. She takes no medications. On examination, she exhibits 2+ ankle edema. Her sitting BP is 150/80. You take repeated BP readings after she arises, and by 1 minute after standing erect she has a BP of 130/70. These findings may be explained by any of the following except which one?

(A) Congestive heart failure

(B) Pericarditis

(C) Adrenal insufficiency

(D) Nausea or vomiting and diarrhea

(E) Diabetes insipidus

15 A 48-year-old patient has hypertension that is controlled reasonably well with sustained-release verapamil and residual poliomyelitis that has left him with weakness of his left leg. He now complains of atypical chest pain, consisting of rather vague substernal pain that is not associated with walking upstairs but that occasionally wakes him during dream sleep. You determine that you should order stress testing but realize that a normal treadmill test is not possible for this patient because of his postpolio status. Which of the following would be the most reasonable next step for investigating the presence of CAD as the cause of the patient's symptoms?

(A) Treadmill EKG stress testing

(B) Treadmill EKG and thallium stress testing

(C) Resting EKG

(D) Dipyridamole–thallium stress test

(E) Coronary angiography

16 A 28-year-old white male patient rushes into his doctor's office in a panic, demanding to see a doctor. He complains of heart palpitations and the doctor manages to examine his heart with a stethoscope to find a regular rate of 160. An EKG shows a supraventric-

ular tachycardia. Which of the following methods, when effective, is the simplest way for differentiating paroxysmal atrial tachycardia with block (PAT) from atrioventricular nodal reentry tachycardia (AVNRT)?

(A) Osler maneuver

(B) Orthostatic versus sedentary BPs

(C) Digoxin level

(D) Carotid sinus massage

(E) Presence or absence of anginal symptoms

17 A 24-year-old law student complains of dyspnea on exertion and syncope and near syncope with light-headedness. There is no orthopnea. These symptoms have been coming on over the last several weeks, first noted during an intramural football game in warm weather. Upon examination you note a remarkable two-pointed steep carotid pulse, a harsh crescendo–decrescendo ("diamond shaped") systolic murmur loudest along the lower left sternal border, and an S_4 gallop. The murmur is decreased with performance of the Valsalva maneuver. Which of the following conditions most likely accounts for the findings?

(A) Aortic insufficiency

(B) Mitral stenosis

(C) Hypertrophic cardiomyopathy

(D) Ventricular septal defect

(E) Mitral insufficiency

18 A 45-year-old man is seen in the emergency department with chest pain radiating into the left arm. He has no atherosclerotic risk factors personally (except his sex) and has no family history of CAD in members prior to the age of 70 years; he does not smoke and has no chronic cough or other respiratory symptoms. Further history reveals that he complains of a sore throat and fatigue that started 10 days ago. BP is 130/85 and the systolic pressure drops by 12 mm Hg during inspiration. Examination finds nontender cervical adenopathy; there is no chest wall tenderness. The heart shows systolic and diastolic murmurlike sounds. The cardiac percussible silhouette is enlarged to beyond the left midclavicular line. An EKG shows ST elevation across the entire precordium. White blood cell count is 3,500 with 60% lymphocytes and is otherwise not remarkable. Which of the following accounts for the described clinical picture?

(A) Acute MI

(B) Acute pericarditis

(C) Dressler syndrome

(D) Acute bronchitis

(E) Tietze syndrome

19 A 48-year-old diabetic man weighs 220 lb (100 kg) at a height of 5 ft 11 in. (1.8 m) and comes to you with the complaint that, for the last 6 weeks, he experiences pain in the calves after walking two city blocks. He smoked 25 pack-years until 3 years ago. He has a BP of 155/105. On examination you fail to find popliteal, posterior tibial, and dorsalis pedis pulses in either lower extremity. The patient admits to symptoms of claudication of the legs (tightening calf pain after walking two blocks) and that he made the appointment hoping that an exercise prescription would result in his being able to walk greater distances. He has been taking 5 mg of glyburide qid (four times per day) and hydrochlorothiazide/triamterene. His glycohemoglobin result returns and is 9%. All but which of the following would be reasonable measures to take at this time?

  (A) Place him on a 1700-calorie American Diabetes Association diet

  (B) Add 500 mg of metformin bid (twice daily)

  (C) Order a treadmill–thallium stress test

  (D) Add an angiotensin-converting enzyme blocking agent (ACEI)

  (E) Obtain ankle-brachial BPs

For Questions 20 through 24, match the lettered types of orthostatic hypotension with the numbered causes. A clinical type may apply to more than one cause.

20 Pericarditis

21 Alcoholic polyneuropathy

22 Fever

23 Hypertensive on beta-blocker

24 Venous pooling after hot shower

  (A) Neurogenic hypotension

  (B) Nonneurogenic hypotension

  (C) Drug-related hypotension

  (D) Supine hypotension

  (E) Septic hypotension

For Questions 25 through 29, match the lettered descriptions of heart sounds to the numbered cardiac diagnoses.

25 Aortic stenosis

26 Mitral regurgitation

27 Hypertrophic cardiomyopathy

28 Mitral valve prolapse

29 Aortic regurgitation

  (A) Holosystolic, low pitch; apex radiates to axilla

  (B) Diastolic decrescendo

  (C) Crescendo–decrescendo; radiates to carotids

  (D) Midsystolic, late systolic, or pansystolic; click

  (E) Crescendo–decrescendo; decreases with squat

For Questions 30 through 34, match the lettered effects with the numbered maneuver that may influence murmurs.

30 Inspiration, squatting

31 Expiration, standing

32 Valsalva phase 3 (release)

33 Valsalva phase 4 (rebound)

34 Handgrip

  (A) Decreases venous return

  (B) Raises systemic vascular resistance, heart rate, and cardiac output

  (C) Increases venous return

  (D) Decreases arterial BP

  (E) Raises arterial BP; slows heart rate

Examination Answers

1. The answer is B. This patient depicts diastolic heart failure (DHF). The name refers to the fact that the ventricular wall is stiff and does not fully relax during diastole. Ejection fraction is not compromised and is generally >50%, though the stroke volume is below normal. The most common causes of this type of failure are age and uncontrolled hypertension. Distended neck veins are more likely to occur with systolic heart failure, wherein the ventricles are flabby and whose contractions are weaker. Likewise pulmonary passive congestion, though not absent in DHF, is more likely in systolic failure and its reduced ejection fraction. Both S_3 and S_4 gallops are found in a strong minority of DHF cases but are found in a majority of systolic failure cases. Hepatomegaly may be found in 15% of cases of either type of failure.

2. The answer is D. Atrial fibrillation is more likely in the presence of a stiff ventricular wall, as occurs in DHF, and is also more likely in an older patient.

3. The answer is A. Although each of the other choices except one is unassailable in the treatment of any form of heart failure, in DHF, lowering the BP to normal levels (<139/<90) and controlling the heart rate are fundamental. The hypertension is the major contributing cause of the heart failure and tachycardia (or even fast normal rates) aggravates the stiff ventricles' slowness to relax and permit adequate ventricular filling. Morphine injections are used in pulmonary edema caused by heart failure, usually of the systolic type.

4. The answer is B. Mitral stenosis produces a rumbling diastolic murmur at the apex, which in its classic presentation is associated with an "opening snap," marking the end of the murmur sound component until the next systolic cycle. The virtually sole cause of mitral stenosis is rheumatic heart disease, which is an increasing rarity. However, patients in the age range of the case presented in the vignette are still around. Many of them decompensated with pulmonary passive congestion, symptomatically very similar to that of left ventricular heart failure, and underwent mitral commissurotomy in the 1950s and 1960s. Later cases were treated by total valve replacement. The murmur of aortic regurgitation is a high-pitched diastolic murmur that starts immediately on the A_2 second

sound, falling off in a decrescendo much like the sound of waves crashing on rocks. Aortic stenosis produces a systolic murmur loudest at the aortic auscultatory area. Dilated cardiomyopathy may produce mitral insufficiency and its systolic murmur, which is due to dilation of the mitral valve ring. Ventricular septal defect is a congenital lesion that causes a harsh crescendo–decrescendo left parasternal murmur.

5. The answer is C. This combination of BP levels is typical of congenital coarctation of the arch of the aorta. An arteriovenous shunt causes a widened pulse pressure (e.g., 150/60) that is distributed symmetrically throughout the vascular system. Abdominal aortic coarctation results in elevated BP levels in the upper extremities and lower BP levels in the lower extremities. Atherosclerotic blockade could occur in any part of the vascular system to produce any of the aberrations of BP discussed. However, atherosclerotic obstruction is highly unlikely in a 17-year-old patient. Although subclavian obstruction is a not rare phenomenon of atherosclerosis in likely candidates, congenital stenosis is not as likely as coarctation of the arch aorta.

6. The answer is A. This is the murmur of aortic stenosis, associated with a congenital bicuspid aortic valve (as well as with rheumatic valvulitis). This congenital lesion is present in 46% of cases of coarctation of all types. None of the other murmurs has a particular association with coarctation. The apical murmur radiating to the left axilla is that of mitral insufficiency. The murmur associate with the hepatojugular reflex is that of tricuspid insufficiency (compression of the liver produces a wave of distention of the jugular veins). The decrescendo diastolic murmur loudest at the left second interspace on the left sternal border is typical of aortic insufficiency. The systolic–diastolic murmur is, of course the murmur of patent ductus arteriosus. Although the latter may be associated with aortic coarctation, that lesion is nearly always diagnosed and treated surgically in infancy.

7. The answer is E. The presence of prosthetic cardiac valves, including bioprosthetic and homograft valves, is an indication for antibiotic prophylaxis before dental procedures, as is the presence of mitral valve prolapse with demonstrable mitral insufficiency. Other indications include having past history of bacterial endocarditis, history of rheumatic fever with valvular dysfunction, surgical systemic-pulmonary shunts, congenital and postsurgical valve deformities, and hypertrophic cardiomyopathy. Answers A, B, and D are examples of heart conditions without valvulitis, and answer C (status postcardiac pacemaker) does not represent a disturbance of the endocardium.

8. The answer is C. Mitral valve replacement (for mitral regurgitation) is the valve surgery fraught with the highest mortality rate. The challenge in limiting the perioperative mortality rate is met by keeping a careful eye on left ventricular size by echocardiography.

9. The answer is D. Smoking, with a prevalence of 25% in 1997, conveys a 3.5 relative risk of CAD; the next most powerful factor, family history, has a relative risk of 3.0. Having HDL <35 mg/dL is associated with a 2.0 relative risk. Obesity, with prevalence in the United States of 30% and rising, brings a relative risk of 1.4. Only central obesity constitutes a risk factor and is associated with the metabolic syndrome. These figures imply certain assumptions of degrees of intensity of the factor in question. For example, smoking as a risk factor probably finds correlation because smokers tend to be compulsive and the great majority smoke a pack or more per day.

10. The answer is E. All three choices, C, D, and E, should occur more or less simultaneously in a case of highly probable MI as this vignette presents. The main point to be made is that the patient should be transported straight away, as few primary care offices are prepared by equipment and currency of training to cope as well with the critical first minutes and hours of evolution of an acute MI. Onset of ventricular tachycardia followed by ventricular fibrillation is most likely to occur within the first 24 hours and accounts for the majority of deaths during that period. The patient should not be allowed to drive himself because of that danger. An aspirin can be crucial in preventing progression of a thrombotic process. Starting an intravenous line, if it is secure, can be helpful, but the paramedics are generally very practiced and quick to achieve this once they arrive.

11. The answer is D. Creatinine phosphokinase–MB and troponin enzymes become positive within 4 to 6 hours and troponin levels remain elevated for 4 to 5 days after the onset of MI (eliminating the need for the less specific later- and longer-persisting enzymes such as LDH). The only "false positive" elevations of any significance occur in cases of angina, a syndrome of CAD of great seriousness in its own right.

12. The answer is C. Thrombolytic therapy, if started within 3 hours of onset of MI and when applied in cases with 0.1 mm or more ST segment elevation on electrocardiogram, reduces mortality from acute MI.

13. The answer is B. Silent MI, although more likely to occur in diabetics, does not carry a worse prognosis because of that characteristic; however, an MI suffered in a diabetic appears more likely to result in sudden death, with or without symptoms. Deep Q waves in leads II, III, and aVF are characteristic of posterior or inferior MI, and during the acute phase an ST elevation is likely to be seen in those same leads. In the acute phase, inferior MI is more likely to present with epigastric pain and even pain that mimics "heartburn" than with the classic squeezing or pressing chest pain that radiates into the left neck or left arm.

14. The answer is D. This setting for orthostatic hypotension, defined as a drop in systolic pressure of ≥20 mm Hg or diastolic ≥10 mm Hg, is likely to have a cardiovascular or endocrine medical cause. A patient with gastroenteritis, losing fluids without recouping fluids, would not have peripheral edema. In the latter situation, hypovolemia is present and relative pooling of the decreased venous volume would tip the balance of orthostatic hypotension.

15. The answer is D. Chemical (nonexercise) stress testing allows evaluation of patients who cannot exert for noncardiac reasons, such as significant arthritis of the lower extremities or physical weakness as in this case. Resting EKG is not sensitive enough for seriously ruling out coronary artery insufficiency. Both treadmill EKG tests, with or without thallium scanning, employing ambulatory exercising as they do, are not suitable for the patient in the vignette. Coronary angiography is the gold standard but should not be the first step in diagnosis.

16. The answer is D, carotid sinus massage. This maneuver has no effect on PAT except to increase the block temporarily, which is signified by temporary prolongation of the PR interval. In the case of atrioventricular nodal reentry tachycardia, it will either have no effect or result in converting the rhythm to regular sinus. The Osler maneuver consists of testing for palpability of a pulseless radial artery with the BP cuff pressure raised above systolic BP. If present, it explains systolic pseudohypertension. Digoxin level may be helpful in differentiating the two because digoxin toxicity is a cause of PAT. However, it is a "soft" association and serves only as a basis for ruling out toxicity before evaluating the dysrhythmia further. Orthostatic BP levels have no particular value in differentiating the two rhythms but either may be associated with orthostatic symptoms, as circulation may be significantly compromised in either case as a result of the excessive rates involved.

17. The answer is C. This condition, hypertrophic cardiomyopathy, was formerly called idiopathic hypertrophic subaortic stenosis. Although it is the leading cause of sudden death during athletic exertion, most cases present with more gradual symptomatology. A reduced stroke volume makes the patient susceptible to hypovolemia as occurs in dehydration and during the Valsalva maneuver. In some cases, mitral insufficiency exists on a secondary basis and its murmur is added to that of the primary lesion (though the low-pitched holosystolic murmur radiating to the left axilla is not described in this case). Mitral stenosis and aortic insufficiency both manifest diastolic murmurs. Ventricular septal defect, although causing a diamond-shaped murmur, does not manifest the described symptoms. Medical treatment is aimed at reduction of the ventricular outflow gradient (difference between the intraventricular and the aortic pressures during systole). This is accomplished by use of beta-adrenergic blocking agents and calcium channel blockers, which serve to increase diastolic compliance.

18. The answer is B. Pericarditis is the cause of the symptoms. Chest pain may resemble that of MI, including radiation into the left arm. The EKG shows ST elevation across the precordium, more than would be seen with virtually any anterior-wall acute injury in MI. (Nevertheless, the patient would be admitted to the coronary care unit and MI would be ruled out by serial cardiac enzymes.) The drop of 12 mm Hg in systolic BP with inspiration is referred to as paradoxical pulse and is a typical finding with effusive pericarditis. It may occur also in chronic lung disease, but the patient in this vignette shows no evidence of that condition. The most common causes of acute pericarditis are viruses, including the Epstein–Barr virus (infectious mononucleosis). Nontender cervical adenopathy in the face of severe sore throat is typical, as is the leukopenia found in this case. The systolic–diastolic friction rubs may be difficult to distinguish from murmurs. The lack of chest wall tenderness rules out Tietze syndrome, a postviral costochondritis. Dressler syndrome is a postinfarction autoimmune form of pericarditis that is typically delayed by about 10 days after the MI. The enlarged cardiac percussible silhouette is caused by the fluid accumulation in the pericardial sac. Acute bronchitis neither produces EKG changes nor causes radiation of chest pain.

19. The answer is C. A treadmill test is inappropriate in a patient with symptoms of claudication of the calves after walking limited distances. His diabetes is in poor control (hemoglobin A1C >6.5). Metformin will potentiate the effectiveness of his endogenous insulin production. The American Diabetes Association diet is an obvious choice for improved control and weight loss. ACEIs are excellent additions for both control of BP and for protection of renal function in a diabetic. Holding hydrochlorothiazide may remove an agent that in some patients increases insulin resistance. Ankle-brachial BPs are necessary baseline data for evaluating peripheral vascular insufficiency (see chapter 6).

MATCHING THE CONDITIONS WITH THE PHYSIOLOGIC TYPES OF ORTHOSTATIC HYPOTENSION

20. Pericarditis: The answer is B, nonneurogenic hypotension. Presence of pericardial fluid or a constrictive membrane reduces the ability of cardiac stroke volume to compensate for venous pooling that occurs with orthostasis.

21. Alcoholic polyneuropathy: The answer is A, neurogenic hypotension. The neurologic pathways involved in peripheral vasomotor recovery from venous pooling fails and postural compensation is compromised.

22. Fever: The answer is B, nonneurogenic hypotension. Various possible aspects of orthostatic hypotension include dehydration and hypovolemia.

23. Hypertensive on beta-blocker: The answer is C, drug related hypotension. Beta-blockers (and several other vasodepressive drugs) block the normal neurologic pathways for response to orthostasis.

24. Venous pooling after hot shower: The answer is B, nonneurogenic hypotension. Physiologic vasomotor response to heat involves arterial and venous dilatation that overwhelms the normal neurologic response to orthostasis.

MATCHING THE LETTERED DESCRIPTIONS OF ABNORMAL HEART SOUNDS WITH THE NUMBERED CARDIAC CONDITIONS

25. Aortic stenosis: The answer is C. This lesion causes a diamond-shaped (crescendo–decrescendo) systolic murmur at the aortic auscultatory area that radiates to the carotid arteries.

26. Mitral regurgitation: The answer is A. Mitral regurgitation (mitral insufficiency) causes a low-pitched holosystolic murmur loudest at the apex that radiates to the left axilla.

27. Hypertrophic cardiomyopathy: The answer is E. This crescendo–decrescendo decreases when the patient squats, as a result of an increase in venous return that allows greater diastolic filling in this condition in which diastolic dysfunction is a part of the pathophysiology.

28. Mitral valve prolapse: The answer is D. Midsystolic, late systolic, or pansystolic click is produced. If there is accompanying mitral insufficiency, then there is the additional murmur thereof, as described in the answer to Question 27.

29. Aortic regurgitation: The answer is B. This lesion causes a high-pitched soft diastolic decrescendo murmur that "crashes" off the second aortic sound and rapidly falls off in a decrescendo.

MATCHING THE LETTERED EFFECTS WITH THE NUMBERED MANEUVERS THAT MAY INFLUENCE MURMURS

30. Inspiration, squatting: The answer is C. This maneuver increases venous return and thus increases mitral regurgitation when present (see Question 28).

31. Expiration, standing: The answer is A. Expiration and standing erect decrease venous return and effect an increase in the prominence of a mitral click.

32. Valsalva phase 3: The answer is D. This is the release phase and produces a rapid decline in arterial BP.

33. Valsalva phase 4: The answer is E. This is the rebound phase after Valsalva and it produces a rise in arterial BP and bradycardia.

34. Handgrip: The answer is B. This produces a rise in systemic vascular resistance, heart rate, and cardiac output.

References

Bradley JG, David KA. Orthostatic hypotension. *Am Fam Physician.* 2003; 68:2393–2398.

Eaton CB, Cannistra AJ. Common cardiac problems in family practice. In: Rudy DR, Kurowski K, eds. *Family Medicine: House Officer Series.* Baltimore: Williams & Wilkins; 1997:71–96.

Gutierrez C, Blanchard D. Diastolic heart failure: Challenges of diagnosis and treatment. *Am Fam Physician.* 2004; 69:2609–2616.

Maisel AS, Zoorob R. B type natriuretic peptide in congestive heart failure. *CME Bull (Am Acad Fam Physician).* 2004; 3:1–4.

Wiviott SD, Braunwald E. Unstable angina and non-ST-segment elevation myocardial infarction: Part I. Initial evaluation and management and hospital care. *Am Fam Physician.* 2004; 70:525–532.

chapter 6

Peripheral Vascular Disease

Examination questions: *Unless instructed otherwise, choose the ONE lettered answer or completion that is BEST in each case.*

1 A 35-year-old man complains of pain and swelling of his right leg (calf, lower leg) of 3 days' duration. History reveals that, 8 weeks ago, he was bedridden for 4 days for a severe bout of influenza. He has had no surgery requiring general anesthesia, he has never been diagnosed with cancer, and he does not have any neurologic disability. Vital signs are normal. Examination finds 1+ pitting edema and redness and diffuse swelling of the right leg. The patient has also a slight, thin, grayish discharge from the edge of his right great toenail. There are no visible superficial veins. A D-dimer test was within normal limits. Which of the following is least appropriate for the clinical disposition at this point in time?

(A) Empirically prescribe an antibiotic effective against infection in the lower half of the body

(B) Prescribe warm compresses and elevation of the affected extremity

(C) Draw a white blood cell count and differential

(D) Order a venous Doppler study of the right leg

(E) Order culture and sensitivity test of the toe discharge

2 A 55-year-old woman who 3 months ago underwent cancer chemotherapy following surgery for breast cancer complains of left calf pain, swelling, and tenderness. The entire left leg (below the knee) is swollen with 1 to 2+ pitting edema, and there is tenderness along the distribution of the deep vein path. The D-dimer serum level is elevated. Venous Doppler study is negative for evidence of deep vein thrombosis (DVT). Which of the following is the best approach at this time?

(A) Venography

(B) Serial ultrasonography

(C) Surgical exploration

(D) Bone scan for metastatic breast cancer disease

(E) Prescribe cefadroxil

3 A 60-year-old male smoker complains of the acute onset of pain in the right leg. Examination shows coldness of one-third of the extremity below the knee distally. Popliteal, posterior tibial, and dorsalis pedis pulses are nonpalpable. With no additional information, which of the following is the most likely source of this arterial insufficiency?

(A) Abdominal aortic aneurysm

(B) Myocardial infarction

(C) Acute thrombosis of the right femoral artery

(D) Atrial fibrillation

(E) Mitral stenosis

4 Which piece of the following information would suggest thrombosis instead of embolization as the cause of a patient's acute arterial occlusion?

(A) Patient had previously been experiencing claudication in one of the calves upon walking two blocks.

(B) Patient has atrial fibrillation.

(C) Patient has mitral stenosis.

(D) The patient has no collateral circulation around the occlusion and suffers greater distal necrosis because of it.

(E) The patient has a known carotid stenosis and hypercholesterolemia and continues to smoke.

5 Regarding the patient in Questions 3 and 4, if his occlusion were chronic instead of acute, which of the following would be the *most sensitive* (i.e., earliest) indicator of chronic occlusive disease involving a patient's legs?

(A) There is an audible bruit over the femoral artery.

(B) There are symptoms of claudication after a brisk walk of half a block, which is relieved by rest.

(C) There is a decrease in the ankle-to-brachial systolic blood pressure (A/B) ratio.

(D) The patient has a 30 pack-year smoking history.

(E) There is skin atrophy and hair loss over the dorsal feet.

6 In the foregoing patient, what A/B ratio would suggest *severe* arterial occlusive disease at rest?

(A) >2.0

(B) <1.0

(C) <0.9

(D) <0.8

(E) <0.4

7 A 40-year-old man complains of 3 days of anterior and posterior chest pains. His blood pressure is 138/84, his pulse is 74 and bounding, his temperature is 98.5°F, and his respiratory rate is 16. His trachea is midline. His lungs are clear to auscultation and percussion. His cardiac examination reveals a new diastolic murmur over the right second intercostal space. A chest x-ray shows dilatation of the ascending aorta, and a computed tomography (CT) scan of the chest confirms that there is a 4-cm aneurysm of the ascending aorta. Which of the following is the most likely cause of this patient's aneurysm?

(A) Medial cystic necrosis

(B) Cigarette smoking

(C) Alcohol abuse

(D) Atherosclerosis

(E) Trauma

8 A 58-year-old male former smoker is treated by you for postviral bronchitis that has not responded to empiric antibiotics in the 10 days since the onset of coryza. Although this does not surprise you after a viral upper respiratory tract infection because the patient had been a smoker, you order a chest x-ray. Although the radiologist finds no evidence of infiltration or heart failure, there is an incidental finding of an ascending aortic aneurysm. Which of the following data would most favor an early consultation with a vascular surgeon?

(A) Smoking history

(B) Presence of a 6:1 ratio of total cholesterol to HDL cholesterol

(C) Family history of ruptured aortic aneurysm

(D) Aneurysm with 6-cm diameter

(E) Poorly controlled hypertension

9 On routine physical examination, a 65-year-old man reveals an expanding pulsatile mass in the midline hypogastrium. A thorough review of the patient's medical history is undertaken and a duplex sonographic study is ordered. Of the following, which is the best criterion for defining a patient with an abdominal aortic aneurysm as a potential surgical candidate?

(A) Aneurysm has 2-cm diameter.

(B) Aneurysm has 4-cm diameter.

(C) Aneurysm has 5-cm diameter.

(D) There is coexisting coronary artery disease.

(E) There is associated claudication of the legs.

10 The man in Question 9 is now 1-week status post-elective surgical repair of his abdominal aortic aneurysm. In a consideration of preventive issues in this patient, which of the following is most likely to cause his death within the next 5 years?

(A) Aneurysm rupture

(B) Wound infection

(C) Stroke

(D) Postsurgical pancreatitis

(E) Coronary artery disease

11 Regarding the patient in Question 9, which of the following, besides its diameter, would put him most at increased risk of rupture of this aneurysm?

(A) Obesity

(B) Age of patient >65 years

(C) Chronic obstructive pulmonary disease

(D) Chronic hepatitis

(E) Diabetes mellitus

12 You have decided to use a medical approach (as opposed to surgical consultation) with your 65-year-old ex-smoking patient with claudication of the right calf and an A/B ratio of 0.9. Which of the following best describes some of the mechanisms of pentoxifylline (Trental) that are of benefit to patients with symptomatic mild claudication?

(A) It improves hemoglobin oxygen saturation within the red blood cells.

(B) It reduces peripheral atherosclerotic plaque.

(C) It decreases the development of thrombi in already partially occluded arteries.

(D) It improves venous return and cardiac output.

(E) It increases red blood cell flexibility.

13 A 65-year-old woman complains of new onset of swelling of her right lower leg and ankle. There is deep calf tenderness. Which of the following would be of the most assistance in quickly determining whether there may be DVT without resorting to venogram or venous Doppler study? Her vital signs are normal, and she does not complain of dyspnea.

(A) D-dimer serum level

(B) Complete blood count

(C) A/B measurements

(D) Serial creatine kinase levels

(E) Sedimentation rate

14 Regarding the patient in Question 13, the test you ordered is reported positive for suggestion of DVT. Along with a confirmatory venous Doppler study, you wish to rule out pulmonary embolism. Which of the following is the most sensitive and specific method, assuming no medical contraindications?

(A) Electrocardiogram

(B) Plain chest x-ray in the interest of time

(C) Spiral CT scan of the chest

(D) Ventilation–perfusion (V/Q) scan of the chest

(E) Arterial blood gas test

15 You find the patient in Questions 13 and 14 has a serum creatinine level of 2.0. With that information in hand, which method of ruling out pulmonary embolism would you now choose?

(A) Electrocardiogram

(B) Plain chest x-ray in the interest of time

(C) Spiral CT scan of the chest

(D) V/Q scan of the chest

(E) Pulmonary arteriogram

16 The patient in Questions 13, 14, and 15 has proven DVT, and pulmonary embolus has been satisfactorily ruled out. The patient demurs on the option of hospitalization. You decide to commit the patient to 6 months of anticoagulation therapy. Which of the following is the most approved method?

(A) Administration of subcutaneous (SQ) heparin every 6 hours based on partial thromboplastin times (PTTs) for 5 days, and immediate initiation of warfarin

(B) Initiation of warfarin, and regulation of its dosage based on daily prothrombin times (PTs) over the first 5 days, followed by daily warfarin and frequency of PT determined by the results and stability of follow-up

(C) Home administration of SQ low-molecular-weight heparin (LMWH), with dosage to be regulated according to PTT follow-up

(D) Home administration of SQ LMWH for 5 days, initiating warfarin orally on day 2 of the LMWH, regulated according to serial PT

(E) Administration of SQ LMWH daily or twice daily for 6 months

17 Relevant to the preceding vignettes, once a patient with DVT has been diagnosed, stabilized, and anticoagulated, one should consider investigating the patient for all except which of the following issues?

(A) Occult malignancy

(B) Deficiency of protein C

(C) Deficiency of protein S

(D) Raynaud phenomenon

(E) Deficiency of antithrombin III

18 For the patient in Question 13, now assume the venous Doppler study was negative for DVT but that superficial leg veins are thrombosed, "ropy," and inflamed. Which of the following would be management of the patient within the community standard?

(A) LMWH

(B) Topical heat application

(C) Surgical division and ligation of the vein

(D) Bed rest

(E) Warfarin

19 A 58-year-old female patient was referred back to you, her family physician, by an ophthalmologist she consulted for an episode of blindness of her left eye (only) lasting about 2 minutes that occurred 2 days ago. She denies visual disturbance since the episode and has no areas of focal weakness or numbness, nor does she have problems of mental concentration or memory. Which of the following segments of the physical examination is likely to furnish the most helpful immediate findings?

(A) Funduscopy

(B) Cardiac segment

(C) Lung fields

(D) Neck

(E) Abdominal segment

20 A 60-year-old man without specific complaints is undergoing a routine complete physical examination by you. He has not been in since his last annual examination 1 year ago. As is your custom on any patient older than 40 years, after auscultation of the heart you place the diaphragm of the stethoscope over the carotid arteries and hear a bruit over the left carotid. The pulses are palpable. No goiter is present. Further history review confirms that he has had no neurologic symptoms, including visual disturbance or motor and somatic sensory symptoms. The remainder of the history and examination are normal, and the patient is taking no ongoing medications. Which of the following should be the proximate disposition of the case?

(A) Refer for carotid angiogram

(B) Start aspirin 85 mg daily

(C) Order carotid Doppler studies

(D) Order cardiac stress testing

(E) Refer for coronary angiography

21 A 60-year-old man has recurrence of symptomatic stenosis of the left iliac artery after undergoing successful balloon angioplasty of the lesion 6 months earlier. Of all the following listed therapeutic interventions, which one is *not* indicated?

(A) Smoking cessation by the patient

(B) Repeat balloon angioplasty

(C) Mechanical atherectomy

(D) Stent placement

(E) Streptokinase infusion

Examination Answers

1. The answer is D. Although DVT lies within the differential diagnosis of this case, the vignette places the patient in the 0% to 13% probability by the Wells clinical decision rules (CDRs). The Wells CDRs, with a maximum point number of 9, show this patient to have 2 points. After 2 points are subtracted for the possibility of another diagnosis (cellulitis) that could account for the findings, the net score is 1. This confers a 0% to 13% possibility of DVT (see Table 6–1). Therefore, the patient may be followed expectantly while he is treated symptomatically or empirically. This patient may well have a case of cellulitis secondary to an infection of the great toe, for which culture, white blood cell count and differential, empiric prescription of antibiotics, and warm compresses would be appropriate. Another strong factor in a case like this, ignored in the Wells criteria, is the normal D-dimer. The latter is sensitive for the presence of intravascular thrombosis, though insignificantly specific.

2. The answer is A. According to the Wells CDR scale, this patient has a score of 4, placing her in the high-probability category for DVT (Table 6–1). Even in the face of negative ultrasonographic studies a venogram should be ordered, although if the Wells score were in the moderate category, then serial ultrasonography would be

TABLE 6–1 Wells Clinical Decision Rule

Clinical Characteristic	Score
Active cancer (within 6 months)	1
Paralysis, paresis, or recent plaster immobilization of lower extremities	1
Recently bedridden for more than 3 days or had surgery within 12 weeks	1
Localized tenderness along the distribution of deep veins	1
Entire leg swollen	1
Calf swelling to 3 cm more expected for symptomatic side	1
Pitting edema confined to the symptomatic leg	1
Collateral superficial veins	1
Previously documented DVT	1
Alternative diagnosis at least as likely as DVT	−2

To determine the probability of DVT, calculate the score and place the patient in one of the following categories: 0 = low probability (0% to 13%); 1 to 2 = moderate probability (13% to 30%); ≥3 = high probability (49% to 81%). Modified from Smucny J. and Cohania R., *American Family Physician* (2004; 70:565).

acceptable. Prescribing cefadroxil (Duricef) would be a good choice for infection below the waist, but there is no evidence for infection in the vignette. Surgical exploration is inappropriate, and checking for metastatic disease has a secondary priority at this point.

3. The answer is D. Atrial fibrillation is the most common cause of acute peripheral arterial blockage. Acute obstruction is virtually always embolic in origin. Thus, acute thrombosis as a cause of acute arterial obstruction is unusual, and when it occurs it implies pre-existing atherosclerotic disease with superimposition of a thrombotic process. All other choices are valid causes of peripheral arterial embolism but not in the incidence of embolism that is due to atrial fibrillation. Myocardial infarction is the second-ranking cause of acute occlusion. When the latter occurs, it can be inferred that there is a significant portion of ventricular wall that is relatively flaccid, adjacent to which there is relative stagnation of blood flow.

4. The answer is A. The patient had previously been experiencing claudication in one of his calves when he walked two blocks. Patients with acute arterial thrombosis typically have some risk factors (including male gender) for the development of atherosclerosis and signs or symptoms of *chronic* arterial occlusive disease such as claudication.

5. The answer is C. A decrease in the A/B systolic blood pressure ratio is the earliest and most sensitive indicator for peripheral arterial occlusion. To obtain the A/B ratio, one obtains a systolic blood pressure reading on the posterior tibial artery and divides this by the systolic blood pressure reading in the brachial artery. Cigarette smoking is the strongest risk factor for peripheral arterial occlusive disease development, but is not an indicator for it. Symptoms, bruits, and skin changes and loss of distal pulses occur later as the occlusive disease progresses.

6. The answer is E, <0.4. A ratio of >1 is normal, as systolic blood pressure is normally slightly higher in the legs than in the arms. A ratio <0.9 is consistent with some degree of arterial occlusive disease and <0.4 would indicate severe disease.

7. **The answer is A.** Descending aortic aneurysms are usually caused by atherosclerosis, although some are caused by trauma. Ascending aneurysms such as presented here are usually secondary to cystic medial necrosis or syphilis.

8. **The answer is D.** The chance that an ascending aortic aneurysm will rupture if the diameter lies in the range of 5 to 10 cm is 11.5%. Above 10 cm the risk of rupture rises precipitously and averages 44%. Smoking history, uncontrolled hypertension, and dyslipidemia are risk factors for aneurysm formation but do not bear directly on risk of rupture.

9. **The answer is C.** As the diameter of an abdominal aortic aneurysm exceeds 5 cm, the chances of rupture rise from 3% to 12% at 4 to 5 cm to 25% to 41% for over 5 cm. Coexisting coronary artery disease is common coexisting pathology, as is claudication of the legs. However, these factors have no direct bearing on the chances of rupture. Note that the abdominal aorta, being "downstream" in the blood distribution from the thoracic aorta, is normally of a smaller diameter and thus is a smaller diameter tolerated in aneurysmal dilatation.

10. **The answer is E,** coronary artery disease. This is the reason aggressive search for underlying coronary artery disease is indicated prior to elective abdominal aortic aneurysm repair. If coronary artery bypass is indicated, it should be done prior to repair of the aneurysm.

11. **The answer is C,** chronic obstructive pulmonary disease. Rupture of an abdominal aortic aneurysm is associated with larger-diameter aneurysms, hypertension, and chronic obstructive pulmonary disease. Advanced age and possibly diabetes mellitus correlate with an increase in the incidence of abdominal aortic aneurysm but are not identified risk factors for rupture.

12. **The answer is E.** It increases red blood cell flexibility. Pentoxifylline improves tissue oxygenation in patients with chronic peripheral arterial occlusive disease by decreasing blood viscosity and increasing compliance in red blood cells.

13. **The answer is A.** D-dimer is quite sensitive for significant thrombus formation. However, it is not greatly specific because it may be elevated in the presence of soft-tissue injury. Complete blood count and sedimentation rate give no specific information regarding an inflammatory process. A/B blood pressure readings are helpful in determining the presence and severity of arterial insufficiency (see Question 6). Creatine kinase enzyme levels are elevated in myocardial infarction.

14. **The answer is C.** For accuracy and speed the spiral CT has become the community standard in most areas. A plain film has nothing to offer in the acute phase, although it may show a recognizable infiltrate after a few days—too late in many cases to prevent further embolism. An electrocardiogram shows nonspecific changes in 70% of cases (e.g., sinus tachycardia and nonspecific T-wave changes). Only 5% may show more specific right-sided changes, such as the new appearance of right-axis deviation, right ventricular hypertrophy, or P pulmonale. Thus, these are found only in cases of large emboli. A V/Q scan depends on lack of uptake of macroaggregates of radioactive albumin in embolized areas of the lung, while the ventilation is unaffected. In lung disease, wherein ventilation is obstructed to affected segments of the lung, parenchyma perfusion may or may not be affected. This test was the standard diagnostic approach until the last 5 years. It is not specific enough, though quite sensitive in high-risk cases. Arterial blood gases may show hypoxia and respiratory alkalosis that is due to hyperventilation, when present in severe cases. The gold standard is pulmonary arteriography. It is 97% sensitive. Routine use of this study is somewhat controversial but is indicated in the following situations: intermediate or high pretest probability when other studies leave doubt of the diagnosis; nondiagnostic V/Q scans; and when diagnosis must be established with certainty, as when there are relative contraindications to anticoagulation.

15. **The answer is D.** The V/Q scan, although imperfect, would be the wisest choice. Both spiral (sometimes called helical) CT scan and pulmonary arteriogram involve dye that is relatively strongly contraindicated in the presence of renal insufficiency. The other choices have been addressed as inadequately accurate. Most DVTs are not detected, but fortunately only about 30% to 40% of patients with these go on to pulmonary embolism and only 10% of these patients die from it.

16. **The answer is D.** Anticoagulation of the patient with DVT and without pulmonary embolus for 6 months reduces the risk of recurrence of DVT and pulmonary embolism by 80% to 90%. The points of this question to be appreciated are the following. First, LMWH (e.g., Lovenox, enoxaparin) is as effective as intravenous therapy for this type of case and has a therapeutic onset of action comparable thereto and requires no monitoring of PTT. Second, warfarin therapy needs several days to be

brought into therapeutic levels as regulated according to PT values, and it must be started virtually concurrently with the LMWH; some believe that warfarin should be started 1 day later because of the possibility of initial increase in coagulability caused by warfarin before its anticoagulation effect takes hold.

17. The answer is D. The Raynaud phenomenon is an arteriolar process involving vasospasm in the manual digits that results in color changes to white, bluish purple, and red, usually cycling over a relatively short period of minutes. If it is an isolated phenomenon, it is called Raynaud disease. Otherwise it is associated with vasospastic phenomena attendant to autoimmune diseases. DVT may be associated with occult (or overt) malignancy (20% of cases, of which 25% are lung cancer) and deficiency of proteins C or S and of antithrombin III. In addition, it may be associated with factor V Leiden mutation, homocystinuria, and paroxysmal nocturnal hemoglobinuria. Mutation in factor V causes a poor anticoagulant response to activated protein C. This defect will not be detected in standard activated PTT, PT, or protein C assays.

18. The answer is B, topical heat application. Anticoagulants are not indicated when extension into the deep venous extension has not occurred. Bed rest is feared to *promote* extension into the deep venous system. Nonsteroidal anti-inflammatory agents and topical heat are usually all that is required in treatment.

19. The answer is D. The patient in this vignette has had a classic bout of amaurosis fugax (transient blindness), always in one eye. The vast majority of cases are due to small emboli from ipsilateral carotid artery stenosis, exceptions being in (usually) young people without vascular disease. In those cases amaurosis may be caused by choroidal or retinal artery vasospasm. The amaurosis associated with carotid artery disease may be partial (e.g., in the form of a quadrantanopsia), though often in medical school the syndrome is described as a complete loss of vision in one eye. Examination of the carotid arteries nearly always reveals auscultatory bruits. With or without a bruit the carotids must be subjected to Doppler studies or carotid artery angiography. Such examination should be done on an urgent basis concurrently with vascular surgery consultation. This syndrome is classified under transient ischemic attack. Timely carotid endarterectomy (CEA) markedly reduces the chances of stroke. Funduscopy would be abnormal only in cases of retinal vasospasm. The remainder of the physical examination, albeit always a worthy endeavor, is not particularly relevant to the complaint.

20. The answer is C. A carotid Doppler study should be done. If the stenosis is ≥60%, then a firm indication for CEA exists. This case is different from that of Question 18 in two main regards: Whereas the patient in Question 18 was symptomatic, this patient is asymptomatic. The symptomatic patient with a transient ischemic attack secondary to carotid disease, male or female, merits urgent CEA. However, as an asymptomatic man this patient deserves a more aggressive therapeutic approach than would an asymptomatic woman. The Asymptomatic Carotid Atherosclerosis Study showed that for ≥60% stenosis, interdictive CEA reduces the odds of stroke from roughly 11% over 10 years (≥2% per year) by roughly 53% (≈1% per year) for the population at large. It has been estimated that about 50% of strokes are due to extracranial pathology, accessible to the surgical knife. If men are considered separately, stroke reduction by preemptive CEA is an impressive 66%. However, if asymptomatic women are considered separately, the results are inconclusive. Carotid angiography is reserved for cases in which surgical indication is less than clear. Daily aspirin is a normal part of secondary prevention (and primary prevention for disease-free adults over the age of 50 or so), for the inhibition of platelet aggregation. Before any vascular surgery is to be performed, studies of the coronary circulation are a part of preoperative evaluation but not a part of the specific diagnosis of bruits or amaurosis.

21. The answer is E. A streptokinase infusion has no place in the treatment of an established plaque, whereas it may be employed in treatment of an acute thrombosis.

References

Chestnut M, Prendergast TJ. Lung disorders of the pulmonary circulation. In: Tierney LM, McPhee SJ, Papadakis MA, eds. *Current Medical Diagnosis and Treatment.* 43rd ed. New York: McGraw-Hill/Appleton & Lange; 2004:212–305.

Ebell MH. Evidence-based initiation of warfarin (Coumadin). *Am Fam Physician.* 2005; 71:763–770.

Executive Committee for Asymptomatic Carotid Atherosclerosis Study. Endarterectomy for asymptomatic carotid artery stenosis. *JAMA.* 1995; 273:1421–1428.

Formon JJ, Kurzweg FT, Broadway RK. Aneurysms of the aorta: A review. *Ann Surg.* 1967; 165:557–563.

Kurowski K. Peripheral vascular disease. In: Rudy DR, Kurowski K, eds. *Family Medicine: House Officer Series.* Baltimore: Williams & Wilkins; 1997:97–122.

chapter 7

Cerebrovascular Disease

Examination questions: Unless instructed otherwise, choose the ONE lettered answer or completion that is BEST in each case.

1 A 45-year-old white man comes to you for the first time for a "complete physical." He is concerned that both his father and paternal grandfather died in their fifties of stroke; further, a paternal uncle recently had a stroke leaving him left hemiparetic but functional. After a complete review of systems and examination of all sectors he returns to review the results, including those of comprehensive laboratory testing. You have found that he has a blood pressure (BP) of 155/98 averaged over three determinations. His total cholesterol (TC) is 240 mg/dL, his high-density lipoprotein cholesterol (HDL-C) is 35 mg/dL, and his low-density cholesterol (LDL-C) is 140 mg/dL. He has smoked a pack of cigarettes per day for the last 25 years. He is employed in a high-tension occupation, that of stock trader, in which his income depends on his success on behalf of his clients. Which of the above risk factors is most prevalent in cerebrovascular (stroke) disease?

(A) Elevated LDL-C

(B) Reduced HDL-C

(C) Elevated TC

(D) Cigarette smoking

(E) Hypertension

2 Which of these risk factors, if corrected, would most reduce this patient's chances of having a stroke?

(A) Elevated LDL-C

(B) Reduced HDL-C

(C) Elevated TC

(D) Cigarette smoking

(E) Hypertension

3 For the uncle of the patient in Question 1, rendered hemiparetic by a stroke, secondary prevention is a critical aspect of his overall management. Which of the following risk factors, if present and corrected by the specific treatment plans listed, would be the most potent in secondary prevention of stroke?

(A) Antihypertensive drug therapy for hypertension

(B) Statin therapy for TC

(C) Smoking cessation in a one pack per day smoker

(D) Daily dosage of aspirin

(E) Warfarin (Coumadin) anticoagulation therapy

4 Risk of stroke with untreated nonrheumatic (nonvalvular) atrial fibrillation varies greatly according to age, presence of risk factors, and history of prior stroke. With all categories thrown together, what is the average annual risk of stroke in the presence of nonvalvular atrial fibrillation?

(A) 1%

(B) 2.5%

(C) 5%

(D) 10%

(E) 17%

5 In the last 15 minutes, a 67-year-old male patient has had the onset of flaccidity in his right arm and the inability to articulate what he wishes to say. His wife calls for advice. Which of the following is the best choice for the next step in disposition of this case?

(A) Make an appointment with you for the next morning in your office

(B) Give instructions for her to drive the patient to the closest emergency department and for her to tell the doctor on duty to call you after she or he has seen the patient

(C) Tell her you will come immediately to make a house call in order to evaluate the situation

(D) Order the patient to be transported to the nearest fully equipped emergency department and then call through to the physician on duty for activation of a protocol

(E) Explain that the patient will need physical and speech therapy after the acute phase of the stroke has passed

6 If the patient in Question 5 had not been reported to you but the neurologic symptoms had recovered within 2 hours (or up to 24 hours), what would be the chances of that patient having a completed stroke with the next 3 months?

(A) 1%

(B) 5%

(C) 10%

(D) 20%

(E) 30%

7 Each of the following may be included in the differential diagnosis of the patient in Question 5 (besides stroke) if considered within the first few minutes of neurologic symptoms except for which one?

(A) Migraine syndrome

(B) Hypoglycemia

(C) Metastatic cancer

(D) Seizure

(E) Amyotrophic lateral sclerosis

8 Knowing that control of hypertension is the most productive of therapeutic measures available for secondary prevention of stroke, within 48 hours after a patient has an acute cerebrovascular event you would be least aggressive in control of elevated BP in which of the following clinical situations?

(A) BP ≥200/≥120 mm Hg

(B) Concurrent acute myocardial infarction with left ventricular failure

(C) Concurrent renal failure

(D) Acute hemiplegia with a BP of 180/95

(E) Hypertensive encephalopathy

9 A 65-year-old white woman has seen you for her yearly gynecologic examination. You have seized the opportunity to pursue other preventive health measures and draw lipids. On the return visit you note her lipids are at reasonably good levels. She once smoked but you talked her into successful cessation 5 years ago. Her past medical history is significant for stenosis of her left femoral artery secondary to atheroscle-

rosis. She has no history of hypertension or diabetes mellitus. On cardiac auscultation you detect sinus arrhythmia but no murmurs. You do not appreciate any carotid bruits. An electrocardiogram reveals sinus arrhythmia with a rate of about 74 and a left anterior hemiblock. Which of the following features from her history or examination is a risk factor for stroke?

(A) Caucasian race

(B) Femoral artery stenosis secondary to atherosclerosis

(C) Sinus arrhythmia

(D) Female sex

(E) Left anterior hemiblock

10 With regard to stroke prevention, what is the best statement about ticlopidine?

(A) Ticlopidine is the best drug available for inhibition of platelet aggregation.

(B) Ticlopidine functions through a thrombolytic mechanism.

(C) The best application of ticlopidine is for platelet deaggregation in patients who are allergic to aspirin or in whom aspirin is contraindicated.

(D) Ticlopidine therapy must be monitored through serial prothrombin time.

(E) Ticlopidine therapy must be monitored through serial partial thromboplastin time.

11 Which of the following patients listed would most warrant an evaluation for vasculitis and the antiphospholipid antibody syndrome as cause(s) of a stroke as opposed to the more common atherosclerotic or embolic cause?

(A) A 40-year-old woman with an ischemic stroke

(B) A 54-year-old man with known atherosclerosis of his iliac arteries and who has had two myocardial infarctions

(C) A 20-year-old patient who has had an intracerebral hemorrhage secondary to rupture of an arteriovenous malformation

(D) A 60-year-old diabetic patient with hypertension

(E) A 70-year-old patient with chronic atrial fibrillation

12 A 65-year-old white man complains of the worst headache he has ever experienced. The headache had its onset at 3:15 PM today and his wife has brought him to you. The patient can speak and walk and is stable as to cardiorespiratory status. Which of the following tests would you order first?

(A) A noncontrast computed tomography (CT) scan of the head

(B) A CT scan of the head with contrast

(C) A magnetic resonance image (MRI) study of the brain

(D) Skull x-rays

(E) Lumbar puncture to look for red blood cells in the cerebrospinal fluid

13 A 65-year-old hypertensive white man who smokes has developed right hemiplegia and expressive aphasia over a period of 15 minutes while on a hunting trip. The attack occurred 30 hours ago and his condition has not changed in the interim. He had complained of headache at the time of onset. At this time he is unable to communicate his symptoms and seems confused aside from his aphasia. Which of the following features is the most probable cause of this clinical condition?

(A) Thrombotic stroke

(B) Metastatic carcinoma from the lung

(C) Hemorrhagic stroke

(D) Neurologic migraine

(E) Transient ischemic attack (TIA)

14 You suspect clinically an ischemic stroke in the region of the right anterior circulation in a 70-year-old male patient with hypertension, who has otherwise been healthy with no known illnesses. He presented with left hemiplegia. Which of the following tests would *not* be appropriate in the initial management of this patient?

(A) A noncontrast CT scan of the head

(B) A complete blood count

(C) Cardiac enzymes

(D) An electroencephalogram

(E) A serum glucose test

15 Which of the following orders would be most appropriate for a 67-year-old male patient with a BP of 160/95 who suffered an ischemic thrombotic stroke 2 hours earlier and who has a pronounced left hemiparesis, and a noncontrast CT scan of the head that reveals no intracerebral hemorrhage?

(A) Coumadin

(B) A low-salt, low-cholesterol diet

(C) Rapid reduction of his BP with labetalol until it is about 120/80

(D) Ticlopidine

(E) Intravenous tissue plasminogen activator

1° Prevent

(#1) BP control

2° prevention

(#1) Stop tob

#2 ASA ···· BP control

#3 Statin TX

#4 Other anticoagula

Examination Answers

handwritten annotations: RR = 3-5X, RR = 1.8-2.6X, AF → CVA, 5% per year

1. The answer is E. Hypertension is the most prevalent of modifiable risk factors for stroke, as it is present in 25% to 40% of patients who have suffered stroke and confers a relative risk (RR) of three to five times the risk of strike in the population at large. The second most prevalent risk factor in stroke patients is hypercholesterolemia, which occurs in 6% to 40% and confers a RR of 1.8 to 2.6.

2. The answer is E. If BP is elevated, reduction through drug therapy will reduce RR of stroke (both ischemic and hemorrhagic) by 42% (95% confidence interval of 33% to 50%). Reduction of elevated TC reduces RR by 25% (95% confidence interval of 14% to 35%).

3. The answer is C. Smoking cessation is the most powerful tool in secondary stroke reduction (33% RR reduction). Aspirin antiplatelet aggregation therapy is more effective than the more expensive thienopyridine class of drugs, which are designed also as antiplatelet therapy (28% reduction in RR vs. 13%). Antihypertensive therapy is the most powerful modality in risk reduction for primary prevention of stroke (42%; see Question 2). However, it reduces RR by 28% in secondary prevention, similar to aspirin therapy. Statin therapy for hypercholesterolemia (and presumably for the subgroups of dyscholesterolemia, i.e., elevated LDL-C and inadequate levels of HDL-C) reduces RR on average 25%. Warfarin therapy, although the strongest tool in secondary prevention of thromboembolic stroke caused by atrial fibrillation (66% secondary stroke RR reduction), is less effective than aspirin for thrombotic–ischemic stroke. Another special circumstance is that of secondary prevention of cerebrovascular disease after a TIA in a patient with moderate or severe carotid artery stenosis. Preemptive carotid endarterectomy reduces RR for recurrent stroke by 44%, nearly as great as that wrought for primary prevention of stroke in asymptomatic carotid stenosis, which is 50% (see chapter 6). Although it is useful to know the rank order of risk factors and of treatment thereof, it goes without saying that all known risk factors should be aggressively addressed in secondary prevention of stroke.

4. The answer is C. When all risk and demographic categories are thrown together, the overall risk of stroke in untreated nonvalvular atrial fibrillation is 5% per year. When the categories are broken down, patients younger than 65 years of age without risk factors ("low risk") have a 1% chance of stroke per year; those 65 to 75 years of age ("low moderate risk"), 1.5% per year; those 65 to 75 years of age who have diabetes or diagnosed coronary artery disease ("high moderate risk"), 2.5% per year; those of any age younger than 75 years with hypertension or left ventricular dysfunction (LVD) but no other risk factors ("high risk"), 6% per year; and, finally, those >75 years of age with hypertension, left ventricular dysfunction, history of previous stroke, TIA, or systemic embolism ("very high risk") have a risk of stroke of 10% per year. Atrial fibrillation associated with rheumatic or other mitral valve disease carries a 17-fold increase in the risk of stroke over age- and sex-matched control subjects.

These ostensibly dry statistics should be appreciated in their rank order (but not memorized specifically) because of the implications for management. Persons of low and low moderate risk status should be treated with aspirin; those of low moderate risk should be treated either with aspirin or warfarin anticoagulation therapy, with a target international normalized ratio of 2 to 3; high moderate, high, and very high risk patients should be treated with aspirin, warfarin anticoagulation therapy, or both, with a target international normalized ratio of 2 to 3.

5. The answer is D. This patient is having a dominant left hemispheric stroke until proven otherwise. Diagnosis of a thrombotic (as opposed to a hemorrhagic) stroke must be made as soon as possible in order to activate a thrombolytic protocol within 3 hours of the onset. If this is done successfully, the stroke may be reversed. Although there is a certain chance this event turns out to be a TIA, acting with alacrity at this early junction compromises no outcome. A patient with neurological symptoms that are due to brain metastases would not have such an acute onset unless there was hemorrhage into the area involved.

6. The answer is C. The patient in the amended vignette had a TIA by definition. The chance of having a completed stroke within 90 days is 10%. Half of those will occur within the first 48 hours after the TIA event. For this reason, TIAs must not be taken lightly. As noted in the discussion of Question 5, each TIA must be managed in an expeditious way to exploit the possibility that thrombolytic therapy would be indicated.

7. The answer is E. Amyotrophic lateral sclerosis (ALS) would have a gradual onset. There would be motor symptoms only, and, although bulbar paralysis is one of the types of amyotrophic lateral sclerosis, problems speaking involve dysarthria rather than expressive aphasia. Migraine aura may take the form of focal neurologic symptoms, from homonymous scotomata to hemiparesis and nearly any temporary focal neurologic lesion in between. Being a transient syndrome, migraine aura may be difficult to differentiate from TIA. The former is more likely to occur in a younger person than is the latter. Hypoglycemia may present with diplopia along with disturbed consciousness and may be briefly confused with TIA or stroke. Metastatic cancer to the brain, with hemorrhage, may present as indistinguishable from a completed stroke until an MRI or CT with contrast is done. However, metastatic cancer would be expected to present with a more gradual onset of more subtle neurologic symptoms before the acute event associated with the hemorrhage. Seizures may present with focal symptoms, usually with shaking movements.

8. The answer is D. This choice was intended to depict an uncomplicated stroke or TIA in the presence of significant hypertension but with BPs <220/120. Generally, BP level immediately after a completed stroke is lower than the previous baseline, sometimes even in the normotensive range, often not recovering the previous level for up to 2 weeks. For this reason and because cerebral and coronary arterial circulation may depend on elevated pressures, generally BP should be treated rather gingerly immediately after stroke or TIA, allowing for "resetting" of autoregulatory mechanisms in the cerebral circulation. A TIA may even be precipitated by an orthostatic drop in BP. Thus, only when BP ≥220/120 (or if there is concomitant renal failure, acute myocardial infarction with left ventricular failure, or hypertensive encephalopathy) should it be aggressively lowered within the first few days after stroke or TIA.

9. The answer is B. Femoral artery stenosis secondary to atherosclerosis is a risk factor for stroke, as would be known coronary artery disease. African American race is a risk factor, but neither Caucasian nor Asian race is a risk factor. As to sex, maleness is a risk factor. Other risk factors for stroke have been discussed in previous questions and their answer sections.

10. The answer is C. While ticlopidine functions as an inhibitor of platelet aggregation to prevent intravascular thrombus formation, it is not superior to aspirin and by some reports is inferior in that regard. No monitoring of clotting functions is required. Its best indication is for substitution for aspirin in patients who cannot take aspirin.

11. The answer is A. In a 40-year-old normotensive woman (especially one with no strong family history of atherosclerotic disease), an ischemic stroke is a definite "outlier." In other words, this is a person one would normally place in a low risk status for stroke. A workup for vasculitis or antiphospholipid antibodies is normally reserved for patients who have other features of these disorders (e.g., evidence of systemic lupus), or those who are on medications that are associated with these disorders (such as procainamide), or those who have suffered ischemic strokes at a young age (age <45) with no risk factors for atherosclerosis and no other explanation (such as an atrioventricular malformation) for this stroke.

12. The answer is A, a noncontrast CT scan of the head. This patient has a classic presentation for subarachnoid hemorrhage (SAH). Ninety percent of SAH cases will show intraventricular blood on a noncontrast CT. Contrast adds nothing to the sensitivity of this study for SAH and takes more time and is more expensive. Contrast also requires assurance that the patient's renal function shows no elevation of serum creatinine; the latter may not be assumed in people with atherosclerotic vascular disease, which is the most common cause of SAH in the group of individuals who are 50 years of age or older. Cerebrospinal fluid is obtained only if the CT scan is negative in the face of suspected SAH and shows no lesions that could cause herniation when the cerebrospinal fluid is withdrawn. Skull x-rays are of no value. A CT scan is more sensitive and faster than an MRI.

13. The answer is C. Headache in the presence of rapid onset of neurologic symptoms is a prominent feature of hemorrhagic stroke and may be severe. The mechanism for this is the edema and swelling that develops in response to the hemorrhage and the resultant increase in intracranial pressure. Vomiting and a clouded sensorium are also typical features. Ischemic strokes do not produce this marked edema and produce either no headache or a very minimal headache. In the latter case the onset is usually not so rapid unless the cause is an embolic thrombus. Brain metastases are always a possibility in a long-time smoker. However, the onset of symptoms is not likely to be rapid. A TIA by definition does not last 30 hours (it is less than 24 hours, usually 1 to 2 hours). Although migraine may be heralded by a neurologic aura (neurologic migraine), the aura is short lived, a matter of minutes to an hour, followed by neurologic recovery and, only then, the headache.

14. The answer is D. An electroencephalogram would not add useful information because the telltale changes would only confirm what is obvious, electrical attenuation denoting reduction of functional brain tissue. A complete blood count, electrolytes, glucose, blood urea nitrogen and creatinine, protein and activated partial thromboplastin time, cholesterol, and liver function tests are typically ordered as baseline studies. Serial cardiac enzymes are ordered because of the frequent concurrence of stroke and myocardial infarction. A noncontrast CT of the head is ordered at presentation to rule out a hemorrhagic stroke.

15. The answer is E, intravenous tissue plasminogen activator. Acute use of warfarin or ticlopidine, although used in tertiary prevention of stroke, is not effective in acute stroke. Tissue plasminogen activator will decrease the neurologic defect if given within the first 3 hours after ischemic stroke, but it increases the risk of hemorrhagic stroke development. Patients should initially be allowed nothing by mouth because of the frequency of associated swallowing difficulties and risk for aspiration. Rapid reduction of BP is contraindicated because this may drastically compromise cerebral blood flow. BP is lowered gradually so that homeostatic mechanisms may readjust to the new systolic pressures. Low salt and low cholesterol are primary and secondary prevention strategies but have no place in acute care of stroke.

References

Aminboff J. Nervous system. In: Tierney LM, McPhee SJ, Papadakis MA, eds. *Current Medical Diagnosis and Treatment.* 43rd ed. New York: McGraw-Hill/Appleton & Lange; 2004: 941–1,000.

Coletta EM. Cerebrovascular disease and brain injury. In: Rudy DR, Kurowski K, eds. *Family Medicine: House Officer Series.* Baltimore: Williams & Wilkins; 1997:123–132.

Solenski NJ. Transient ischemic attacks: Part I. Diagnosis and evaluation. *Am Fam Physician.* 2004; 69:1665–1674.

Solenski NJ. Transient ischemic attacks: Part II. Treatment. *Am Fam Physician.* 2004; 69:1681–1688.

chapter 8

Cardiovascular Problems in Children

Examination questions: *Unless instructed otherwise, choose the ONE lettered answer or completion that is BEST in each case.*

1 On a routine well child examination of a 9-year-old boy, you hear a grade III/VI systolic murmur along the left sternal border. You believe it is a functional murmur. Which of the following would assist you in making that determination by decreasing the intensity of a functional murmur?

(A) Temperature of 102°F

(B) Hemoglobin level of 8

(C) Anxiety

(D) Performing a Valsalva maneuver

(E) Cutaneous vasodilatation

2 A 4-year-old boy is brought to you for routine well child examination after his family moved into the area, seeking a new physician for their care. The boy has manifested normal growth and development. He has normal energy output, playing outdoors with his age peers without difficulty. He manifests no cyanosis. On examination you notice a grade IV/VI smooth-sounding (i.e., not harsh) systolic murmur, which is loudest at the pulmonic auscultatory area. The second sound has a fixed split, not varying with inspiration. Which of the following is the most likely diagnosis of this murmur?

(A) Pulmonic stenosis (PS)

(B) Ventricular septal defect (VSD)

(C) Functional murmur

(D) Atrial septal defect (ASD)

(E) Patent ductus arteriosus (PDA)

3 Regarding the patient in Question 2, which of the following is the most significant complication,

besides congestive heart failure (CHF), that may result from late diagnosis?

(A) Frequent and severe upper respiratory infections

(B) Right ventricular CHF

(C) Shunt reversal

(D) Clubbing of the fingernails

(E) Left ventricular CHF

4 A 15-year-old girl complains of chest pains and palpitations. Her mother is concerned that the girl may have mitral valve prolapse (MVP). In what position(s) is a click that is attendant to MVP most likely to be heard upon auscultation?

(A) Supine

(B) Sedentary

(C) Standing

(D) Prone

(E) Reverse Trendelenburg position

5 You are examining a 4-year-old boy for routine well child care. You hear a soft grade I/II murmur loudest in the left second intercostal space. Which of the following would most reassure you and the parents that this is a venous hum and *not* the murmur of pulmonic valvular stenosis?

(A) A venous hum has only a diastolic component.

(B) A venous hum has a coarse, harsh sound.

(C) The murmur stops with compression of soft tissue.

(D) With PS, cyanosis is present.

(E) In venous hum, S_2 is normal.

6 While examining a 3-week-old male infant for his first well child visit, you notice that he has a harsh, pansystolic loud murmur at the lower left sternal border. There is also a heave over the left precordium. The child has been eating normally and the family has not observed any episodes of cyanosis or dyspnea. You find no cyanosis. You had examined this child at birth and before his discharge from the newborn nursery and did not discern any murmurs during these examinations. S_2 is normally split (increases with inspiration). Which of the following lesions is the most likely to account for the murmur?

(A) Tetralogy of Fallot

(B) ASD

(C) PDA

(D) VSD

(E) Venous hum

7 Regarding the child in Question 6, for which of the following complications is the child at risk?

(A) Heart failure

(B) Eisenmenger syndrome

(C) Bacterial endocarditis

(D) Failure of the defect to spontaneously close

(E) All of the above

8 You detect a grade III/VI harsh murmur over the left sternal border and second right intercostal space in a 13-year-old adolescent boy. He has no dyspnea, orthopnea, syncope, or chest pains. You suspect he has congenital aortic stenosis. Each of the following findings on physical examination correlates with that diagnosis, except which one?

(A) There is radiation of the murmur to the neck.

(B) There is presence of an ejection click.

(C) The murmur is loud and harsh both at the base and left sternal border.

(D) There is radiation of murmur to the left axilla.

(E) There is presence of a palpable thrill in the suprasternal notch.

9 Regarding the patient in Question 8, on the basis of his age group, which of the following types of congenital aortic stenosis is likely to be present in his case?

(A) Unicuspid valve

(B) Bicuspid valve

(C) Tricuspid with partially fused leaflets

(D) Subvalvular stenosis

(E) Supravalvular stenosis

10 Diminished blood pressure readings are found in an adolescent's legs, relative to that found in the upper extremities. You suspect coarctation of the aorta. Each of the following may be associated with coarctation except for which factor?

(A) This may be an XO female patient.

(B) There may be notching of the ribs seen on x-ray.

(C) A delay in the femoral pulse may be found.

(D) Cyanosis of the lips and clubbing of the fingernails may be observed.

(E) The patient is more likely to be male than female.

11 A 16-year-old boy is brought to you for the first time by his parents, complaining of increasing fatigability. Auscultation of the heart reveals a grade III/VI systolic ejection murmur and thrills at the right second intercostal space and in the suprasternal notch. S_2 is not split, either in inspiration or in expiration. The murmur is heard neither over the carotid arteries nor in the left axilla. Which of the following lesions explains these findings?

(A) PS

(B) Aortic stenosis

(C) ASD

(D) VSD

(E) MVP

12 A baby is born prematurely, at a weight of 3.64 lb (1.65 kg). What is the treatment of choice for a hemodynamically significant PDA in this infant that persists for longer than 48 hours?

(A) Observation for clinical deterioration

(B) Thrombosing the patent ductus via cardiac catheterization

(C) Surgical ligation

(D) Vasodilators

(E) Indomethacin

13 You hear a carotid bruit in a 3-year-old girl who has otherwise been healthy and has been growing and developing appropriately for her age. She is on no medications. Which of the following would you recommend?

(A) Aspirin 325 mg by mouth each day

(B) Persantine by mouth three times each day

(C) A carotid Doppler study

(D) A cerebral angiogram

(E) Observation only

14 You have seen a newborn boy within a few hours of birth. His weight was 8.5 lb (3.85 kg). You heard a loud murmur along the lower left sternal border. You delay his discharge home with the mother, pending evaluation of the cardiac status. On day 3 the nursery reports that the baby manifests cyanosis. Which of the following most likely accounts for this picture?

(A) PDA

(B) Transposition of the great vessels

(C) Coarctation of the aorta

(D) ASD

(E) Hypoplastic left heart syndrome

15 On a routine newborn examination of a 12-hour-old male infant, you hear a grade III/VI systolic murmur heard best along the left mid to upper sternal border. The baby, weighing 7 lb (3.2 kg), was born at term via a normal spontaneous vaginal delivery. There were no prenatal or perinatal complications. The child has been eating well. On examination his color is good and there is no tachypnea or cyanosis. His pulse rate is normal and his lungs are clear. Which of the following would you recommend?

(A) Blood pressure readings in the right arm and a leg

(B) Observation only for 1 to 2 days

(C) Chest x-ray and electrocardiogram

(D) Two-dimensional echocardiogram with Doppler study

(E) Indomethacin

16 After following the newborn baby in Question 15 for 2 days more, you find that the murmur has not disappeared; there is no other change in the baby's status. What is now the best choice among the following for the disposition of the case?

(A) Blood pressure readings in the right arm and a leg

(B) Discharge the baby for return and re-examination in 2 weeks

(C) Chest x-ray and electrocardiogram

(D) Two-dimensional echocardiogram with Doppler study

(E) Indomethacin

Examination Answers

1. The answer is D. Performing a Valsalva maneuver will reduce the intensity of functional murmurs. Functional murmurs increase in intensity in situations that increase cardiac output, such as with fever, anemia, anxiety, or cutaneous vasodilatation. The Valsalva maneuver diminishes end diastolic left ventricular volumes and diminishes cardiac output, and it either diminishes the murmur or produces no change in the murmur.

2. The answer is D. ASD is a not uncommon congenital anomaly. It is characterized by a systolic murmur located at the pulmonic auscultatory area and fixed split second heart sound. The murmur is caused not by flow through the ASD but by increased flow through the pulmonary artery outflow tract; thus, the murmur sounds very much like that of PS. VSD is the most common congenital heart defect. Like ASD, PDA, and PS, it is a noncyanotic condition because the shunt is left to right in ASD, VSD, and PDA and PS is not characterized by a shunt of any kind (though in advanced cases there may be cyanosis). ASD usually causes no symptoms until the second decade, except in the complete form. In the latter there is not only an ostium primum defect but a VSD and mitral insufficiency as well. Such cases are usually symptomatic in childhood. In any event, the diagnosis needs to be made in order to effect repair before CHF compounds the issue.

3. The answer is C, shunt reversal (from left to right toward right to left) that produces cyanosis. Right ventricular CHF and ultimately cyanosis and nail clubbing are direct results of shunt reversal. Left ventricular CHF usually does not occur in this disease. Frequent upper respiratory tract infection and even pneumonia are early complications of ASD and other left-to-right shunts, but they are not the most dire consequences.

4. The answer is C. Either standing or squatting positions are the most likely to allow auscultation of the MVP click. MVP in adolescents is most likely to occur in thin girls. Chest pains and palpitations are reported with MVP, but it has not been proven that these symptoms are more common in MVP patients than in the population at large. In the Trendelenburg position the patient is supine with head tilted upward; the reverse Trendelenburg position

has the patient prone with the head end tilted down. The latter is a quick treatment for neurogenic hypotension in order to increase cerebral circulation.

5. The answer is C. A venous hum is blocked by compression of the soft tissue just cephalad to the maximum point of audibility of the murmur. One accomplishes this by placing one or two fingers in a transverse position in the aforementioned position. The murmur also is said to dissipate when the child lies supine, but this is not reliable. Further, the venous hum often dissipates with the turning of the child's head. The quality of the murmur is soft, not harsh. The murmur tends to be both systolic and diastolic in timing; that is, it is machinerylike. Neither PS nor venous hum may manifest cyanosis with the exception that, in the case of PS, cyanosis may occur in advanced and symptomatic cases (this patient manifested no other signs or symptoms). S_2 is normal in venous hum, of course, but also in mild to moderate cases of PS. Jugular venous hum occurs after the age of 2 years, often in preschoolers, but never as late as adolescence.

6. The answer is D. VSDs account for 30% of congenital heart defects and are the most common type. Tetralogy of Fallot manifests cyanosis early on, as there is a right to left shunt from the beginning. ASDs cause a murmur that is located more cephalad, at about the second left intercostal space near the left sternal border, and is characterized by a fixed split second sound. Patent ductus is characterized by a continuous murmur that is loudest in systole (the machinery murmur). Venous hum has been described. It does not make an appearance until after about 2 years of age.

7. The answer is E, all of the above. Patients with VSD may develop several complications, most of which relate to the increased pulmonary blood flow. This can lead to pulmonary hypertension, the more likely the larger the defect. The latter, of course, leads to a reversal of the shunt, then becoming right to left (the Eisenmenger syndrome). Smaller VSDs often spontaneously close in the first few years of life, but this is less likely with larger defects and in older children. Patients with VSD are prone to bacterial endocarditis, and prophylaxis is recommended.

8. The answer is D. Radiation of a systolic murmur to the left axilla is virtually pathognomonic of mitral insufficiency. The murmur of aortic stenosis is loud and harsh, both at the base and at the left sternal border, and radiates to the carotids. There may be palpable thrills in the suprasternal notch, the right base (point of S_2), and over the carotid arteries. The intensity of the suprasternal notch thrill best correlates with the size of the gradient across the area of stenosis. An ejection click is common (thus, not all clicks are caused by MVP). Of all cases, 75% are of the valvular stenosis type, 23% are subvalvular, and 1% to 2% are supravalvular.

9. The answer is C. Of cases of congenital aortic stenosis, 75% is of the valvular type and the patient is in his teens; chances are that he will have tricuspid leaflets that are partially fused. Those cases that are discovered in infancy usually have a unicuspid situation with a diaphragmlike effect and no defined fissures. Those that are discovered in the preschool years usually have a bicuspid valve. Subvalvular stenosis, presenting as a membrane with a hole in it, comprises 23% of congenital aortic stenosis. Supravalvular stenosis is relatively uncommon (1% to 3% of cases) and consists of two types, both of which may be familial. One type manifests abnormal facies and mental retardation.

10. The answer is D. Cyanosis of the lips and clubbing of the fingernails will not be observed in coarctation. Male individuals are significantly more often affected than female individuals. However, if a phenotypic female is affected, she is quite likely to be an XO genotype. The femoral pulse delay and collateral formation are usually not evident in children. Although delayed femoral pulses are not usually found in children, by the age of adolescence this finding is common. Also, by adulthood, rib notching is commonly found in coarctation. The most common locus of coarctation is the thoracic aorta just distal to the origin of the left subclavian artery.

11. The answer is A. PS occurs most often as valvular stenosis, comprising 10% of congenital heart disease lesions. In mild to moderate cases, an opening click may be heard more prominent during expiration than inspiration. In severe cases, S_2 is not heard at all and hence no split is discernible. In the most severe cases there is early cyanosis, often caused by right to left shunting through a patent foramen ovale. Other cases do not become symptomatic until later in life, constituting an indication for balloon valvuloplasty and occasionally valve replacement, which is best accomplished before the individual reaches the age of 20 years. Aortic stenosis, 75% of which cases are of the valvular type, do not become symptomatic until the

fourth or fifth decades, if ever. The murmur radiates to the carotids. ASD manifests a fixed split S_2. VSD exhibits a systolic ejection murmur, loudest along the lower left sternal border. MVP murmur radiates to the left axilla.

12. The answer is E, indomethacin. Most hemodynamically significant PDAs in premature infants will close with the use of intravenous indomethacin if they do not spontaneously close within the first 2 days with supportive care. Indomethacin is dosed orally at 0.1 to 0.3 mg/kg every 8 hours or intravenously at 0.1 to 0.3 mg/kg every 12 hours. Indomethacin does not usually effect closure of PDA in full-term infants. If indomethacin is not successful, then surgical ligation is indicated.

13. The answer is E, observation only. Carotid bruits are a common physiologic murmur in children and can be heard in conjunction with a Still murmur.

14. The answer is B. Transposition of the great vessels accounts for delayed onset of cyanosis in a newborn. Transposition of the great vessels presents with cyanosis early in life. A patent ductus is necessary along with the transposition to allow any oxygenated blood to reach the systemic circulation. Without either a patent ductus or other pathway for shunting of oxygenated blood into the left side of the heart, the condition is incompatible with life. The ductus arteriosus serves the purpose but closes within a few days. Those cases that are associated with VSD (thus the loud murmur typical of that lesion) begin shunting unoxygenated blood into the right ventricle, and mixed systemic oxygenated and unoxygenated blood goes into the systemic circulation. When transposition is associated with ASD, there is only a soft murmur but cyanosis occurs at about the same time. Although an isolated ASD could be associated with cyanosis, the cyanosis would not occur in infancy. Rarely in adulthood, pulmonary hypertension can develop, which then can change the shunt to a right to left shunt and produce cyanosis, but this is much less likely to be seen in ASD as it is in VSD or if a patent ductus persists. Whether associated with ASD or VSD, cyanosis is worse when there is also PS. Hypoplastic left heart is not characterized by a shunt and therefore is not associated with cyanosis. Transposition of the great vessels occurs in male to female infants 3:1 and tends to occur in larger than average-sized babies. Repair through reversal of the great vessels surgically must occur within the first 7 days.

15. The answer is B, observation only with no testing or treatment if the murmur disappears in the next 1 or 2 days. In newborns, evidence of cyanosis, tachypnea, increasing supplemental oxygen needs, poor pulses, and hypotension are more indicative of hemodynamically significant congenital heart disease than whether or not a murmur is present. This is probably the common transitional murmur. *Transitional murmur* is a nonspecific term for benign and transient functional murmurs often present in newborns within minutes to hours (but not at the moment) of birth, one of which may be the PDA.

16. The answer is A. Blood pressure in the right arm should be compared with that of either leg to rule out coarctation of the aorta (the most common locus of which is the thoracic aorta just distal to the origin of the left subclavian artery; see Question 11). If the arm systolic pressure exceeds that of either leg by 15 mm Hg or more, or if the femoral pulses are difficult to palpate, then the baby should be referred for evaluation of possible coarctation. If the blood pressure comparisons are within normal limits, then the child can be discharged and re-examined in 2 to 3 days for signs of congestive failure. Then, if all signs are normal except that the murmur persists, the baby can be observed another 2 to 4 weeks before being referred for elective evaluation. If in the foregoing there is then congestive failure or cyanosis, the patient should be referred for cardiological evaluation as soon as possible. If the murmur were continuous, it would be due to transient patency of the ductus arteriosus, usually not persisting beyond a few days and then more likely in underweight premature newborns. In the latter case indomethacin is an often successful medical option for effecting closure (see Question 12).

References

Bricker JT, Anderson JC. Cardiovascular problems in children. In: Rudy DR, Kurowski K, eds. *Family Medicine: House Officer Series.* Baltimore: Williams & Wilkins; 1997:133–144.

Tilo EH, Rosenberg AA. The newborn infant. In: May WW, Levin MJ, Sondheimer JM, et al., eds. *Current Pediatric Diagnosis and Treatment.* 17th ed. New York: McGraw-Hill; 2005.

Yetman AT, Miyomoto SD, Sondheimer HM. Cardiovascular diseases. In: May WW, Levin MJ, Sondheimer JM, et al., eds. *Current Pediatric Diagnosis and Treatment.* 17th ed. New York: McGraw-Hill; 2005.

chapter 9

Hypertension

Examination questions: Unless instructed otherwise, choose the ONE lettered answer or completion that is BEST in each case.

1 You have been following a 35-year-old Caucasian man for 5 years as his primary care physician. During those years the patient has "spiked" his blood pressure (BP) several times to such levels as 150/100 when he first arrived at the office, most often when he was on a tight schedule. Usually the BP has subsided to 110–120/70–80. However, over the past year, more and more time elapses after the patient's arrival at the office before the BP subsides to normal range, and over the past 2 months the lowest systolic BP level you have found has been 145 and the lowest diastolic BP level has been 98. This has occurred despite the patient's compliance with your prescribed no-salt-added diet. The patient denies headaches, focal weakness, numbness, and bouts of confusion. The man weighs 165 lb (74.74 kg) at a height of 5 ft 10 in (1.77 m). Which of the following medication classes would be the least likely to be effective as single drug therapy?

(A) Thiazide diuretic

(B) Angiotensin-converting enzyme inhibitor (ACEI)

(C) Beta-blocking agent

(D) Angiotensin-converting enzyme (ACE) receptor blocking agent

(E) Verapamil (calcium channel blocker, or CCB)

2 Regarding the patient in Question 1, which of the following aspects of the physical examination is least important to complete before initiating drug therapy for the patient?

(A) Eyes

(B) Abdomen

(C) Neck

(D) Heart

(E) Neurological portion

3 A 48-year-old African American man has manifested BP levels of 150/100, 145/95, and 170/105 on consecutive separate days over a 3-week period. He has a family history of deaths by stroke and renal failure. Which of the following may be the single most propitious choice for the first drug to be prescribed?

(A) Hydrochlorothiazide

(B) Lisinopril (an ACEI)

(C) Propranolol (beta-adrenergic blocker)

(D) ACE receptor blocking agent

(E) Hydralazine (vasodilator)

4 Normal BP is presently defined as <140/<90. However, therapeutic targets vary with special circumstances. Regarding the patient in Question 3, a black male patient with hypertension, what should be the targeted therapeutic level of BP?

(A) ≤100/50

(B) ≤139/89

(C) ≤130/80

(D) ≤125/75

(E) ≤100/60

5 Regarding the patient in Question 3, which of the following has the most special significance in ancillary studies to obtain *before* starting the patient on the chosen drug therapy?

(A) Electrocardiogram (EKG)

(B) Blood urea nitrogen (BUN), creatinine

(C) Electrolytes

(D) Complete blood count

(E) Liver function battery

6 Hypertension is the most potent risk factor for which one of the following conditions?

(A) Myocardial infarction

(B) Peripheral vascular disease

(C) Stroke

(D) Lung cancer

(E) Renal failure

7 A 75-year-old woman is seeing you for the first time; it is the first time she has seen any doctor for the past 30 years. She had three random, consecutive BP determinations over a 1-week period that were measured at 180/80, 170/75, and 183/85. You decide that her isolated systolic hypertension should be treated with a pharmaceutical agent. Which of the following would be the best first-line drug?

(A) Hydrochlorothiazide

(B) Lisinopril (an ACEI)

(C) Propranolol (beta-adrenergic blocker)

(D) ACE receptor blocking agent

(E) Verapamil (CCB)

8 Regarding the patient in Question 7, assuming no vascular complications in evidence at the time of the institution of the drug of choice, which of the following is the most specifically indicated in follow-up?

(A) EKG

(B) Serum lipid screen

(C) Serum homocystine screen

(D) Serum potassium screen

(E) Serum iron screen

9 A 52-year-old obese man has a BP of 160/100; he has been under treatment for the past 25 years, presently consisting of an ACEI and a CCB, and he has a creatinine level of 2 mg/dL and a BUN level of 38 mg/dL. Although he has a brother with diabetes mellitus type II, his 2-hour postprandial blood sugar is 90 mg/dL. You ordered a C-peptide test and find that the level is elevated. In discussion of his renal function, you must teach the patient what he must do to retard the accelerated reduction of renal function. You begin by telling him that which of the following diseases is the leading cause of end-stage renal disease (ESRD)?

(A) Diabetes

(B) Pyelonephritis

(C) Hypertension

(D) Chronic glomerulonephritis

(E) Polycystic kidney disease

10 A 45-year-old white man with a multiple family history of hypertension weighs 180 lb (81.54 kg) at a height of 5 ft 10 in. (1.77 m) and presents with a BP of 145/95. You place the patient on a no-salt-added diet with a resultant fall in BP to 130/85 that is consistent for the next 6 months. The BP then rises again as the patient gains weight to 195 lb (88.33 kg) and lapses on the low-salt diet. This time the BP responds dramatically to hydrochlorothiazide/triamterene. As first-line drugs for therapy in essential hypertension, thiazide diuretics are effective in approximately what percentage of cases of hypertension in white individuals?

(A) 10% to 20%

(B) 20% to 30%

(C) 30% to 40%

(D) 40% to 50%

(E) 60% to 70%

11 A 35-year-old woman presents to you with BP readings of 150/100, 145/98, and 160/95 on three successive days. A routine metabolic profile shows normal BUN, creatinine, blood sugar, sodium, chloride, and bicarbonate but a potassium level of 2.8 mEq/L. She denies diarrhea, vomiting, past or present fistulae or enterostomy, or taking any prescription medications. Which of the following types of hypertension is most likely present?

(A) Essential hypertension of the vasoconstrictive type

(B) Essential hypertension of the salt-retentive type

(C) Pheochromocytoma

(D) Primary aldosteronism

(E) Renovascular hypertension

12 Which of the following may be an important part of making the diagnosis in the case of Question 11?

(A) 24-hour urine catecholamine levels

(B) 24-hour urine vanillylmandelic acid (VMA) levels

(C) 8 AM supine overnight and 12 PM upright serum aldosterone levels

(D) BP levels sitting followed by BP levels standing every 15 seconds for 2 minutes

(E) Urinary metanephrine levels

13 Each of the following statements regarding pheochromocytoma is true except which one?

(A) Patients with paroxysms of anxiety are often tested for pheochromocytoma.

(B) Ten percent of cases are bilateral (found in both adrenals).

(C) Familial cases tend to be bilateral.

(D) Sensitivity and specificity for 24-hour urine metanephrine, free catecholamine, and VMA levels are sufficient alone to diagnose pheochromocytoma.

(E) Virtually all cases are curable through surgery.

14 You have followed a 45-year-old Asian hypertensive man. Only recently has control been reasonably established on a combination of verapamil (CCB), lisinopril (ACEI), and the combination diuretic hydrochlorothiazide/triamterene. BP levels have averaged 130–145/78–90 over the past 3 weeks. Prior to that time the patient had been erratic in follow-up, but you have educated him to the importance of consistency and compliance. Routine serum urea nitrogen and creatinine levels are found to be 30 mg/mL and 1.9 mg/mL, respectively, and urinalyses show proteinuria. You place the patient on a protein-restricted diet, 0.75 g/kg. After 2 weeks you embark upon a more comprehensive evaluation. Relative indications for 24-hour urine studies in hypertensive patients in a primary care situation include all but which of the following?

(A) Creatinine excretion for measurement of creatinine clearance

(B) Method to rule out chronic glomerulonephritis

(C) Measurement of protein excretion to diagnose microalbuminuria

(D) Urinary excretion of salt for estimation of salt intake

(E) Measurement of urinary urea nitrogen (UUN) for estimation of dietary protein balance

15 In hypertensive patients with no other risk factors (e.g., diabetes) and who are not ethnically African Americans, which of the following is the therapeutic target for BP levels?

(A) ≤120/80

(B) ≤130/85

(C) 130–140/≤89

(D) 140–159/90–99

(E) ≤210/≤120

16 A 29-year-old woman has become hypertensive and BP levels are difficult to control. You have her on 10 mg of lisinopril twice daily, hydrochlorothiazide/triamterene once daily, and 80 mg of verapamil three times daily. BP levels run 160/105 despite the foregoing. Serum potassium was normal before therapy was started. The 24-hour urine studies for VMA, metanephrine, and free catecholamines were within normal limits. Which of the following may be helpful in further elucidating the diagnosis?

(A) EKG

(B) Liver function profile

(C) Lipid screen

(D) Abdominal examination

(E) Complete blood count

Examination Answers

1. The answer is A. This patient manifests the characteristics of hypertension based on elevated peripheral resistance as a preponderant mechanism. The patient's vignette suggests a person sensitive to or responsive to sympathomimetic mechanisms (i.e., the "hot reactor"). As such, the patient's BP is more likely to respond to ACEIs, ACE receptor blockers, beta-blockers, or CCBs rather than to diuretics. Failure of the patient to respond to salt restriction supports the theme, as diuretic responsive hypertension is based on salt and water retention that increases volume. Thirty-five percent of whites and Asians, if hypertensive, respond to diuretics, particularly thiazides. All others respond to the other drugs to varying degrees, often in combination with the other classes mentioned. Ultimately, many cases manifest mixed pathophysiology, because homeostatic mechanisms tend to protect BP on the low side with the passing of time.

2. The answer is E. The neurological examination in the vignette has a small chance of being positive and is not particularly relevant in hypertension that is uncomplicated. Eyes should be examined for funduscopy to rule out papilledema or other hypertensive retinopathic findings. The abdomen should be examined for renal artery bruit in order to rule out renal artery stenosis and renal hypertension by either fibrous band or atherosclerotic plaque. The neck should be examined for goiter to rule out thyrotoxicosis, a cause of systolic hypertension. The heart should be examined for signs of left ventricular hypertrophy (by percussion) and for gallop sounds of early congestive heart failure.

3. The answer is A. Hydrochlorothiazide, a thiazide diuretic, is the best first single drug trial for an African American with the story in the vignette. Some two-thirds of African Americans respond to diuretics, as their hypertension is based on salt retention and volume dependency. African Americans also may respond well to CCBs and to labetalol, the alpha-beta-adrenergic blocker.

4. The answer is D. All hypertensive patients must have their BP levels controlled to normal levels not only to reduce stroke and other atherosclerotic disease risk status but also for protection of renal function over time. However, African Americans, along with diabetics, among others, have renal function that is more vulnerable to deterioration with elevated BP levels, even at high normal levels; 125/75 is calculated to a mean arterial pressure (MAP) of 100. Nephrologists actually recommend that African Americans' BP levels (MAP) be controlled to an MAP of 98 mm Hg.

5. The answer is C. Electrolytes should be checked before starting a hypertensive patient on any drugs, but particularly a diuretic. The reason for this is that one of the causes of secondary hypertension is primary aldosteronism. It causes not only hypertension of a salt-retentive type but also hypokalemia. Once the diuretic is started, the serum potassium is unreliable for several days. The other studies mentioned, except for the liver function battery, are all part of a proper database for initiation of therapy in hypertension but may be obtained after the drug therapy has begun.

6. The answer is C. Hypertension is the most powerful risk factor for stroke, including both hemorrhagic and thrombotic types. Of course, hypertension is a contributing risk factor for all the atherosclerotic diseases as well, but it is not a risk for lung cancer.

7. The answer is A. Hydrochlorothiazide is the best single first drug therapy for aged individuals with isolated systolic hypertension, as it is in a majority of African Americans at any age. Elderly people with hypertension, too, have a tendency for salt-retentive, volume-dependent hypertension. In the case of elderly persons, this is frequently reflected in isolated systolic BP elevations.

8. The answer is D. Thiazides should never be used in elderly individuals without following serum potassium. Most clinicians would "cover" serum potassium by adding supplemental potassium and monitoring serum potassium or prescribing a combination thiazide with a potassium-sparing agent such as spironolactone (e.g., Aldactazide) or triamterene (e.g., Dyazide, Maxzide). Older people are more susceptible to orthostatic hypotension with diuretics and especially so in the face of hypokalemia (<3.5 mEq/L). The other choices, except for serum iron, although relevant to anyone with vascular disease, are not specific to thiazide diuretics.

9. The answer is A. Diabetes is the chief cause of ESRD, accounting for up to 50% of cases, whereas hypertension is the cause in 27% of cases of ESRD. The pathophysiological mechanisms of diabetes type II are underway for years before the onset of hyperglycemia occurs. This is a result of insulin resistance and resultant hyperinsulinemia. C-peptide levels are directly related to endogenous insulin levels. So this patient, being a prediabetic (elevated C-peptide) with imperfectly treated hypertension, has a double dose of risk factors and must get immediately to work toward preservation of renal function (see chapter 17).

10. The answer is C. As mentioned in a variety of ways in this publication, about 35% of whites, Asians, and most other ethnic groups in the United States (but 65% of African Americans) with hypertension have a primarily salt- and water-retention mechanism and thus respond to both salt restriction and diuretic therapy.

11. The answer is D. Hypertension in the face of hypokalemia and in the absence of diuretic medication or gastrointestinal or other pathologic loss of potassium is primary aldosteronism until proven otherwise.

12. The answer is C. In primary aldosteronism, the serum baseline aldosterone level is >20 µg/dL. The level does not rise after 4 hours of erect posture. A 24-hour urine study for aldosterone is also measured and indicates hyperaldosteronism when the excretion is >20 µg/24 hours. VMA, catecholamines, and metanephrine are measured to diagnose pheochromocytoma. Sitting and standing BP levels are done to diagnose orthostatic hypotension.

13. The answer is E. Only about 75% to 80% of cases are cured. Not only are 10% of cases bilateral but another 10% have metastases at the time of diagnosis. The majority of patients presenting to the primary care physician with paroxysms of anxiety have a phobic reaction or anxiety neurosis by other names; however, many of these individuals have elevated BP levels during attacks of anxiety and are logically evaluated for pheochromocytoma. Sensitivity and specificity for 24-hour urine metanephrine levels alone are not sufficient to diagnose pheochromocytoma. However, if the specimen is tested also for free catecholamines and VMA, then they are sufficient, provided the symptoms occur on the day of the collection or the tumor excretes norepinephrine, which appears on a constant basis. Familial cases tend to occur in association with multiple endocrine

neoplasia, types II A and II BF, and the familial cases tend to be bilateral.

14. The answer is B. Chronic glomerulonephritis is diagnosed by urinalysis specifically for red cell casts and by kidney biopsy, not by 24-hour assessment of any urinary parameters. Creatinine excretion must be known for measurement of creatinine clearance (requires a simultaneous serum creatinine level) and for validation of the adequate length of time of collection. Measurement of protein excretion is needed to diagnose microalbuminuria (specifically albumin content) and nephrotic syndrome. If the former is present, a change in drug choices is in order so as to preserve renal function as well as to prescribe a diet restricted in protein (e.g., ACEIs, reduction of protein from the average of 1.25 g/kg to 0.75 g/kg). Measurement of UUN for estimation of dietary protein intake allows a check on baseline as well as follow-up protein intake (or to prove to yourself or the patient whether he is or is not complying with the dietary protein restriction); urinary excretion of salt is accomplished for estimation of salt intake, usually to be restricted in hypertension, and can also function as a check-back on salt-restriction compliance. The formula for calculation of protein intake from UUN is as follows (also see chapter 17):

Dietary protein in grams = UUN in grams/24 hr + (0.31 × lean body weight in kilograms) × 6.25

15. The answer is B. The BP target for therapy and follow-up of essential hypertension is ≤130/85. This is true only for nondiabetic individuals and persons who are not African American. The upper limit of normal systolic BP is 139; the pressure definition of stage 4 hypertension is ≥210/≥120 mm Hg, according to the Joint National Committee on Detection, Evaluation and Treatment of High Blood Pressure.

16. The answer is D. The patient should be examined for an abdominal bruit, specifically a bruit deep in one flank that could be generated by renal artery stenosis. Essential hypertension, be it volume dependent or based more on peripheral vascular resistance, usually has its clinical onset in a person's late thirties or forties. Hypertension significantly earlier or that which comes on after a person reaches the age of 60 must be evaluated for other causes, of which renovascular type is one. When a person is at a younger age, the cause is most likely due to a congenital fibrous band, which has a 2:1 female-to-male occurrence ratio. After a person reaches the age of 60, the cause is more likely an atherosclerotic one, which has a 2:1 male-to-female occurrence ratio. None of the other choices has any specific relevance to the diagnosis of the pathophysiology of hypertension.

References

Initial therapy of hypertension. *Med Lett.* 2004; 46:53–56.

Joint National Committee on Detection, Evaluation and Treatment of High Blood Pressure (JNC-V). *Arch Intern Med.* 1993; 153:161.

Rudy DR. Hypertension. In: Rudy DR, Kurowski K, eds. *Family Medicine: House Officer Series.* Baltimore: Williams & Wilkins; 1997:145–168.

US Preventive Services Task Force. Recommendations and rationale: Screening for hypertension. *Am Fam Physician.* 2003; 68:2019–2022.

SECTION III

Neurology

chapter 10

Neurology in Primary Care

Examination questions: *Unless instructed otherwise, choose the ONE lettered answer or completion that is BEST in each case.*

1 You are shopping for sports equipment at a sporting goods store and your eye catches a young man practicing rock climbing at about 25 ft (7.6 m) above the main floor. You notice that his weight is resting on his right foot in a toe hold. The foot manifests a tremor at about 3 Hz and because of this his heel is oscillating at that rate. This is an example of which of the following tremors?

(A) Parkinsonian tremor

(B) Rest tremor

(C) Isometric tremor

(D) Intention tremor

(E) Action tremor

2 A 65-year-old white man complains that he has a tremor of the right hand. It is best displayed when he reaches for a pen and is manifested easily in the finger-to-nose test. In which of the following locations is the lesion?

(A) Right brachial plexus

(B) Right cerebellum

(C) Left motor cortex

(D) Left cerebellum

(E) Left basal ganglia

3 Regarding Question 2, each of the following processes may be the cause except for which one?

(A) Stroke

(B) Brainstem tumor

(C) Multiple sclerosis (MS)

(D) Chronic alcoholism

(E) Amyotrophic lateral sclerosis (ALS)

4 A 16-year-old boy has developed a movement disorder. When he abducts his arms, they begin to flap like beating wings. Which of the following disease processes is likely to be the cause?

(A) Hemochromatosis

(B) Drug-induced tremor

(C) ALS

(D) Wilson disease

(E) Essential tremor

5 A 67-year-old man has had a gradual onset of a rest tremor over the last 2 years. On examination you note a 4- to 6-Hz flexion–extension tremor at the elbow and pronation–supination movement of the forearm. This patient may manifest each of the following additional findings except for which one?

(A) Tremor worsens with stress.

(B) Tremor diminishes with volition of the movement.

(C) Tremor improves with alcohol ingestion.

(D) Patient exhibits bradykinesia (slow, shuffling gait and decreased arm swinging).

(E) Patient exhibits cogwheel rigidity.

6 A 68-year-old white woman has been a patient of yours for 2 years and is a lively conversationalist. She has had unexpected falls recently and complains of "weakness" of her legs. As she enters the office for the first time in 3 months, she manifests a wide-based gait that you have not noted in the past. She complains also of urinary urgency incontinence. She answers questions correctly but often takes long to speak and is not as spontaneous in her responses as she had been in the past. She can carry out sequential tasks upon request. Which of the following conditions explains these findings?

(A) Subdural hematoma

(B) Multiple-infarct dementia

(C) MS

(D) Normal pressure hydrocephalus (NPH)

(E) Alzheimer disease (AD)

7 Regarding the patient in Question 6, which of the following is the mainstay of therapy?

(A) Ventriculoperitoneal shunt

(B) Glucocorticoid therapy

(C) Nonsteroidal anti-inflammatory drug therapy

(D) Physical therapy

(E) Aspirin 85 mg daily

8 A 25-year-old white female patient of German and Danish descent had an episode 3 months ago consisting of several days of urinary hesitancy, blurred vision in the left eye, and some difficulty in sureness of gait. She was visiting away and waited for her family's return so as to be able to consult you, her primary physician. However, by the time she had returned from vacation the symptoms had disappeared. Now, these symptoms are recurring in a slightly different form. She now complains of diplopia, hypesthesias, paresthesias, and an electrical sensation down the spine when she flexes her neck. Her gait is again disturbed and she manifests hyperreflexia on the left lower extremity along with a Babinski sign. Which of the following is the most sensitive test for diagnosing her condition?

(A) Computed tomography scan of the head

(B) Lumbar puncture

(C) Serologic test for Lyme disease

(D) Test for vitamin B_{12} blood level

(E) Magnetic resonance image (MRI) of the brain

9 Regarding the patient in Question 8, each of the following is an approved disease-modifying drug for the condition *except* for which one?

(A) Interferon 1a

(B) Interferon 1b

(C) Glatiramer

(D) Infliximab

(E) Mitoxantrone

10 A 78-year-old woman is brought by her family for gradual loss of the ability to care for herself. Although she is fully ambulatory and her level of consciousness is full, she has left her kitchen stove on without knowing it and has lost total control of her checkbook, whereas in the past she had been assidu-

ous in the management of her financial affairs. The family wishes to know if there is a cause that can be treated satisfactorily. Which of the following lists of ancillary studies would be the most propitious for diagnosing reversible causes of her dementia?

(A) Complete blood count, thyroid-stimulating hormone, noncontrast computed tomography scan of the head, mental status examination

(B) Serum electrolytes, liver function battery

(C) Chest x-ray, upper endoscopy

(D) Liver biopsy and serum iron, total iron-binding capacity, and ferritin levels

(E) Carotid angiogram

11 A 67-year-old man is brought to you by his family because of rigid gait and lack of facial expression coming on over a period of several months. You suspect Parkinson disease (PD). Many aspects of PD can mimic other neurological syndromes. Which *one* of the following features is seen in patients with PD?

(A) Choreiform movements

(B) A resting tremor that is unilateral at its onset

(C) A loud, widely variable tone speech

(D) Spastic gait

(E) A bilateral resting tremor

12 You are examining a 65-year-old patient with PD. She is on no medication. Although she has some features of bradykinesia and demonstrates some cogwheeling on physical examination, she states that her tremor is the only feature that disturbs her functioning. Which of the medications listed here would be most likely to improve her tremor?

(A) Amantadine

(B) Carbidopa/levodopa

(C) Orphenadrine

(D) Selegiline

(E) Amitriptyline

13 A 48-year-old man had suffered from a gastroenteritis-like syndrome 3 weeks before experiencing a rapid onset of paralysis that began with his lower extremities and progressed to involve the upper extremities as well. He complains also of fingertip numbness and hypesthesias. As you hospitalize him for close monitoring, you obtain no history of recent industrial toxin exposure, recent ingestion of any canned foods or shellfish, or recent tick bite. The patient's vaccine immune status is totally up to date. This syndrome is an example of which of the following pathologic processes?

(A) Chronic inflammatory neuropathy

(B) Combined upper and lower motor neuron disease

(C) Neuropathy associated with malignant disease

(D) Autoimmune polyneuropathy

(E) Mononeuropathy

14 A 72-year-old man who remains athletic, boats in the summer, and skis in the winter comes to you 2 weeks after his latest winter vacation. He complains of increasing fatigue and drowsiness. His daughter urged him to come in when she found him increasingly difficult to arouse. Although he admits to taking several falls, he is unaware of any head injury. Further, his neurological examination discloses no lateralizing or focal findings. Head and scalp examinations are negative for focal tenderness and deformity. Plain x-ray of the skull is negative. Complete blood count and comprehensive chemical profile as well as thyroid-stimulating hormone levels are within normal limits. Which of the following is the likely diagnosis?

(A) Postconcussion syndrome

(B) Chronic subdural hematoma

(C) Medical condition

(D) Subarachnoid hemorrhage

(E) Stroke

15 An 18-year-old man en route to a morning of water sports with peer-group friends fell from the back of a truck bed and struck his head on the pavement. He was confused for 5 minutes and could not remember his phone number. He then spent most of the rest of the day with his friends, though did not enjoy himself. He asked to be taken home to his parents' house at 3 PM. Within an hour his parents noted that he was becoming confused and drowsy. Which of the following accounts for this picture?

(A) Postconcussion syndrome

(B) Subdural hematoma

(C) Nonneurological medical condition

(D) Stroke

(E) Epidural hemorrhage

UMN → affect contralateral side: Hyperreflexia
spasticity → clonus

LMN → ↓ flaccidity

Examination Answers

1. The answer is C. An isometric tremor is produced by muscle contractions in opposition to a steadily applied force. One can reproduce it by asking the patient to hold a heavy object. The implication is that the person is not accustomed to the isometric exercise by the set of muscles in play (i.e., he or she not in condition for the activity or is anxious about the activity).

2. The answer is B, right cerebellum. Intention tremors, examples of kinetic tremor, originate in the cerebellum, ipsilateral to the symptomatic extremity, unlike what occurs in upper motor neuron lesions in the cortex. Of course, upper motor lesions do not produce tremors but do produce spasticity as well as hyperreflexia on the contralateral side, the latter resulting on occasion in clonus. Right brachial plexus lesions, being peripheral neuropathic, would produce flaccid paralysis. Basal ganglia lesions are the site of parkinsonian tremor.

3. The answer is E. ALS is a degenerative process involving a combination of upper and lower motor lesions (i.e., spasticity and flaccidity). There is no tremor. However, at the onset there is frequently twitching or fasciculations of muscle fiber groups as they are denervated by the progression of the disease. An exception can occur if the more selective form, primary lateral sclerosis, occurs, a purely upper motor neuron disease. As mentioned in the explanation for Question 2, this may result in sustained or unsustained clonus, especially demonstrated in the ankle jerk. All the other processes mentioned may affect the cerebellum and cause intention tremor, including chronic alcoholism.

4. The answer is D. Wilson disease is caused by abnormally elevated gastrointestinal absorption and decreased hepatic excretion of copper, resulting in liver buildup as well as depositions in the brain, cornea, and kidney. The wing beating tremor is a classic sign. Hemochromatosis causes liver damage but not tremor. Drug-induced tremors vary with the type of drug involved and may be fine tremors of sympathomimetic enhancement, resembling a benign essential tremor; mimic in some ways athetoid tremors, as in tardive dyskinesia; may be rest tremors, associated with neuroleptics, metoclopramide, or phenothiazines; or the intention tremors of

alcoholism. ALS does not cause tremor per se (see discussion of Question 3).

5. The answer is C. Benign essential tremor improves with alcohol ingestion. The patient has Parkinson's disease (PD) and manifests the tremor typical of that condition (although 10% to 20% of cases show no tremor while manifesting all the other findings mentioned in the vignette). Classically, PD exhibits the rest tremor described (decreasing with consciously intended movements of the involved extremity), the cogwheel rigidity, and bradykinesia.

6. The answer is D. NPH is within the differential diagnosis of dementia. Classically and fairly reliably, the triad of gait instability, urinary incontinence, and dementia distinguishes this condition as opposed to AD (positive predictive value, 65%). The dementia is usually not the presenting complaint and is characterized by lack of spontaneity, inattention, and latency in response. Correctness of statements and fact recall are not usually positive findings in NPH, problems that are encountered in AD. Gait abnormality is a later finding in AD, as is urinary incontinence, and AD more often involves agnosia, aphasia, and apraxia, abnormalities that are not encountered in NPH. Apraxia refers to discoordination of learned movements such as strike, step, and arm swing in gait. In addition, AD features difficulty with word formation and failure to interpret stimuli within an appropriate context. Chronic subdural hematoma may manifest symptoms of dementia, headache, and drowsiness but not usually urinary incontinence. Multiple-infarct dementia mimics AD.

7. The answer is A. The only therapy that may change the course of the disease is ventriculoperitoneal shunt to decompress the cerebrospinal fluid (CSF; however, part of the definition of NPH is a "normal" pressure of CSF). Success is best achieved when the symptoms have been of relatively short duration such as in the presented case. Even then, estimates of success vary widely, from 33% to 90%.

8. The answer is E. This clinical picture in a young woman of Northern European descent, that of scattered neurologic findings that exacerbated and remitted and recurred 3 months later, fits the classic picture of MS.

Females are affected twice as frequently as males. The MRI of the brain is nearly completely sensitive, though not perfectly specific. The MRI performed with a high-field magnet (≥ 1.5 T) should show areas of high signal in the white matter of the brain and spinal cord on T2-weighted images, characteristic of demyelinating lesions in MS. Therefore, the demyelinating process affects both sensory and motor fibers. Lumbar puncture is also very helpful in disclosing CSF immunoglobulin G concentration increased relative to other CSF proteins, such as albumin with oligoclonal bands (90% sensitive and less specific than MRI). Lyme disease and subacute combined degeneration (as in pernicious anemia) should be entertained and ruled out, the latter by the B_{12} level, but they have no value in the diagnosis of MS per se. Other tests that address diseases in the differential diagnosis include thyroid-stimulating hormone, sedimentation rate, antinuclear antibodies, and a serologic test for syphilis. A more refined list would address more rare conditions, not likely to be relevant in the early stages of this syndrome encountered in primary care.

9. **The answer is D.** Infliximab is a tumor necrosis factor inhibitor used in rheumatoid arthritis and other autoimmune diseases. Of interest is that fact that, as understanding of MS has developed, it has emerged as an autoimmune disease. The other drugs mentioned are all capable of a roughly one-third reduction in the rate of exacerbation of the disease and appear to address the autoimmune aspects of MS. A most promising drug, not yet approved, is natalizumab (Antegren), whose early studies indicate a 90% reduction in acute activity and 50% reduction in number of relapses.

10. **The answer is A.** Reversible causes of dementia include pernicious anemia, hypothyroidism (especially in the elderly population), and depression. Serum electrolytes would diagnose hyponatremia, a cause of stupor, not dementia; liver function blood tests or biopsy would diagnose hepatic coma; carotid angiogram would elucidate cerebral arterial blood flow, which is important in focal neurological symptoms as in transient ischemic attack or stroke. The other modalities and tests offer no significant information for diagnosing dementia or disturbance of consciousness.

11. **The answer is B.** The tremor in PD is initially unilateral, only later involving both sides. Choreiform movements are rapid, purposeless movements that occur in Huntington chorea (wormlike movements) and Sydenham chorea (jerky movements of the extremities, particularly hands and feet), but not in PD. About 20% of PD patients eventually develop a dementia, and autonomic features including orthostatic hypotension are common. Constipation and impotence can also be seen. The gait is shuffling with little arm swing. The speech is very soft and monotonal but delirium is not a part of the picture.

12. **The answer is C.** Orphenadrine (Disipal, Norflex) is an anticholinergic medication. This class of drugs is most helpful when the main goal of therapy is to control rigidity and tremor. Other examples of this class used in PD include benztropine mesylate (Cogentin), biperidin (Akineton), procyclidine (Kemadrin), and trihexyphenidyl (Artane). Although other medications are superior in improving the rigidity and bradykinesia of PD, the anticholinergics are more effective in diminishing the tremor. Amantadine improves all aspects of the disease but not if they are severe. Levodopa alleviates all aspects of PD but does not alter the progression of the disease. Sinemet is a fixed combination of carbidopa and levodopa. Selegiline is a monoamine oxidase inhibitor that is sometimes used as an adjunct to levodopa to control the fluctuations in its effect. Amitriptyline is an antidepressant with strong anticholinergic side effects; is not used in the treatment of PD.

13. **The answer is D.** This patient has Guillain-Barré syndrome (GBS) which is thought to be based on an autoimmune process. The condition is also called demyelinating polyradiculoneuropathy. Twenty percent of cases appear to have links with *Campylobacter jejuni* infection. Most other cases have followed apparent viral gastroenteritis, viral upper respiratory tract infection, or influenza by about 1 to 3 weeks. The disease, though potentially life threatening (3% to 5% case mortality) because of involvement of respiratory and deglutition functions, is usually self-limited and reverses within a few weeks. The differential diagnosis includes botulism, intermittent porphyria, diphtheria, Lyme disease, poliomyelitis, heavy metal poisoning, and tetrodotoxin poisoning from contaminated shellfish. Chronic inflammatory demyelinating neuropathy is similar in symptomatology and signs except that it is chronic, remitting, and exacerbating. Combined upper and lower motor neuron disease is a description of ALS. Both sensorimotor and pure sensory polyneuropathies can occur as nonmetastatic complications of malignancies. On some occasions this syndrome may precede the diagnosis of cancer. Therefore, occult malignancy must be considered initially in the differential diagnosis of Guillain-Barré syndrome as well. Mononeuropathies involve just one peripheral nerve, for example cranial nerve VI palsy occurring in diabetes, usually type I.

14. **The answer is B.** This history fits that of chronic subdural hematoma from acceleration–deceleration forces that cause tearing of bridging veins in a closed head injury. Such injuries are more likely to occur in older people and often without a definite history of head injury. Whether they should be evacuated surgically depends on the clinical situation and the thickness of the hematoma. Postconcussion syndrome presents similarly clinically but would hardly be expected to be devoid of a clear history of head trauma, complete with a healing scalp contusion. Medical conditions should be part of the differential diagnosis but diabetes, anemias, renal and hepatic failure, and hypothyroidism have been ruled out. Subarachnoid hemorrhage is arterial and as such is sudden and dramatic (see chapter 7). Strokes virtually always result in focal and lateralizing neurological findings; also, their onsets are rapid, not subtle.

15. The answer is E. The acute injury, with or without concussion, has caused a skull fracture that parts the middle meningeal artery on one side on the other. After the "lucid interval" the patient begins to exhibit signs of increasing intracranial pressure and presents a neurosurgical emergency. This generally forces a decision within 24 to 72 hours. Postconcussion syndrome unfolds over much more time, as does a subdural hematoma (see Question 14) and medical conditions. Stroke causes focal rather than diffuse neurological symptoms and signs.

References

Aminoff MJ. Nervous system. In: Tierney LM, McPhee SJ, Papadakis MA, eds. *Current Medial Diagnosis and Treatment.* 43rd ed. New York: McGraw-Hill/Appleton & Lange; 2004: 941–1,000.

Calabresi PA. Diagnosis and management of multiple sclerosis. *Am Fam Physician.* 2004; 70:1935–1944.

Rowland LP, ed. *Textbook of Neurology.* Baltimore: Williams & Wilkins; 1995.

Smaga S. Tremor. *Am Fam Physician.* 2003; 68:1545–1552.

Verrees M, Selman WR. Management of normal pressure hydrocephalus. *Am Fam Physician.* 2004; 70:1071–1078, 1085–1086.

- Subdural hematoma
- epidural hematoma
- SAH
- Postconcussion syndrome

SECTION IV

Problems of the Respiratory Tract in Primary Care

chapter 11

Acute and Chronic Lung Disease

Unless instructed otherwise, choose the ONE lettered answer or completion that is BEST in each case.

1 A mother brings her 11-year-old boy to you to discuss his recent onset of seasonal wheezing. She says the boy has symptoms on average about three times per week and at least one night per month. After examining his lung fields you diagnose asthma. Based on the history as given by the mother, in what classification (stage) of asthma is this boy's disease?

(A) Mild intermittent
(B) Mild persistent
(C) Preclinical
(D) Moderate persistent
(E) Severe persistent

2 Regarding the patient in Question 1, which of the following would be an appropriate therapeutic plan for long-term control?

(A) High-dose inhaled corticosteroids
(B) Short-acting inhaled beta-2 agonists
(C) Systemic corticosteroids
(D) Cromolyn or nedocromil
(E) Daily inhaled beta-2 agonists

3 A 45-year-old male, 30-pack-year smoker complains of exertional dyspnea and dry cough increasing over the past year. He denies orthopnea. He has been a schoolteacher all his adult life, was athletic in his twenties and thirties, and has lived in homes built after 1975. You ordered spirometry testing. The results are as follows: forced vital capacity (FVC), 40% of expected FVC for age and weight (normal 80% to 120%); forced expiratory volume in 1 second (FEV$_1$), 90% of expected; FEV$_1$/FVC, 95% of the

predicted ratio. Which of the following conditions accounts for these findings?

(A) Acute asthma
(B) Chronic obstructive pulmonary disease (COPD)
(C) Restrictive lung disease
(D) Pneumonia
(E) Mesothelioma

4 A 58-year-old man who has smoked all his adult life at the rate of one pack per day (38 pack-years) complains of acute dyspnea. He has had a cough producing half a cup (118.26 mL) of sputum each morning. After the onset of a bout of coryza, on the third day he became short of breath. Physical examination reveals no definite wheezes, but rather just a reduced percussible diaphragmatic excursion; the patient purses his lips during expiration. His spirometry results are as follows: FVC, 90% of expected FVC for age and weight (normal 80% to 120%); FEV$_1$, 50% of expected; FEV$_1$/FVC, 50% of the predicted ratio. Which of the following conditions best explains these spirometry findings?

(A) Acute asthma
(B) COPD
(C) Restrictive lung disease
(D) Pneumonia
(E) Mesothelioma

5 A 55-year-old man and his wife complain that for a year he has been constantly clearing his throat and frequently coughs just as he is falling off to sleep or on occasion while asleep. He has never smoked and is on no prescription medications, and he has not seen other doctors for the cough. Which of the following is the least likely cause of this problem?

(A) Postnasal drainage drip (PND)

(B) Incipient asthma

(C) Gastroesophageal reflux disease (GERD)

(D) Eosinophilic bronchitis

(E) Bronchiectasis

6 Regarding the patient in Question 5, assume he had smoked 20 pack-years but quit 15 years ago. Which of the following would be least appropriate after finding a normal chest examination and chest x-ray?

(A) Inquire regarding atopic disease (personal or family history of allergic rhinitis, asthma) or heartburn and nocturnal gastric eructation

(B) Inquire and check the office record as to prescription and nonprescription medication use

(C) Order a computed tomography (CT) scan of the chest

(D) If the patient does not prove to have any of the "pathogenic triad," check spirometry and if normal treat as needed with cough suppressants at night and expectorants by day

(E) Start an empiric trial of omeprazole

7 A 65-year-old woman complains of dyspnea with exertion of low intensity but gradually becoming worse over the past several months. She had smoked for 20 years but quit 25 years ago. She has also a history of asthma but has exhibited no wheezing at the times of examination in the office. She has a history of atopic disease in her younger adult years. Presence of paroxysmal nocturnal dyspnea has been difficult to assess because the patient has slept with two pillows since childhood and preferred that position before she became symptomatic. Cough is not a significant complaint and she manifests no peripheral edema. Spirometry testing indicates obstructive airway disease but her symptoms have only partially responded to beta-2 agonists and inhaled glucosteroids. Which of the following would be most helpful in determining whether congestive heart failure (CHF) plays a significant part in her symptoms?

(A) Brain natriuretic peptide (BNP) levels

(B) History of distance in brisk walking before the onset of symptoms

(C) Resting electrocardiogram (EKG) testing

(D) EKG–treadmill stress testing

(E) Methacholine challenge

Match the findings in the numbered items with the lettered causes of acute dyspnea (adapted from Karnani).

8 Intermittent breathlessness; triggering factors exist; allergic rhinitis; prolonged expiratory phase

9 Smoker; barrel chest; prolonged expiratory phase

10 History of hypertension, coronary artery disease, diabetes; orthopnea, paroxysmal nocturnal dyspnea; pedal edema, jugular venous distention

11 History of generalized anxiety, panic disorder, sighing breathing

12 Postprandial dyspnea

(A) Gastroesophageal reflux, aspiration, or food allergy

(B) Anxiety disorder, hyperventilation

(C) CHF

(D) COPD

(E) Asthma

Unless instructed otherwise, choose the ONE lettered answer or completion that is BEST in each case.

13 A 55-year-old male cancer patient has a 1-week history of cough and low-grade fever. There are rales at both bases, but the chest is resonant to percussion in all lung fields. A chest x-ray is negative for lung infiltrates. Which of the following situations may best explain a false-negative chest x-ray for pneumonia in this patient?

(A) There is coexistent CHF.

(B) *Streptococcus pneumoniae* is the causative organism.

(C) Pneumonia is secondary to obstructing endobronchial tumor.

(D) *Mycoplasma pneumoniae* is the causative organism.

(E) The patient has a profound neutropenia.

14 A 25-year-old man who was previously healthy has a rapid onset (over 10 hours, starting during midmorning) of severe sharp, stabbing, chest pain and a temperature of 102°F when he consults you at 6 PM. He has otherwise been in good health, does not smoke, and denies any high-risk activities for HIV acquisition. He has no allergies. Physical examination reveals a temperature of 102°F, a pulse of 110, and a blood pressure of 124/82. He appears to be in great distress, being both toxic and in much pain with each inspiration. Chest examination reveals bronchophony, egophony, and dullness to percussion in the right posterior chest. There are some "sticky" rales in this area also. There is no accessory muscle use, clubbing, or cyanosis, but there is definite splinting of the right lung field with inspiration. A sputum Gram stain reveals gram-positive diplococci. Chest x-ray reveals a right lower lobe infiltrate. Which of the following therapeutic interventions is the most likely to benefit this patient the most?

(A) Penicillin

(B) Trimethoprim/sulfamethoxazole

(C) Postural drainage

(D) Tetracycline

(E) Cefadroxil

15 A 19-year-old male college student has experienced a gradual onset of a dry cough over a period of 1 week. He complains of headache. The white blood cell count is 11,500 with normal differential except for three band forms. Chest examination is negative for rales ("crackles") and percussible dullness. The chest x-ray shows patchy bronchopneumonic infiltrates. Which of the following is the most likely cause of this condition?

(A) *S. pneumoniae*

(B) *Klebsiella pneumoniae*

(C) *M. pneumoniae*

(D) Gram-negative sepsis

(E) *Staphylococcus aureus*

16 A 65-year-old man has developed a cough with low-grade fever and comes to see you on the fourth day. He complains of headache and difficulty focusing mentally. His vital signs reveal an apparent sinus bradycardia at 56. A complete blood count shows a low-grade leukocytosis with an unremarkable differential; electrolytes manifest a hyponatremia at 128 mEq/L. Chest x-ray shows diffuse patchy infiltrates weighted toward the bases. Which of the following is the most likely diagnosis?

(A) Pneumococcal pneumonia

(B) Klebsiella pneumonia

(C) Mycoplasma pneumonia

(D) Legionella pneumonia

(E) Viral pneumonia

17 Which of the following scenarios would suggest alertness to the possibility of an anaerobic organism as a cause?

(A) Pneumonia in a long-time smoker with COPD

(B) A stroke patient in the acute phase with bulbar symptoms and dysphagia

(C) A 45-year-old woman who 1 week earlier had an influenza infection

(D) A 30-year-old nonsmoker with a cough who recently traveled to Arizona

(E) A 34-year-old nonsmoker with AIDs

18 In which of the following clinical situations would a determination of alpha 1 protease inhibitor (formerly called alpha-1 antitrypsin) level be most appropriate?

(A) There is a 75-year-old patient with severe emphysema and cor pulmonale. The person is now home bound and on continuous O_2 with an FEV_1 of 0.9 L; the patient has marked hypoxemia, mild CO_2 retention, and a 35-pack-year smoking history.

(B) There is a 70-year-old male patient with increasing shortness of breath for 10 years and a 30-pack-year smoking history.

(C) There is a 32-year-old patient with mild shortness of breath with heavy exertion for 1 year and with a 1-pack-year smoking history.

(D) There is a 48-year-old male patient with mild shortness of breath with exertion for 1 year and a 40-pack-year smoking history.

(E) There is a 55-year-old patient with shortness of breath for 5 years who has a 20-pack-year history of smoking, but who quit 5 years ago. Her husband smokes two packs of cigarettes per day in the house.

19 Assuming no contraindications, which of the following medications is the first-line pharmacologic agent of choice in treating mild to moderate COPD?

(A) Inhaled corticosteroids

(B) Oral corticosteroids

(C) Inhaled beta-agonist

(D) Oral theophylline

(E) Inhaled ipratropium bromide

Examination Answers

1. The answer is B, mild persistent, according to the National Education and Prevention Program. This system of definitions provides treatment guidelines. Mild persistent asthma is defined as occurring more than twice per week and more than two nights per month but less often than daily and no more than one night per month. Mild intermittent classification is any asthma less severe than mild persistent, that is, two bouts per week or less and two nights per month or less. Expected spirometry findings, in both mild intermittent and mild persistent asthma, should be 80% or more of predicted function, that is, peak expiratory flow (PEF) and FEV_1.

2. The answer is D. Cromolyn and nedocromil are basophil-stabilizing agents. Although mild intermittent asthma requires no maintenance medication, the other three levels of severity are indications for long-term pharmacologic agents. Mild persistent cases may be maintained on low-dose corticosteroids (glucocorticoids) or basophil stabilizers. Medium- and high-dose inhaled glucocorticoids are reserved for moderate persistent and severe persistent severity, respectively. Quick-relief agents such as rapidly acting beta-2 agonists are to be used only as rescue medications, not for long-term therapy. Moderate persistent and severe persistent cases are indications for the alternate agents, long-acting bronchodilators as well. Systemic glucocorticoids are to be used only in severe persistent cases (see Table 11–1).

3. The answer is C. The reduced FVC, the amount one can exhale in one breath after full inspiration, defines restrictive lung disease. FEV_1 is the proportion of the FVC (as a percentage) that can be exhaled in 1 second and can be normal in restrictive lung disease. FEV_1/FVC is normal if 95% of the predicted ratio is achieved (i.e., 75% of the FVC exhaled within 1 second). Poor effort is not a likely explanation in this case, as the patient has a history of athleticism and determination. The chronicity rules out pneumonia. Both acute asthma and COPD manifest prolonged FEV_1 on spirometry, not reduced FVC. Mesothelioma occurs virtually solely in people who have worked around and have inhaled dust from asbestos. Pulmonary fibrosis has several causes, among which are respiratory bronchiolitis associated interstitial lung disease. It occurs in this age group in heavy smokers. It remits in 20% of cases and may respond to glucocorticoids. The median life expectancy with the diagnosis is more than 10 years. Smoking cessation is necessary. The other major cause is idiopathic pulmonary fibrosis, a disease that comes on in a person's late fifties, has no known treatment, and whose prognosis is approximately 3 years after diagnosis.

4. The answer is B. The reduced FEV_1 and FEV_1/FVC ratio are indicative of COPD. Actually, the spirometry findings are also compatible with acute asthma, as both conditions are characterized by reduced capacity to exhale air. The clinical information given in the vignette rules against asthma in the chronicity, the absence of wheezing, and the pursed lips during expiration, a nearly pathognomonic finding for COPD. (Although advanced and critically severe asthma may not exhibit wheezing, that combination occurs in association with far advanced and acute illness compared with the case presented.)

TABLE 11–1 Classification of Severity of Asthma

	Mild I	Mild P	Mod P	Severe P
Symptoms	$\leq 2 \times$/wk ≤ 2 nights/mo	$> 2 \times$/wk > 2 nights/mo	$< 1 \times$/day > 1 night/wk	Constant night (often)
Pulm tests	FEV_1,PEF $\geq 80\%$ predicted	FEV_1,PEF $\geq 80\%$	FEV_1 or PEF $> 60\%$, $< 80\%$	FEV_1 or PEF ≤ 60
Meds	None daily	Low dose Inh corticost or cromolyn or nedocromil	Medium dose Inh corticost LA Br LA beta-2 agonist	High Inh corticost LA Br LA beta-2 agonist Systemic corticost

Notes: Mild I, mild intermittent; Mild P, mild persistent; Mod P, moderate persistent; Severe P, severe persistent; Inh corticost, inhaled corticosteroid; LA, long-acting; Br, bronchodilator.

5. The answer is D. Eosinophilic bronchitis, though not a rare disease in pulmonary clinics, is uncommon in primary care practice. PND, asthma, and GERD, the "pathogenic triad of chronic cough," account for a significant majority of chronic cough in nonsmoking, immunocompetent cases. There may be two causes in 18% to 62% of cases. Chronic cough is defined as persistent for more than 8 weeks. Bronchiectasis is a strong fourth cause. In smokers, of course, chronic bronchitis and COPD come to the fore. Angiotensin-converting enzyme inhibitors cause a cough in 5% to 20% of cases. PND appears to have an atopic basis and may respond to an H1 antihistamine. PND may be associated with sinusitis; sinus x-rays may be negative in some 20% to 40% of cases. It should be appreciated that asthma may manifest cough without wheezing in up to 57% of cases. A methacholine challenge test is recommended in possible asthma cases as being virtually 100% sensitive so that a negative test effectively rules out asthma. Although a 24-hour esophageal pH monitor is the gold standard for diagnosis of GERD, empiric treatment with H+ pump blocking agents such as omeprazole is a more practical approach. Chest x-ray is abnormal in 87% of cases of bronchiectasis, although a CT scan of the chest is superior.

6. The answer is C. This early in the evaluation phase, empiric trials are more appropriate than going straight to a CT scan. The possibility of bronchogenic carcinoma cannot be ignored, even after 15 years lapsed time since the person quit smoking. A CT scan of the chest is nearly as sensitive as bronchoscopy and is an acceptable method of investigating for this cancer that is not diagnosable early enough to cure in the present state of the art. Spirometry findings have no direct linkage to lung cancer, though many lung cancer patients will have chronic lung disease. Inquiring or treating empirically for PND, GERD, or asthma is entirely appropriate and probably more likely to yield the diagnosis than investigating for lung cancer, because lung cancer usually is asymptomatic when in early stages while the chest x-ray remains negative. Inquiring for the medication history would bring out such factors as angiotensin-converting enzyme inhibitor drugs. Still, failure to reach a conclusion with that approach warrants evaluation for lung cancer in the ex-smoker.

7. The answer is A. A BNP level >100 pg/mL is 83% sensitive and 99% specific for congestive heart failure. The present, somewhat involved vignette was designed to illustrate the occasional diagnostic dilemma presented when a patient has known lung disease but may or may not have CHF in addition. Higher cutoff levels of BNP convey a lower sensitivity but greater specificity. Degree of exertion to result in dyspnea is a quantitative tool of assessment but is not specific for either pulmonary or cardiac disease. Resting or stress EKG testing may diagnose coronary insufficiency but tells nothing of the state of cardiac compensation. Methacholine challenge may confirm the presence of reactive airway disease (asthma), but a normal result does not rule out CHF in the present case.

8. The answer is E. Intermittent breathlessness and the existence of triggering factors, allergic rhinitis, and a prolonged expiratory phase describe asthma. Unlike with COPD, the prolonged expiratory phase is caused by a dynamic spasm of the bronchiolar musculature and is reversible by medication.

9. The answer is D, being a smoker and having a barrel chest and prolonged expiratory phase. COPD is evidenced by these findings and is statistically likely, given the history of smoking. Both asthma and COPD exhibit a prolonged expiratory phase of respiration.

10. The answer is C. In this situation (history of hypertension, coronary artery disease, diabetes; orthopnea, paroxysmal nocturnal dyspnea; and pedal edema, jugular venous distention), CHF is a statistical probability; however, the cause of dyspnea is not diagnosed by the symptomatology given.

11. The answer is B. For history of generalized anxiety, panic disorder, and sighing breathing, the cause is anxiety disorder, hyperventilation. The attendant respiratory alkalosis aggravates the symptoms of anxiety.

12. The answer is A. For postprandial dyspnea, the cause is gastroesophageal reflux, aspiration, or food allergy. Always there would be an accompanying cough.

13. The answer is E. When the patient has a profound neutropenia (as occurs perhaps in a patient who is undergoing anticancer chemotherapy or is for other reasons immunoincompetent), infiltration formation, dependent in part on invasion of the area by neutrophiles, may not form as expected. False-negative chest x-rays for pneumonia are unusual, except when done within the first day or two after onset of a bronchopneumonia, but they can be seen in cases of dehydration, profound neutropenia, or if *Pneumocystis carinii* is the causative organism. CHF shows typical findings that are distinguishable from infection. Pneumococcus (*S. pneumoniae* or *Diplococcus pneumoniae*) causes the most typical and recognizable infiltrate visible in a lobular or lobar distribution, except in unusual circumstances. Obstructing tumors in the lung not only typically cause visible infiltrates distal to the tumor but also are dense enough to mask the tumor itself. Thus, in those cases, follow-up chest x-rays are important in smokers. Mycoplasma pneumonia causes what has been called "atypical pneumonia," in that its roentgenographic findings are out of proportion to the clinical picture, which tends to be rather mild.

14. The answer is A. Penicillin remains the drug of choice in this typical community-acquired case in a previously healthy person with lobar pneumonia. The etiologic agent maybe assumed to be caused by *S. pneumoniae*. Because of the acuteness of the case, this patient will need to be hospitalized for a day or two but should respond dramatically. Trimethoprim/sulfamethoxazole (Bactrim, Septra), although theoretically effective against the gram-positive side of the spectrum, is bacteriostatic, not bacteriocidal. If the patient is allergic to penicillin, then most clinicians would employ a macrolide antibiotic, such as clarithromycin. In this acutely ill patient who is to be hospitalized, levofloxacin would act more rapidly. Postural drainage has no place in acute pneumonitides. Tetracycline is not powerful enough for this clinical situation. However, in subacute progression of a lower respiratory infection, where mycoplasma may be considered, both the tetracyclines and the macrolides may be better choices than penicillin. Cefadroxil is classified as a first- generation cephalosporin but is generally more effective against the gram-negative spectrum and usually considered in "below the waist" infections.

15. The answer is C. Mycoplasma pneumonia has been named one of the atypical pneumonias, based on x-ray findings out of proportion to clinical findings. Headache is a hallmark of mycoplasmal respiratory infection. The course is slow and symptoms fairly mild, although mycoplasmal infections may be associated with a multitude of extrapulmonary involvements, such as the Raynaud phenomenon, related to cold agglutinins present during the acute infection and cardiac involvement in dysrhythmias, CHF, and EKG abnormalities. Streptococcal (pneumococcal) pneumonia is classically the opposite of the picture presented here (i.e., rapidly developing course, discrete or lobar x-ray findings, significant leukocytosis and fever). Pneumonia from *K. pneumoniae* is uncommon, being a gram-negative infection that produces lobar pneumonia in its classic form, found as an opportunist in people immunologically defenseless such as diabetics, alcoholics, and COPD patients. *S. aureus* is also found as a pathogen in the lungs only as an opportunist. Gram-negative sepsis is, of course, a systemic critical condition in which pneumonia is not particularly a prominent finding.

16. The answer is D, Legionella. The case illustrates several points: Bradycardia is common and headache and stupor not uncommon in Legionella disease; early laboratory findings are nonspecific. However, diagnosis is ultimately made by the 3- to 5-day growing culture in buffered charcoal yeast extract agar or less often by acute and convalescent antibody titers in a fourfold rise to 1:128, requiring 4 to 12 weeks for the change, earlier for immunoglobulin M and later for immunoglobulin G types; hyponatremia is often out of proportion to the clinical severity of the disease. Viral pneumonia is characterized by one of the most severe nonproductive coughs encountered in primary care medicine. The other choices have been discussed elsewhere.

17. The answer is B. The stroke patient with bulbar signs and symptoms is at risk of aspiration pneumonia. Aspiration pneumonia is usually produced by aspirated oral anaerobes. Neurologic deficits that are associated with dysphagia, level of consciousness, seizures, drug overdose, alcoholism, and recent dental procedures may all cause aspiration. Influenza pneumonic complications are most likely to be pneumococcal or staphylococcus. The Southwest U.S. traveler must be considered to have coccidioidomycosis. AIDs patients may have any of the pneumonitides discussed, depending on their clinical status, but their specific susceptibility is to *P. carinii*.

18. The answer is C, a 32-year-old with mild shortness of breath with heavy exertion for 1 year and with a smoking history of 1 pack-year. The question emphasizes that not all COPD is caused by smoking. When COPD presents in the absence of a severe smoking history or significant other environmental air pollution history, alpha 1 protease inhibitor deficiency must be considered as an etiology. If present, the enzyme can be given exogenously.

19. The answer is E. Inhaled ipratropium bromide, an anticholinergic agent, is the first-line drug therapy for COPD. Recent reports indicate that it may be surpassed by a new member of the family, tiotropium, because it has some incremental advantages, such as once-daily dosing and a marginal therapeutic edge as measured by amount of supplemental beta-2 agonists and Transitional Dyspnea Index scores. All of the listed agents are sometimes used in COPD patients (although inhaled corticosteroids have been shown to have little effect), but inhaled ipratropium bromide or another member of that family should be the starting agent because of its better therapeutic profile.

References

Holmes RL, Fadden CT. Evaluation of the patient with chronic cough. *Am Fam Physician.* 2004; 69:2159–2166, 2169.

Karnani NG, Reisfield GM, Wilson GR. Evaluation of chronic dyspnea. *Am Fam Physician.* 2005; 71:1529–1537, 1538.

Lipsky MS, Sternbach M. Pneumonias, bronchitides and chronic lung disease. In: Rudy DR, Kurowski K, eds. *Family Medicine: House Officer Series.* Baltimore: Williams & Wilkins; 1997:185–200.

Mintz M. Asthma update: Part I. Diagnosis, monitoring and prevention of disease progression. *Am Fam Physician.* 2004; 70: 893–898.

National Asthma Education and Prevention Program. Expert Panel Number 2. Washington, DC: National Institutes of Health/National Heart, Lung, and Blood Institute; 1997. NIH publication 97–4951.

chapter 12

Respiratory Diseases in Infants and Children

1 A 2-week-old full-term baby boy has developed a cough and exhibits fever, cyanosis, and tachypnea. Which of the following organisms should be considered in the choice of antibiotic therapy of this community-acquired pneumonia (CAP)?

(A) *Streptococcus pneumoniae* and beta-hemolytic streptococci

(B) *Staphylococcus aureus* and Hemophilus organisms

(C) Chlamydia organisms and *Staphylococcus albus*

(D) Group B streptococci and coliform bacteria

(E) *Chlamydia trachomatis* and *Mycoplasma pneumoniae*

2 A 2-month-old baby girl who has lived at home since her normal birth and delivery has respiratory distress, although she manifests no fever. You suspect pneumonitis. Which of the following is the likely best choice of antibiotics, assuming the girl has a CAP and is to be treated as an outpatient?

(A) Penicillin

(B) Azithromycin

(C) Amoxicillin

(D) Ceftriaxone

(E) Ampicillin

3 A previously healthy 1-year-old child has a rapid onset of a rattling cough without preceding coryza. Temperature is 101°F. He has a dull facial expression. Which of the following is the best first choice of antibiotic for this CAP in an outpatient setting?

(A) Penicillin V potassium

(B) Amoxicillin

(C) Erythromycin or other macrolide antibiotic

(D) Gentamycin

(E) Methicillin

4 A 7-year-old boy is diagnosed with pneumonia. Which of the following is the least likely among expected bacterial causes to be considered?

(A) *Chlamydia pneumoniae*

(B) *M. pneumoniae*

(C) *S. pneumoniae*

(D) *Hemophilus influenzae* type B

(E) *C. trachomatis*

5 It is a well-accepted practice to forego sputum cultures in diagnosis of CAPs that are presumed to be treatable in the outpatient setting. This is because the sputum is more likely to be of oral rather than pulmonary origin, and such specimens are likely to contain a preponderance of oral bacteria. However, there are occasions when it appears to be worthwhile to attempt to obtain a sputum sample for culture in that circumstance. Which of the following criteria would allow confidence that the sputum sample was valid for study?

(A) Cough is clearly productive.

(B) Patient has a temperature >101°F.

(C) The specimen is obtained from the nasopharynx.

(D) The ratio of white blood cells to epithelial cells in the specimen is greater than 1:1.

(E) The patient has not suffered from recent vomiting.

6 Which of the following agents is the cause of the vast majority of cases of bronchiolitis?

(A) Influenza A

(B) Influenza B

(C) Adenoviruses

(D) Respiratory syncytial virus (RSV)

(E) *S. pneumoniae*

7 Which of the following is the most likely age range of an infant with an incidence of bronchiolitis?

(A) 3 to 6 months

(B) 6 to 9 months

(C) 1 to 12 months

(D) 6 to 15 months

(E) 12 to 24 months

8 Which of the following is the peak season of RSV infection?

(A) May through June

(B) July through August

(C) November through March

(D) March through May

(E) April through June

9 Which of the following is an accepted method of prophylaxis against RSV in the present state of technology?

(A) Vaccination with live attenuated RSV

(B) Vaccination with killed RSV preparation after exposure

(C) Pooled gamma globulin

(D) Monoclonal antibody given monthly

(E) Amoxicillin through the peak season

10 Which of the following is established as effective in hospitalized RSV infection?

(A) Nebulized furosemide

(B) RSV immune globulin (RSV-IG)

(C) Aerosolized ribovirin

(D) Supportive care and supplemental oxygen

(E) Antibiotics

11 Which of the following organisms accounts for the vast majority of cases of croup (laryngotracheobronchitis, laryngotracheitis, or laryngotracheobronchopneumonitis)?

(A) RSV

(B) Parainfluenza viruses

(C) Mycoplasma organisms

(D) Chlamydia organisms

(E) Ureaplasma organisms

12 Which of the following best differentiates, by history, laryngotracheobronchitis (croup) from epiglottitis?

(A) Temperature

(B) Presence of inspiratory stridor

(C) Length of time from onset to defining symptom

(D) Lung field auscultation

(E) Presence or absence of dyspnea

13 What is the most likely age range of an infant or child with an incidence of croup?

(A) Birth to 3 months

(B) 3 months to 6 months

(C) 6 months to 12 months

(D) 12 months to 6 years

(E) 6 months to 12 years

14 The parents of a 6-year-old boy report that he has developed rapidly a temperature of 103°F at the same time as he complains of dyspnea, drooling, inability to swallow well, and soft inspiratory stridor. On examination he manifests intercostal retractions. You have the child taken to the emergency department and met by an otolaryngologist to examine the patient in the operating room, where a tracheotomy could be performed as the epiglottis and larynx were to be examined. After the emergency has been dealt with, which of the following antibiotics is appropriate?

(A) Penicillin

(B) Amoxicillin

(C) Clarithromycin

(D) Ceftriaxone

(E) Dihydrostreptomycin

15 In the first 6 years of life, children are exposed to and infected by a variety of viruses. Some of these carry more serious implications than others. Repeated infection with which of the following organisms may result in subsequent asthma?

(A) Influenza A organisms

(B) RSV

(C) *S. aureus*

(D) *Klebsiella pneumoniae*

(E) *Moraxella catarrhalis*

Examination Answers

1. The answer is D. Group B streptococci and coliform bacteria are the flora to be expected in pneumonia of the newborn within the first 3 weeks. The antibiotic of choice is amoxicillin and the patient should be admitted to a hospital.

2. The answer is B. Azithromycin is the antibiotic of choice for respiratory disease of the infant between the ages of 3 weeks and 3 months. This is based on the fact that the most likely organisms to be encountered in a CAP in this age group are *C. trachomatis* and *S. pneumoniae*. *C. trachomatis* is significant in its involvement of the eyes. Thus, empiric coverage must be designed to cover that organism as well as *S. pneumoniae*.

3. The answer is B. Amoxicillin is recommended as the empiric choice in this age group, even though *C. pneumoniae* is one of the two most commonly found etiologic agents, along with *S. pneumoniae* (amoxicillin is not effective with chlamydia). Chlamydial pneumonia is more slowly developing, and the second tier of likely agents to be found in this age group includes *H. influenzae* type B and Moraxella organisms. Thus, especially in acutely developing illness, amoxicillin is a wiser first choice here than a macrolide.

4. The answer is E. *C. trachomatis* has virtually disappeared from the pathogenic flora by the time a child reaches the age of 4 years, whether as a cause of pneumonia or of other infections. From the age of 5 years into adolescence, the most common organisms to found in pneumonia in the outpatient setting are *C. pneumoniae*, *M. pneumoniae*, and *S. pneumoniae*. *H. influenzae* type B is a less common cause and much more so as increasing numbers of children are immunized against this organism in the first year of life.

5. The answer is D. If white blood cells in the sputum specimen are greater than 25/low-power field and epithelial cells less than 25/low-power field, one can have confidence in the validity of a sputum specimen. A productive cough is a more propitious situation than a less productive one for obtaining a sputum sample, but that fact does not guarantee a valid sample. Fever has no predictive value in obtaining a specimen. No authorities have related recent vomiting to sputum validity, either positive or negative. A nasopharyngeal source is less secure for validity than is an oral source because the bacteria that colonize the nasopharynx are no more likely than oral sources to reflect the pulmonary contents.

6. The answer is D. RSV is the predominant cause of bronchiolitis, though other organisms that may be implicated are mycoplasma, chlamydia, ureaplasma, and pneumocystis. Bronchiolitis may be responsible for chronic lung disease in children and life-threatening disease in children under 3 months of age, especially those who were born at gestational ages of ≤28 months. Although case fatality is less than 1%, the mean length of illness is 12 days and in 10% of cases the illness lasts longer than 4 weeks.

7. The answer is C. Bronchiolitis occurs in children throughout the first year and even up to age 2, though most serious disease occurs within the first 3 months. The mean age range for hospitalization is 3 months. Patients for whom hospitalization must be considered are those younger than 3 months, those with gestational age at birth <34 weeks, and those with comorbid cardiopulmonary disease or immunodeficiency.

8. The answer is C. November through March, the typical winter season, is the annual span of disease from RSV.

9. The answer is D. The monoclonal antibody given monthly throughout the season of RSV is palivizumab. Another method of prophylaxis is intravenous RSV immune globulin (RSV-IG), such as RespiGam.

10. The answer is D. Supportive care and supplemental oxygen are effective according to research evidence. None of the others are proven to be effective in hospitalized children with RSV disease. Of interest is that RSV-IG, although recommended for prophylaxis, is not felt to be effective in acute disease. Said to be "possibly effective" are nebulized ipratropium with or without a beta-2 agonist (e.g., albuterol); oral, inhaled, or parenteral glucosteroids; and nebulized epinephrine. Confounding the question of efficacy of glucosteroids and epinephrine is that many patients who respond may have atopic disease with an asthmatic component.

11. The answer is B. Parainfluenza viruses (human parainfluenza viruses 1, 2, and 3 account for 75% of all cases). Of interest is the fact that parainfluenza viruses have exhibited a pattern of biennial epidemics during the autumn months of odd-numbered years since 1973.

12. The answer is C. Croup, a viral illness with subglottic involvement, typically exhibits the symptoms of inspiratory stridor only after 12 to 24 hours of coryza, typical of a viral "cold." Epiglottitis, a much more serious condition, begins suddenly. Epiglottitis is caused by bacterial infection with supraglottic involvement, classically *H. influenzae* but also by *S. aureus* and *Corynebacterium diphtheriae*. Although epiglottitis is characterized more by high fever than is croup, this appears to be a weak factor on which to base a preliminary diagnosis. Whereas croup virtually always includes a cough, epiglottitis rarely does so. Epiglottitis typically includes dysphagia while croup does not. The child with croup is comfortable in all positions whereas the patient with epiglottitis will be sitting forward with the mouth open. Both conditions are characterized by dyspnea.

13. The answer is E. Six months to 12 years is the wide range of age within which a child can be afflicted with croup. In contrast, epiglottitis can affect infants, older children, or adults. In adults, epiglottitis is not the potentially life-threatening disease it is in younger people.

14. The answer is D. The vignette describes typical epiglottitis, a respiratory emergency. Of note is the fact that the stridor of epiglottitis is not as dramatic as that of croup. Examination to confirm the diagnosis must be made by an expert who will recognize the cherry red epiglottis and erytenoids. The antibiotic must be chosen to be effective against *H. influenzae* type B. Ceftriaxone is the antibiotic of choice.

15. The answer is B. RSV infection in children under the age of 5 years may result in subsequent wheezing in 30% to 40% of patients, which is essentially asthma or at least reactive airway disease.

References

King MS. Respiratory diseases in infants and children. In: Rudy DR, Kurowski K, eds. *Family Medicine: House Officer Series*. Baltimore: Williams & Wilkins; 1997:201–216.

Ostapchuk M, Roberts DM, Haddy R. Community acquired pneumonia. *Am Fam Physician*. 2004; 70:899–908.

Steiner RWP. Treating acute bronchiolitis with RSV. *Am Fam Physician*. 2004; 69:325–330.

SECTION V

Problems of the Gastrointestinal Tract

chapter 13

Medical Problems of the Gastrointestinal Tract

Examination questions: *Unless instructed otherwise, choose the ONE lettered answer or completion that is BEST in each case.*

1 A 35-year-old man has complained of abdominal pain and variably changing bowel habits consisting of cramps and diarrhea alternating with constipation or bloating for about 5 years. Associations between dietary intake and either diarrhea or constipation are highly inconsistent from day to day. He has not lost weight and his height and weight are as expected, given his parents' anthropometrics. He has no family history of colorectal cancer and flexible sigmoidoscopy has been negative on two occasions, the latest being 1 year ago. He denies hematochezia. Which of the following is the most likely diagnosis?

(A) Carcinoma of the ascending colon

(B) Sprue

(C) Carcinoma of the descending colon

(D) Zollinger–Ellison syndrome

(E) Irritable bowel syndrome (IBS)

2 Which of the following is *best* known about the condition found in Question 1?

(A) Antidepressants (e.g., amitriptyline, clomipramine, desipramine) are effective in symptomatic relief independent of effects on psychological symptoms.

(B) Smooth muscle relaxants (cimetropium, hyoscine, otilonium) are effective against symptoms.

(C) Tegaserod (Zelnorm), a 5HT4 antagonist, is effective against diarrhea symptoms of this condition.

(D) People with IBS have a greater likelihood of having undergone cholecystectomy or hysterectomy than the population at large.

(E) Increasing fiber in the diet is effective in control of symptoms.

3 Which of the following parasites is capable of causing intestinal malabsorption?

(A) *Enterobius vermicularis*

(B) *Giardia lamblia*

(C) *Ancyclstoma duodenale*

(D) *Necator americanus*

(E) *Entamoeba histolytica*

4 A 75-year-old white woman with presumptive recurrent pneumonia was readmitted to the hospital where she had been kept for 2 weeks as a result of her prolonged course. She had been discharged on levofloxacin. After a period of recovery she began to have fever again plus weakness, dyspnea, and watery diarrhea with mucus. Upon readmission she was placed on moxifloxin and doxycycline, based on x-ray findings of pneumonia. A complete blood count showed a leucocytosis level greater than that which had been found on the previous admission, 30,000/mm^3 with a neutrophilia and a left shift toward young cells (band nuclei). Which of the following is the likely cause of her illness?

(A) Recurrent pneumonia

(B) IBS

(C) Pseudomembranous colitis

(D) Carcinoma of the descending colon

(E) Ulcerative colitis

5 Which of the following is the most powerful risk factor for *acquisition* of *Clostridium difficile*?

(A) Staying in the hospital for 4 weeks or longer

(B) Having multiple underlying diseases

(C) Sharing a hospital room for 2 days with a patient infected with *C. difficile*

(D) Being on immunosuppressive therapy 3 months ago

(E) Being on antibiotic therapy just completed after 2 weeks

6 Which of the following is the best choice of therapeutic agents among those presented for the treatment of pseudomembranous colitis?

(A) Clindamycin

(B) Third-generation cephalosporin

(C) Amoxicillin-clavulanate

(D) Metronidazole

(E) Doxycycline

For Questions 7 through 11, match the numbered causes of occult gastrointestinal (GI) bleeding with the lettered settings in which the cause is most likely to be found.

7 Carcinoma of the colon

8 Vascular ectasia (angiodysplasia)

9 Blue rubber bleb nevus syndrome

10 Celiac sprue

11 Kaposi sarcoma, cytomegalovirus colitis

(A) Chronic renal failure

(B) Cutaneous hemangiomas

(C) Chronic diarrhea, abdominal pain

(D) Age ≥ 50 years

(E) Acquired immunodeficiency disease

For Questions 12 through 16, match the numbered conditions commonly associated with nausea and the lettered recommended pharmacologic agents or combinations for treatment thereof.

12 Migraine headache

13 Vestibular nausea

14 Pregnancy-induced nausea

15 Gastroenteritis

16 Postoperative nausea, vomiting

(A) Dopamine antagonists (DAs), serotonin antagonists (SAs)

(B) DAs, SAs, dexamethasone

(C) Metoclopramide, prochlorperazine

(D) histamine 1 blocker, anticholinergics

(E) Ginger, vitamin B_6, promethazine

Resume choosing the one lettered answer or completion. A nausea treatment choice may be used for more than one cause of nausea.

17 A 74-year-old man being treated for chronic renal failure has the rapid onset of hematochezia consisting of frequent maroon-colored stools. Upper endoscopy was negative to the ligament of Treitz, as was colonoscopy except for bleeding brisk enough to obscure visibility. Radioisotope-tagged red cell scan (Technetium 99) revealed a small bowel source. Which of the following is the most likely cause of brisk GI bleeding, given the foregoing scenario?

(A) Meckel diverticulum

(B) Lymphoma

(C) Crohn disease

(D) Angiodysplasia

(E) Jejunoileal diverticulum

18 The patient in Question 17 has not stopped bleeding and you consider angiography as a therapeutic approach. Which of the following is the most significant disadvantage with that plan?

(A) It is specific only for a bleeding Meckel diverticulum.

(B) There is a risk of intestinal infarction with embolization.

(C) There is no intervention capability.

(D) It misses mucosal lesions.

(E) Physician interpretation is time consuming.

19 A 35-year-old male graduate student complains of intermittent difficulty swallowing for the last 3 months. He notes that this happened 6 years ago and lasted for about 7 months. Which of the following symptoms would most enable you to reassure the patient that he does not have an organic basis for the dysphagia?

(A) Rapidly progressing dysphagia with weight loss

(B) Slowly progressing dysphagia, over months or years

(C) Intermittent acute symptoms or even acute obstruction

(D) Dysphagia for both solids and liquids

(E) Odynophagia

20 Ulcerative colitis is a systemic disease and involves many extraintestinal processes. They include all of the following except which one?

(A) Uveitis

(B) Sclerosing cholangitis

(C) Arthropathies

(D) Pyoderma gangrenosum

(E) Erythema nodosum

Examination Answers

1. The answer is E. This vignette perfectly describes IBS. IBS is defined as a chronic noninflammatory condition characterized by abdominal pain, altered bowel habits (diarrhea or constipation), or bloating without known organic basis. Although it is true that alternating constipation and diarrhea is a red flag for consideration of colorectal carcinoma (CRC), CRC is highly unlikely considering chronicity alone. In the event of that presentation of CRC, the tumor would likely be in the descending colon and often associated with hematochezia. Also ruling against CRC is lack of family history in a person well under the minimum age of appearance of the vast majority of sporadic CRC, which is 50 years. Sprue or adult celiac disease is a condition of malabsorption that is characterized more by diarrhea than by changing bowel habits and nearly in all cases by muscle mass wasting and weight loss. Zollinger–Ellison syndrome is characterized by chronic diarrhea associated with adenomas, classically present in the pancreas. Both celiac disease and Zollinger–Ellison syndrome are minimally prevalent, in contrast to the common prevalence of IBS.

2. The answer is D. People with IBS have a greater likelihood of having undergone cholecystectomy or hysterectomy than the population at large. Although some studies have found amelioration of symptoms by antidepressants, it cannot be discerned whether the therapeutic benefit was dependent or independent of depression relief. It appears that smooth muscle relaxants may result in improvement of symptoms of IBS, but studies' results lack statistical significance. The 5HT4 antagonist tegaserod is known to be effective against constipation-predominant IBS in women, not diarrhea-related IBS. Of some surprise, statistical random controlled studies showing effectiveness of dietary fiber are not forthcoming as of early 2005, though dietary fiber is a mainstay of gastroenterologists in the management of IBS. Nevertheless, addition of fiber has other well-known preventive effects, such as prevention of diverticulosis coli.

3. The answer is B. Giardia is a protozoan that causes numerous GI symptoms, including nausea, vomiting, diarrhea, and steatorrhea. Giardiasis is the most common (i.e., prevalent) parasite worldwide and second in the United States after *E. vermicularis* (pinworm). The protozoan is passed by the fecal–oral route and therefore occurs where water processing is less than optimal, such as in developing countries and outdoor camping situations. In the latter scenario it is enhanced in its communicability by its survivability in cold water. The pinworm, whose only host is humans, lives in the large intestine and lays eggs on the perineum. It rarely results in more than perineal pruritus, but occasionally can cause weight loss, urinary tract infection, and appendicitis. The appendicitis risk is due to the possibility of obstruction by the adult forms of the worm (males are 2–5 mm and females are 8–13 mm in length). *A. duodenale* and *N. americanus* are the "Old World" and "New World" hookworms, respectively. Hookworm causes pruritus on occasion and, after attainment of a large worm load in the intestines, may cause microcytic, hypochromic anemia through consumption of host blood. *E. histolytica* is the etiology of amebiasis and acutely causes diarrhea, dysentery, and severe abdominal pain and may ultimately result in chronic systemic disease. Each of the parasites discussed here that are passed through the fecal–oral route are more incident and prevalent in cultures that practice oral–anal sex.

4. The answer is C. Pseudomembranous colitis is the most likely diagnosis in view of the woman's recent and continuing treatment with antibiotics and the watery diarrhea. Although pneumonia may be recurrent or persistent and antibiotics continue to be indicated, the diarrhea and marked leucocytosis require a working diagnosis of pseudomembranous colitis. Neither IBS nor carcinoma of the colon causes watery diarrhea or leucocytosis. Ulcerative colitis is unlikely in view of the clinical setting.

5. The answer is A. A hospital stay of 4 weeks or longer results in a 50% rate of *C. difficile* acquisition, compared with a 3% prevalence of GI colonization in the general population; a 2-week stay appears to present a risk of 13% for acquisition. Sharing a hospital room becomes a greater risk of acquisition after 3.2 days, as does placement of a nasogastric tube and use of antacids. One should appreciate the difference between *acquisition* of the bacterium and *colitis* caused by *C. difficile*. The situations that risk *clinical disease* from *C. difficile*, that is, pseudomembranous colitis and diarrhea related to *C. difficile*, given the intestinal presence of the organism, include recent and prolonged antibiotic therapy, immunosuppressive therapy, multiple underlying diseases, admission to an intensive care unit, and advanced age.

6. The answer is D. Metronidazole is effective against *C. difficile* and is inexpensive; the most important side effects are neurologic. The second choice of antibiotics is vancomycin, the chief caveat being nephrotoxicity. Each of the other antibiotics mentioned is a risk factor for the disease, being broad spectrum and not specifically effective against *C. difficile*. Among the antibiotics, clindamycin is fraught with the greatest risk of *C. difficile* disease. Only 20% of antibiotic-related diarrhea is caused by *C. difficile*, but virtually all cases of pseudomembranous colitis. Pseudomembranous colitis carries a 1% to 2.5% case mortality.

MATCHING QUESTIONS 7 THROUGH 11

7. The answer for carcinoma of the colon is D, age ≥ 50 years.

8. The answer for vascular ectasia (angiodysplasia) is A, chronic renal failure.

9. The answer for blue rubber bleb nevus syndrome is B, cutaneous hemangiomas.

10. The answer for celiac sprue is C, chronic diarrhea, abdominal pain.

11. The answer for Kaposi's sarcoma, cytomegalovirus colitis is E, acquired immunodeficiency disease.

MATCHING QUESTIONS 12 THROUGH 16

12. The answer for migraine headache is A, DAs, SAs.

13. The answer for vestibular nausea is D, histamine 1 blocker, anticholinergics.

14. The answer for pregnancy-induced nausea is E, ginger, vitamin B_6, promethazine.

15. The answer for gastroenteritis is A, DAs, SAs.

16. The answer for postoperative nausea, vomiting is B, DAs, SAs, dexamethasone.

DISCUSSION OF QUESTIONS 12 THROUGH 16

These recommendations are based on the theories of the mechanisms involved in production of nausea associated with the five conditions. The nausea of migraine is associated with the neurotransmitter dopamine, antagonists of which are used for headache with nausea, such as metoclopramide (Reglan) or prochlorperazine (Compazine). For nausea alone in migraine are recommended the same categories as well as serotonin antagonists, such as ondansetron (Zofran). Vestibular nausea is mediated by histamine and by acetylcholine, and hence it is treated by histamine 1 blocking agents ("antihistamines") and by anticholinergic agents. The mechanism of nausea associated with pregnancy is poorly understood but the recommendations made, that is, ginger and vitamin B_6, are based on empiric response and safety for use during the first trimester of pregnancy. Hyperemesis gravidarum is treated by either promethazine (Phenergan) or an SA and, as a second line approach, glucocorticoids. Neurotransmitters associated with gastroenteritis are dopamine and serotonin; therefore DAs are used, as just exemplified. The same applies to postoperative nausea and vomiting.

17. The answer is D. Angiodysplasia may occur throughout the GI tract but is found most frequently in older patients and those with chronic renal failure. All other choices may be sources of small intestinal bleeding but relatively infrequently as compared with angiodysplasia.

18. The answer is B, risk of intestinal infarction with embolization. Angiography functions as a diagnostic tool for brisk GI bleeding by the show of dye that appears in the lumen when the arterial blood supply to the bleeding segment of bowel has been cannulated. It is also a therapeutic tool that works by embolization of the vessel that supplies the bleeding area. The chief danger is that of infarction of the segment that is hemorrhaging. Small bowel barium follow-through is a diagnostic tool for hemorrhage but is failing in that it misses mucosal lesions. The Meckel scan is specific for that purpose and thus is not helpful in finding other sources of bleeding. Neither red cell scan nor capsule endoscopy (swallowed disposable wireless endoscopic capsule) allows intervention along the diagnostic capability. Capsule endoscopy is very time consuming for the interpretation.

19. The answer is D. Dysphagia that is due to an esophageal motor disorder is characterized by symptoms with both solids and liquids. Rapidly progressing dysphagia with weight loss is a cause for suspicion of esophageal cancer. Slowly progressing dysphagia, over months or years, is suggestive of benign stricture; intermittent acute symptoms or spasmodic acute obstruction is characteristic of symptomatic esophageal ring (the Schatzki ring, *at the lower end of the esophagus*); odynophagia, although it is due to other causes, when of recent onset, usually indicates ulcerative esophagitis caused by aphthous disease, or if longer, such ulcerative disease could be due to more serious underlying causes such as immune compromise emanating from such diseases as cancer, blood dyscrasias, cancer chemotherapy, or acquired immunodeficiency disease.

20. **The answer is A.** Extraintestinal processes of *ulcerative colitis* include all of those listed except uveitis. Although the two conditions may coexist, they are not particularly associated. In fact, if uveitis were present it would behoove the doctor to consider a different enteropathy, such as Reiter syndrome. Sclerosing cholangitis, pyoderma gangranosa, and arthropathies are well known to be associated with ulcerative colitis, though the bases for these are poorly understood. Similarly, erythema nodosa is associated but less frequently than the other entities.

References

Flake ZA, Scalley RD, Bailey AG. Practical selection of antiemetics. *Am Fam Physician.* 2004; 69:1169–1174, 1176.

Kennedy TM, Rubin G, Jones RH. Clinical evidence: Irritable bowel syndrome. *Am Fam Physician.* 2005; 71(3):525.

Kucik CJ, Martin GL, Sortor BV. Common intestinal parasites. *Am Fam Physician.* 2004; 69:1161–1168.

Manning-Dimmit LA, Dimmit SG, Wilson GR. Diagnosis of gastrointestinal bleeding in adults. *Am Fam Physician.* 2005; 71:1339–1346.

Mitchell SH, Schaeffer DC, Dubagunta S. A new view of occult and gastrointestinal bleeding. *Am Fam Physician.* 2004; 69:875–881.

Nidiry JJ. Medical problems of the gastrointestinal tract. In: Rudy DR, Kurowski K, eds. *Family Medicine: House Officer Series.* Baltimore: Williams & Wilkins; 1997:217–234.

Schroeder MS. Clostridium difficile-associated diarrhea. *Am Fam Physician.* 2005; 71:921–928.

metachlopramide Reglan → DA
prochlorperazine Compazine → DA
ondansetron Zofran → SA

pRomethazine Phenergan →

migraine nause → dopamine ← GE
              ↳ serotonin ← GE

Vestibular Nausea → histamine / acetylcholine

chapter 14

Surgical Problems of the Gastrointestinal Tract

Examination questions: Unless instructed otherwise, choose the ONE lettered answer or completion that is BEST in each case.

1 Which of the following is true about carcinomas of the upper gastrointestinal (GI) tract?

(A) Incidence of carcinoma of the stomach is increasing in the United States.

(B) Incidence of carcinoma of esophagus and proximal stomach is increasing.

(C) Carcinoma of the stomach is a disease for which routine screening is appropriate.

(D) Vitamin C intake is a risk factor for carcinoma of the stomach.

(E) Excess intake of fruits and vegetables is a risk factor for carcinoma of the stomach.

2 A 56-year-old man is concerned about stomach cancer because of the death of a co-worker from that disease. Each of the following is a risk factor for stomach cancer except which one?

(A) Familial adenomatous polyposis

(B) History of a gastric ulcer that revealed high-grade dysplasia

(C) Atrophic gastritis

(D) *Helicobacter pylori* infection

(E) Hyperplastic polyps

3 Which of the following is the most important, productive, and practical reason to offer or refer for upper endoscopy any patient over 45 years of age with persistent dyspepsia?

(A) To diagnose gastric peptic ulcer

(B) To diagnose gastroesophageal reflux

(C) To diagnose early stomach cancer

(D) To diagnose peptic duodenal ulcer disease

(E) To diagnose atrophic gastritis

4 A 45-year-old man complains of abdominal pain of less than 2 days' duration, located in a periumbilical position, to which was added, after 12 hours, vomiting as well. The bouts of vomiting were not particularly preceded by nausea. Abdominal examination reveals generalized pain aggravated by palpation, without rebound tenderness and neither notable distention nor localization of the tenderness. There has been no particular past history of postprandial discomfort before the onset of the present illness; there have been no specific food intolerances. Which of the following is the most likely diagnosis to account for these symptoms?

(A) Small bowel obstruction

(B) Large bowel obstruction

(C) Acute appendicitis

(D) Acute gastritis

(E) Acute cholecystitis

5 You suspect atypical presentation of appendicitis in a 26-year-old man who has had abdominal pain for 2 days: There is no rebound tenderness, questionable obturator and psoas signs, and a higher white blood cell (WBC) count than is usually encountered in appendicitis. Which of the following may be *least* helpful in determining whether the patient has appendicitis, thus making it less likely for you to commit to unnecessary surgery or missing timely intervention in the event of appendicitis?

(A) Abdominal plain films

(B) Helical computed tomography (CT) scan of the abdomen

(C) CT scan

(D) Ultrasonography

(E) Magnetic resonance image

6 A 40-year-old white man has been treated for peptic ulcer disease (PUD) symptoms for several weeks. The patient also has diarrhea, a problem he had not had in the past. He denies taking nonsteroidal anti-inflammatory medication either by prescription or over the counter. You treated the patient with a 3-week course of the histamine 2 receptor blocking agent (H2 receptor blocker) ranitidine, but the patient's symptoms became only slightly improved and recurred fully within days after discontinuance of the drug. You then prescribed the hydrogen pump blocking agent omeprazole for 3 weeks with similar disappointing results. Esophagogastroduodenoscopy then demonstrated a large ulcer (3-cm diameter) distal to the duodenal bulb. During the procedure, studies were done for *H. pylori* that were negative. Which of the following would be the next logical action?

(A) Draw blood for a gastrin level

(B) Refer for lower endoscopy to rule out ulcerative colitis

(C) Order barium upper GI series with small bowel follow-through to rule out Crohn disease

(D) Order stool cultures for bacterial cause of infectious diarrhea

(E) Order stool studies for ova and parasites

7 A 55-year-old man is alcoholic and has an episode of bleeding esophageal varices. The patient is impressed with your warnings regarding the dangers of alcoholism and vows to visit a local Alcoholics Anonymous chapter and to stop drinking alcohol. Which of the following is a valid medical approach to reduce the chances of repeat bleeding episodes, thus avoiding surgical emergencies caused by hemorrhage?

(A) Calcium channel blocking agent

(B) Beta-selective agonist agent

(C) H2 receptor blocker

(D) Nonselective beta-adrenergic blocking agent

(E) Proton pump blocker

8 A 70-year-old white woman is found to have a hemoglobin level of 4 g/100mL and a macrocytosis. Serum vitamin B_{12} level is abnormally low. The patient denies history of diarrhea. Serum folic acid levels are normal. As you begin treatment of this patient, which of the following procedures comes under the heading of "best practice"?

(A) Barium enema

(B) Barium swallow with small bowel follow-through

(C) Upper GI barium series

(D) Colonoscopy

(E) Upper endoscopy

9 Which of the following sites of colon cancer, upon presentation of symptoms and signs, confers the most favorable prognosis?

(A) Cecum

(B) Ascending colon

(C) Transverse colon

(D) Iliocolic junction

(E) Sigmoid colon

10 A 35-year-old white man has had abdominal pain for the past 36 hours. Examination of the anterior aspect of the abdomen is negative for rebound tenderness, though there is some deep tenderness in the midline below the umbilicus (indication of pain with deep palpation but without true guarding or rebound response upon release). The WBC count is elevated to 19,000 with 80% neutrophiles, of which 30% are bands. Which of the following would be helpful in establishing a diagnosis of retrocecal appendicitis?

(A) Babinski response

(B) Obturator sign

(C) Rovsig sign

(D) Murphy sign

(E) Osler sign

11 A male newborn who is 4 weeks old has begun to vomit over the past 2 days after each feeding and the vomit is blood streaked. Last evening the vomiting became projectile. You notice a peristaltic wave in the upper abdomen moving from left to right. Deep palpation between attacks reveals an olive-sized nodule in the epigastrium. Which of the following is the likely diagnosis?

(A) Acute gastritis

(B) Iliocolic intussusception

(C) Pyloric stenosis

(D) Esophageal atresia

(E) Pneumonia

12 An 11-month-old male infant develops apparent colicky abdominal pain, as he screams and draws up his knees with each bout of pain. Within 12 hours the child exhibits vomiting and diarrhea consisting of bloody mucous stools. Deep palpation reveals a sausagelike mass in the supraumbilical area of the midline abdomen. Which of the following is the most likely cause of these findings?

(A) Meconium plug

(B) Hirschsprung disease

(C) Carcinoma of the colon

(D) Shigellosis

(E) Intussusception

13 A 45-year-old female patient has just been told that her brother, who is 3 years older than her, has been diagnosed with colorectal cancer (CRC). She has no symptoms or change in bowel habits, blood in the stool, or any abdominal discomfort. She wishes to know what measures she should take in order to avoid an encounter with the disease. First, you explain to her that the lifetime risk of carcinoma of the colon is about 2.5% for the average American. What would the corresponding risk figure be for her, a person who has a first-degree relative with colon cancer?

(A) 2.5% to 3%

(B) 7% to 7.5%

(C) 10%

(D) 15%

(E) 20%

14 Regarding the patient in Question 13, you perform flexible sigmoidoscopy and excise a polyp that turns out histologically to be an adenomatous polyp of the tubular type. What is your next advice and disposition for her medical care?

(A) Fecal occult blood testing every year, three stools, two samples per stool, beginning at age 50 years

(B) Dual-contrast barium enema annually starting at 50 years of age

(C) Flexible sigmoidoscopy every 5 years starting at 50 years of age

(D) Colonoscopy now and every 3 years if findings are negative

(E) No need to worry, considering the odds are overwhelmingly in her favor

15 Regarding the patient in Questions 13 and 14, she now has been told that her brother's CRC was confined to the muscularis of the colon, without lymph node involvement. What is the approximate average 5-year survival rate for her brother with CRC?

(A) 90%

(B) 70%

(C) 27%

(D) 5%

(E) 2%

16 A 35-year-old para 3 gravida 4 woman is in her seventh month of pregnancy. She experiences rapidly building onset of acute abdominal pain with a positive Murphy sign. Temperature is 101°F and WBC count is 13,000 with a neutrophilia and leftward shift. There is ultrasonic evidence of numerous gallstones without evidence of a common duct stone. Which of the following is the best course of action?

(A) Laparoscopic cholecystectomy with the first open elective operating day

(B) Cholecystectomy by laparotomy with the first open elective operating day

(C) Cholecystectomy and common duct exploration with the first open elective operating day

(D) Laparoscopic cholecystectomy within 72 hours

(E) Cholecystectomy by laparotomy within 72 hours

Examination Answers

1. The answer is B. Although the overall incidence of carcinoma of the stomach has been decreasing in the United States for years, carcinoma of the proximal stomach, esophagogastric junction, and esophagus is increasing. Most physicians feel this is because of the increased incidence and prevalence of gastroesophageal reflux disease. The latter is related to the increasing prevalence of obesity. Vitamin C intake may be protective. Lack of fruit and vegetables may be a risk factor. Screening of asymptomatic patients of normal risk status for carcinoma of the stomach is not recommended because of the invasiveness of any effective screening method, and the low incidence in low-risk populations.

2. The answer is E. Hyperplastic polyps (of the colon or elsewhere) have no malignant potential and are not associated with gastric carcinoma. However, surveillance for gastric cancer is recommended for individuals with each of the other four risk factors. Familial adenomatous polyposis, noted for CRC development in all persons by the age of 40, is also thought to be a risk factor for adenocarcinomas in other sites, as is the Lynch syndrome (family cancer syndrome II, hereditary nonpolyposis CRC). Gastric ulcer with biopsy evidence of high-grade dysplasia (and also gastric metaplasia, but not benign gastric ulcer) is a risk factor. Pernicious anemia is a risk factor as is atrophic gastritis, without which pernicious anemia does not exist.

3. The answer is C. Perhaps of the greatest surprise, gastric cancer can be a screenable disease. Despite the fact that a large proportion of patients with gastric cancer are asymptomatic, if patients are chosen for high-risk status (see the explanation given for Question 2) and upper endoscopy is utilized aggressively, the cure rate can be as high as 90%. The other choices are fruitful indications for esophagogastroduodenoscopy as well, but a degree of time urgency is conferred for early diagnosis of gastric carcinoma.

4. The answer is A. Vomiting in clinical obstruction signifies an upper GI or small bowel locale, especially at the pylorus, whereas distention as the dominant symptom signifies lower bowel obstruction. The higher or more proximal the location of the obstruction, the more rapid the onset, but this is neither as reliable nor as precisely defined as the choice designated. Presence of occult blood in the stool, although more likely in upper GI obstruction, is neither specific nor sensitive for either type. Appendicitis, perforated viscus, and ischemic bowel disease all are characterized by steady as opposed to intermittent symptoms. Gastritis symptoms are constant, but vomiting is the central rather than secondary symptom and the vomiting is certainly preceded by nausea. Cholecystitis manifests specific right upper quadrant tenderness and a positive Murphy sign.

5. The answer is A. Although plain abdominal x-rays may identify an appendiceal fecalith (appendicolith), that occurs in only 5% of cases. Ultrasonography carries an accuracy of 71% to 97%. CT scanning is also quite accurate, with sensitivity of about 92% and specificity of 97%. A magnetic resonance image is helpful in children and women. A helical CT scan is useful in differentiating appendicitis from salpingitis in women.

6. The answer is A. Association of refractory PUD and diarrhea, especially when one or more ulcers include(s) a lesion larger than usual, located distal to the duodenal bulb, suggests Zollinger–Ellison syndrome. Gastrinomas occur in the pancreas, duodenal wall, or lymph nodes, or, when associated with multiple endocrine neoplasia, type 1, occur in multiples in endocrine organs such as the parathyroid glands. One-third of gastrinomas are malignant. Over 90% of patients with gastrinomas develop PUD and one-third will have watery diarrhea that can be quite severe and, of course, refractory to usual treatment. Although each of the other choices are causes of diarrhea, they would have to coexist with PUD in this case, none of which is found in that association.

7. The answer is D. Nonselective beta-blockers have been shown to reduce the chances of bleeding from esophageal varices to 15% from a 25% rate in placebo-treated control subjects. H2 receptor blockers and proton pump blockers would be good choices for reflux symptoms but are not reported to prevent hemorrhage from varices once they have developed.

8. The answer is E. The patient has pernicious anemia. Treatment consists of parenteral monthly injections of vitamin B$_{12}$. The reason for doing upper endoscopy at the time of diagnosis is to rule out gastric carcinoma.

the risk of which is threefold that of the general population. The *prevalence* of gastric carcinoma is 1% to 3% in pernicious anemia.

9. The answer is E. A sigmoid colon (as with other descending colon) location is most likely to be discovered in Duke stage A (confinement to the mucosa) because the earliest symptom is usually hematochezia, occurring well before the primary tumor encircles or obstructs the colon. This location confers a 5-year cure rate of 90%. Blood from tumors arising from more proximal levels is digested and changed from a visible form in the early stages, thus not alerting the patient until change in bowel habits or even bowel obstruction supervenes. Fecal occult blood screening could, of course, detect early and curable tumors in the more proximal locations. Thirty-two percent of CRCs occur in the descending colon, divided into 25% in the sigmoid and 7% in the remaining descending colon. Males are more likely than females to develop cancer in the left or descending colon whereas females are more likely to develop it in the right colon.

10. The answer is B. The obturator sign is defined as pain upon internal rotation of the thigh with the right hip flexed. When it elicits pain deep in the lower lumbar area (as opposed to the hip joint proper or pain radiating down the anterior thigh), it signifies contact between the internal obturator muscle and an inflammation process, usually a retrocecal appendix. The psoas maneuver is the alternative if retrocecal appendicitis is still suspected and the obturator sign is absent (either one may be performed before the other). With the psoas sign the ipsilateral hip is extended and pain is elicited if there is an inflammatory process touching the psoas muscle. The Babinski sign is an abnormal plantar reflex of the foot and toes in the presence of an upper motor neuron lesion in the opposite side of the brain or any part of the corticospinal tract above the crossover level. The Rovsig sign is the presence of right lower quadrant pain upon release of deep pressure by the examining hand in the abdomen in the presence of classic appendicitis with normal positioning wherein the organ is touching the anterior parietal peritoneum. The Murphy sign is the inhibition of inspiratory effort when the examining hand is deeply placed beneath the right costal margin in the presence of an inflamed gallbladder. The Osler sign is the presence of painful petechia-sized red spots on the hands and feet pathognomonic of subacute bacterial endocarditis.

11. The answer is C. This patient has a typical presentation of pyloric stenosis. A male infant who is 2 weeks to 4 months of age most typifies pyloric stenosis. Male infants are affected four times as frequently as female infants.

12. The answer is E. Intussusception is the most common cause of bowel (as opposed to pyloric) obstruction in the first 2 years of a baby's life. Eighty percent of cases occur in the first 2 years of life, peaking in the time period from 5 to 9 months. Male infants are affected three times as frequently as female infants; presentation includes colicky abdominal pain, "current jelly stools," reflex vomiting, leukocytosis, hemoconcentration, and a palpable mass. Meconium plug is a cause of obstruction in the newborn. Hirschsprung disease is a potentially fatal condition of the newborn in which normal peristalsis is prevented by the segmental absence of ganglion cells of the mucosal and muscular layers of colon or rectosigmoid segments of bowel. Obviously, both are causes of congenital bowel obstruction. Carcinoma of the infant colon is extremely rare. Shigellosis is a form of bacterial dysentery that causes profuse bloody diarrhea.

13. The answer is B, 7% to 7.5%. The lifetime risk of carcinoma of the colon of about 2.5% is roughly tripled for a person who has a first-degree relative with either colon cancer or adenomatous polyp. This translates to a 7% to 7.5% lifetime risk. Because the incidence increases with each decade of life, all the foregoing percentages are multiplied for the upper age groups. For example, the expected incidence of colon cancer of nearly 0.4% per 1,000 year at age 50 would be more than 1.2% per 1,000 in every year for a person with such a first-degree family history.

14. The answer is D. Although A, B, and C are acceptable methods of CRC screening for patients of average risk, beginning at age 50, any patient who has a first-degree family history of CRC should begin such screening at age 40. Because this patient has now been diagnosed with a tubular adenomatous polyp, one of three precancerous types, she should undergo colonoscopy now and this should be repeated every 3 years, assuming the study reveals no cancers (see chapter 45). The presence of a single adenomatous polyp in any segment of the large intestine implies the strong possibility of other polyps throughout the remainder of the colon.

15. The answer is B. CRC confined to muscularis or serosa is classified as Duke stage B. The average 5-year life expectancy is between 60% and 75%.

16. The answer is E. Acute cholecystitis, whose definition is satisfied by the fever and leukocytosis and severity of pain in this case, is an indication for early cholecystectomy. However, acute cholecystitis is a contraindication for the laparoscopic approach. Furthermore, pregnancy also is a contraindication. Other contraindications to laparoscopic cholecystectomy are obesity, advanced age, chronic obstructive pulmonary disease, cirrhosis, and previous abdominal surgery. Biliary pain without signs of acute inflammation, biliary dyskinesia (defined as <50% ejection fraction after gallbladder stimulation by cholecystikinin cholecystoscintigraphy), and calcified gallbladder are each indications for elective cholecystectomy, by laparoscopic approach if the aforementioned contraindications do not pertain. Except for the foregoing caveats, laparoscopic cholecystectomy permits earlier discharge, less morbidity, and lower perioperative mortality.

References

Bellows CF, Berger DH, Crass RA. Management of gallstones. *Am Fam Physician.* 2005; 72:637–642.

Brown CM. Surgical issues of the gastrointestinal tract. In: Rudy DR, Kurowski K, eds. *Family Medicine: House Officer Series.* Baltimore: Williams & Wilkins; 1997:235–254.

Layke JC, Lopez PP. Gastric cancer: Diagnosis and treatment options. *Am Fam Physician.* 2004; 69:1133–1140, 1145–1146.

McQuaid KR. Alimentary tract. In: Tierney LM, McPhee SJ, Papadakis MA, eds. *Current Medical Diagnosis and Treatment.* 43rd ed. New York: McGraw-Hill/Appleton & Lange; 2004: 515–622.

Old H, Dusing RW, Tap W, et al. Imaging for suspected appendicitis. *Am Fam Physician.* 2005; 71:71–78.

chapter 15

Diseases of the Liver

Examination questions: Unless instructed otherwise, choose the ONE lettered answer or completion that is BEST in each case.

1 A 35-year-old woman who admits to intravenous drug abuse has been nauseated and anorectic for about 1 week. You obtain a hepatitis panel. Which of the following sets of laboratory findings make the diagnosis of acute hepatitis B?

(A) Hepatitis B surface antigen (HBsAg) negative, hepatitis B core antibody (anti-HBc) negative, hepatitis B surface antibody (anti-HBs; immunoglobulin G type unless otherwise designated) negative

(B) HBsAg negative, anti-HBc positive, anti-HBs positive

(C) HBsAg negative, anti-HBc negative, anti-HBs positive

(D) HBsAg positive, anti-HBc positive, IgM anti-HBc positive, anti-HBs negative

(E) HBsAg positive, anti-HBc positive, IgM anti-HBc negative, anti-HBs negative

2 Which of the following is the best indicator of a high degree of hepatitis B virus (HBV) replication and hence a marker of "infectivity"?

(A) HBsAg

(B) Hepatitis B core antigen (HBcAg)

(C) Hepatitis Be antigen (HBeAg)

(D) Anti-HBs

(E) Anti-HBc

3 A 28-year-old female patient reports that in the past she was an intravenous street-drug user and once had acute hepatitis B. She now contemplates a relationship with a man whom she believes she may marry, and she wants to know whether she is a carrier of hepatitis B. Her fiancé is a stockbroker and has never been immunized against hepatitis B. Which of the following findings would indicate that she is a carrier and that her fiancé should be immunized?

(A) HBeAg negative, HBc antibody positive, HBsAg positive, and alanine aminotransferase (ALT) and aspartate aminotransferase (AST) levels normal

(B) HBsAg negative, HBV DNA undetectable, anti-HBc positive, anti-HBs positive

(C) HBsAg positive, anti-HBc positive, IgM anti-HBc negative, ALT level elevated 25% above normal, and AST level elevated 20% above normal

(D) HBsAg negative, anti-HBs negative, anti-HBc negative, and ALT and AST levels within normal limits

(E) HBsAg positive, anti-HBc positive, IgM anti-HBc positive, anti-HBc negative, and ALT and AST levels approximately forty times normal

4 In regard to the patient in Question 3, she is tested and the findings are as follows: HBeAg negative, HBc antibody positive, HBs antibody positive, and ALT and AST levels normal. What is your advice to the patient vis-à-vis her fiancé?

(A) He should take the three-injection series of hepatitis vaccine.

(B) He should have hepatitis B immune globulin injection.

(C) The couple should be advised to use a barrier method of contraception for protection of the man from hepatitis B.

(D) There need be no particular protective measures for the woman's fiancé.

(E) The fiancé should take a course of an immune modulator such as recombinant alpha-2b (Intron A).

5 A 56-year-old male patient who had transfusions 20 years ago and contracted hepatitis C comes to you as a new patient. During your examination you notice dilated flank veins, redness of the palms, and suspicion of ascites. From a computed tomography scan you find ascites and conclude that the patient has cirrhosis. Knowing that hepatitis C is a strong risk factor for hepatocellular carcinoma, stronger even than hepatitis B, you decide to begin with a screening baseline test for that disease. Which of the following tests serves that purpose?

(A) Carcinoembryonic antigen test

(B) Alpha fetal protein test

(C) Breast cancer 1, early onset (BRCA1) genetic test

(D) Human chorionic gonadotropin test

(E) Prostate-specific antigen test

6 A 45-year-old white man has undergone a routine periodic physical examination. You note that, for the past 3 years, each hepatic profile testing ordered by your office has shown ALT and AST elevations of up to two to three times normal levels. You decide to investigate in stepwise fashion. Each of the following steps would be appropriate at this time, except for which one?

(A) Inquire as to drinking habits

(B) Inquire as to intravenous street-drug usage

(C) Complete review of the patient's medications

(D) Order an ultrasound study of the liver

(E) Order serologic tests for hepatitides A, B, and C and blood tests for iron studies

7 A 35-year-old woman who has had two pregnancies and is 20% overweight presents with jaundice. Serum conjugated bilirubin level is elevated to twice the upper limit of normal. Unconjugated bilirubin is normal. Which of the following, as a single procedure, is most likely to elucidate a cause of this clinical situation?

(A) Blood draw for hepatitides A, B, and C

(B) Computed tomography scan of the liver

(C) Ultrasound study of the extrahepatic biliary system

(D) Plain x-ray of the abdomen

(E) Blood draw for ALT and AST

8 A 46-year-old woman is evaluated for worsening fatigue and pruritus that have been present for at least 8 years. Recently she has complained of diarrhea with stools that float in the commode. She drinks two to three glasses of wine weekly. On examination you find xanthomas on the extensor surfaces of the

forearms. She also manifests xanthelasmas on the eyelids. There are dilated flank veins on each side of the trunkal area. There is no mass palpable. The comprehensive metabolic profile shows elevated alkaline phosphatase to twice the upper limit of normal and direct-acting (conjugated) bilirubin is elevated to 1.5 times the upper limit of normal. The lipid profile reveals elevated cholesterol to 280 mg/dL and high-density lipoprotein cholesterol at 70 mg/dL. Which of the following is the most likely diagnosis?

(A) Choledocholithiasis

(B) Gilbert disease

(C) Carcinoma of the head of the pancreas

(D) Primary biliary cirrhosis (PBC)

(E) Alcoholic cirrhosis

9 Which of the following is the most likely to be passed by a blood donor?

(A) Hepatitis A

(B) Hepatitis B

(C) Hepatitis C

(D) Hepatitis D

(E) Hepatitis E

10 Which of the following organisms causes the greatest number of cases of transfusion-related hepatitis?

(A) Hepatitis A virus

(B) HBV

(C) Hepatitis C virus (HCV)

(D) Hepatitis D virus

(E) Hepatitis E virus

11 Your patient is a 55-year-old male professor of language at the nearby university. He has been stable in his professional life and as a marital partner and adequately so as a parent. He appears for periodic health profile evaluation. A routine chemistry battery returns with surprise findings of mean cell volume in an otherwise normal hemogram of 97 μm^3 (also 97 fL); gamma glutamyl transpeptidase of 255 U/L (normal is 5 to 40 U/L); serum AST of 199 U/L(formerly SGOT, 1–36); ALT of 101 (formerly SGPT, 1–45); and blood urea nitrogen of 6 mg/dL. Alkaline phosphatase is normal at 75 U/L. Bilirubin levels, conjugated and unconjugated, are normal. What should be your *next* measure?

(A) Order gallbladder untrasound study

(B) Arrange a liver biopsy

(C) Arrange esophagogastroduodenoscopy

(D) Order hepatitis profile (tests of antigens and antibodies of hepatitides A, B, and C)

(E) Obtain further information through an interview of the patient regarding alcohol intake

12 Regarding the patient in Question 11, which of the following approximates his chances of having or developing cirrhosis?

(A) 0%

(B) 15%

(C) 30%

(D) 45%

(E) 75%

13 A 30-year-old white man with a history of ulcerative colitis develops obstructive jaundice, associated with fever. There has been no colicky pain and very little abdominal pain in general. A gallbladder ultrasound study is negative for gallstones. The direct-acting bilirubin level is elevated, as is the alkaline phosphatase level, whereas the indirect-acting bilirubin level is normal. ALT and AST levels are elevated to less than 10% above the upper limits of normal. An empiric course of ciprofloxicin results in rapid subsidence of the fever. Which of the following is the most likely cause of this constellation of findings?

(A) PBC

(B) Primary sclerosing cholangitis (PSC)

(C) Choledocholithiasis

(D) Steatohepatosis

(E) Viral hepatitis

14 A 45-year-old woman presents with fatigue, anorexia, brown urine, and malaise. She denies alcohol intake entirely, illicit drug use, and history of treatment with blood products, and she is on no medications that may cause elevation of hepatocellular enzymes. Examination reveals scleral icterus and mildly tender hepatomagaly. Both AST and ALT levels are elevated to four times normal and smooth muscle antibody (SMA) and antinuclear antibody (ANA) levels are positive. She has a history of Hashimoto thyroiditis but no history suggestive of inflammatory bowel disease. Alkaline phosphatase and gamma glutamyl transpeptidase are both elevated to twice normal limits. A hepatitis profile yields no evidence of hepatitides A, B, C, or E. Which of the following may be the best initial presumptive diagnosis?

(A) PSC

(B) PBC

(C) Viral hepatitis

(D) Choledocholithiasis

(E) Autoimmune hepatitis

15 A 15-year-old girl presents with malaise, fatigue, depression, and clinical evidence of hepatitis in the absence of viral causation. An older sister is awaiting liver transplantation. Which of the following blood studies may be most specifically helpful in establishing the diagnosis?

(A) ANA levels

(B) Anti-SMA levels

(C) Complete blood count

(D) Ceruloplasmin level

(E) Serum iron, total iron-binding capacity, and ferritin levels

Knowledge of incubation periods and portals of entry of the five identified hepatitides is critical for prognosticating and preventing the spread of cases. For Questions 16 through 20, match the numbered hepatitis types with the lettered modes of transmission.

16 Hepatitis A

17 Hepatitis B

18 Hepatitis C

19 Hepatitis D

20 Hepatitis E

(A) Transmitted by body fluids other than gastrointestinal; carries high risk of chronic hepatitis and high risk of sexual transmission

(B) Transmitted mainly by fecal–oral contamination; fraught with no complications except in third-trimester pregnancy

(C) May be transmitted by percutaneous or nonpercutaneous means; requires presence of hepatitis B in order to procreate

(D) Transmitted by body fluids other than gastrointestinal; carries very high risk of chronic hepatitis; prominent in transfusion-induced hepatitis but risk of sexual and accidental needle-stick transmission is relatively low

(E) Transmitted mainly by fecal–oral contamination; fraught with no complications

Examination Answers

1. The answer is D, HBsAg positive, anti-HBc positive, IgM anti-HBc positive, anti-HBs negative. The presence of HBsAg signifies infection. The presence of anti-HBc indicates active immunity, which is not necessarily effective. However, IgM anti-HBc presence occurs only during acute infection, and the IgM antibody is gone after the acute phase and is present neither in chronic disease nor the carrier state of hepatitis B.

HBsAg negative, anti-HBc negative, anti-HBs negative signifies susceptibility, because both types of antibody are absent while surface antigen is absent as well. HBsAg negative, anti-HBc negative, anti-HBs positive signifies immunity through hepatitis B vaccination (the vaccine functions to produce antibodies to surface antigen but not to core antigen). HBsAg positive, anti-HBc positive, IgM anti-HBc negative, anti-HBs negative signifies chronic infection (core antibodies present, IgM antibodies absent but surface antigen also present). HBsAg positive, anti-HBc positive, IgM anti-HBc negative, anti-HBs negative signifies chronic hepatitis B infection.

Finally, the set HBsAg negative, anti-HBc positive, anti-HBs negative (not given as a choice for Question 1) may have four interpretations. First, the patient may be recovering from acute infection. Second, the patient may be distantly immune (testing may miss very low levels of anti-HBs). Third, the patient may be susceptible but exhibit a false-positive anti-HBs finding. Fourth, there may be undetectable levels of HBsAg and the patient is a carrier. The reader is referred to Table 15.4 in Friedman, 2006.

2. The answer is C. HBeAg correlates with a high degree of viral replication. Conversely, HBe antibody correlates with a low rate of replication. HBV DNA also correlates with replication and is used to monitor response to therapy for human papillomavirus infection, especially in cases where an HBeAg mutant has occurred.

3. The answer is A. The combination finding of HBeAg negative, HBc antibody positive, HBsAg positive, and ALT and AST levels normal indicates the presence of virus in equilibrium with immunity and absence of evidence of hepatocellular disruption (i.e., the asymptomatic carrier state).

The finding of HBsAg negative, HBV DNA undetectable, anti-HBc positive, anti-HBs positive indicates immunity that is due to past infection. The finding of

HBsAg positive, anti-HBc positive, IgM anti-HBc negative, ALT level elevated 25 % above normal, and AST level elevated 20% above normal indicates chronic active infection. Note that the acute phase IgM anti-HBc is absent. The finding of HBsAg negative, anti-HBs negative, anti-HBc negative, and ALT and AST levels within normal limits indicates the naïve state of absent infection and susceptibility, which is a similar but slightly different pattern than that alluded to in discussion of Question 1. The finding of HBsAg positive, anti-HBc positive, IgM anti-HBc positive, anti-HBc negative, and ALT and AST levels approximately forty times normal is, of course, the typical picture of acute hepatitis B.

4. The answer is D. The pattern of testing of the patient in Questions 2 and 3, that of no evidence of hepatocellular disease, absence of HBsAg, and positivity of HBc and HBs antibodies, indicates immunity from past infection. No precautions are indicated. Recombinant alpha-2b is employed in chronic active hepatitis.

5. The answer is B. Alpha fetal protein is a marker for hapatoma (hepatocellular carcinoma). Carcinoembryonic antigen is best used for follow-up of progress for treated colorectal carcinoma; the BRCA1 gene is a marker for inherited tendency for breast cancer; human chorionic gonadotropin is a marker found in choriocarcinoma and testicular cancer; prostate-specific antigen is a marker for follow-up of prostate cancer. Not any of these markers are perfectly specific, and thus they are best applied for following the progress of the cancer once diagnosed and treated.

6. The answer is D. Ultrasound of the liver should not be done until the factors included in the other choices have been investigated as well as several others. The latter include presence of uncontrolled diabetes, obesity, and dyslipidemia. Every drug on which a patient has been placed should be perused for possibilities of elevation of liver enzymes, and the list is too long to address in this work. Chronic hepatitides B and C are common. Hemochromatosis is much more common than appreciated decades ago. If the ALT is twice that of the AST, then alcoholism should be suspected. However, that relationship is neither quite sensitive nor specific.

7. The answer is C. Conjugated bilirubinemia (direct-acting bilirubin), when in the absence of unconjugated bilirubin, indicates extrahepatic obstructive jaundice. Ultrasound is more likely to elucidate the cause than computed tomography, the latter generally giving more information regarding the parenchyma of the liver and of the pancreas. The hepatitides cause more often a mixed picture of elevations of both conjugated and unconjugated bilirubin. Plain x-rays are seldom helpful in jaundice. ALT and AST levels may be mildly elevated in obstructive jaundice, but neither confirms nor rules out obstruction; if obstruction is present, no anatomic diagnosis will be made from the test.

8. The answer is D. PBC occurs more often in women than men by a ratio of roughly 4 or 5:1. Steatorrhea is typical, as are xanthelasmas and xanthomas. Patients are asymptomatic for years before beginning complaints of pruritus, a common symptom of biliary obstruction. Along the way, first alkaline phosphatase and then conjugated bilirubin become elevated. Antimitochondrial antibodies are positive in 95% of cases, though the test is not adequately specific. Alcoholic cirrhosis is not characterized by the skin manifestations alluded to and is not characterized by the symptoms of biliary obstruction from early on, as is PBC. Choledocholithiasis, although a cause of biliary obstruction, is neither a slowly progressive process nor insidious in onset. The same can be said for carcinoma of the pancreas. The latter is noted for "painless jaundice" with a palpable gallbladder (the Curvoisier sign). Gilbert disease (or syndrome) is a mild condition in which there is an inherited tendency for intermittent elevation of unconjugated bilirubin levels.

9. The answer is B. Hepatitis B is more transmissible than hepatitis C, though hepatitis C is significantly more likely to cause chronic hepatitis, once passed (75%), cirrhosis (20% within 20 years), and hepatocellular carcinoma (1% to 4% per year). Hepatitis A never becomes chronic nor does it result in a carrier state, nor does hepatitis E. Hepatitis D occurs only in concert with hepatitis B.

10. The answer is B, hepatitis B. Even though HCV has a greater chance of causing hepatitis, once passed, the fact that HBV is much more frequently passed in transfusion results in the greatest number of transfusion-related hepatitis cases being caused by HBV. HCV is the second most common cause of transfusion-related hepatitis.

11. The answer is E. The combination of elevated gamma glutamyl transpeptidase and normal alkaline phosphatase strongly suggests active drinking if there are no laboratory signs of biliary obstruction, the latter being elevated conjugated (direct-acting) bilirubin and elevated alkaline phosphatase to name two tests. The elevation of AST out of proportion (e.g., 2:1) to ALT is also suggestive of alcoholic hepatitis as opposed to viral hepatitis, and a lower than expected blood urea nitrogen level may be found in active alcoholism. Assuming the social history revealed that the patient drinks six to eight glasses of wine or equivalent daily, examining for the stigmata of cirrhosis is appropriate as well (spider angiomata, palmar erythema, testicular atrophy, distended flank veins, etc.) Gallbladder ultrasound study is not indicated in the absence of abdominal pain and biliary obstruction. It is premature to order the other tests and procedures until the results of further inquiry and empiric response to alcohol abstention are known.

12. The answer is B. Despite the seriousness of alcoholism, only approximately 15% of alcoholic individuals will develop cirrhosis, even though one-third will have fatty liver at one time or another. That said, an alcoholic without liver disease frequently pays the huge psychosocial costs of alcoholism in the loss of job, breakup of marriage, and psychological damage to his or her children.

13. The answer is B. PSC is associated with ulcerative colitis or Crohn colitis in two-thirds of cases, though only 1% to 4% of ulcerative colitis cases have coexisting PSC. As in PBC, pruritus and incidental findings of elevated alkaline phosphatase may precede clinical jaundice. The diagnosis is confirmed by endoscopic retrograde cholangiography, which usually shows evidence of extrahepatic ductal inflammatory injury or liver biopsy. PSC is most commonly found in men more so than women at a ratio of 1.5 to 2:1 between the ages of 20 and 30 years. The diagnosis is also confirmed by histopathology in liver biopsy. PSC is commonly complicated by bacterial ascending cholangitis. PBC is noted for xanthomas and xanthelasmas and is found in women between the ages of 40 and 60 years (see Question 8 and explanation). Choledocholithiasis is unlikely in the absence of colic and gallstones in the gallbladder. Steatohepatosis (fatty liver) is common in many asymptomatic conditions such as diabetes, morbid obesity, and alcoholism and in itself would not cause the symptoms in the vignette. Viral hepatitis is not considered during the acute phase without elevations of AST and ALT that are fifty to one hundred times normal.

14. The answer is E. Autoimmune hepatitis is initially a diagnosis of exclusion in a patient who manifests evidence of acute, subacute, or chronic hepatitis without evidence of viral, chemical, infectious, or pharmacological causation. Presence of SMA and ANA as well as other autoimmune diseases (e.g., thyroiditis in this case) lends further circumstantial evidence of autoimmune disease. PSC is less likely because of the absence of colitis.

15. The answer is D. A ceruloplasmin level that is lower than normal may be indicative of Wilson disease. The disease is characterized by copper overload, damaging the liver and kidneys and resulting in central nervous system abnormalities, most commonly depression. SMA and ANA may be connected with autoimmune hepatitis, but the patient is younger than expected for that condition. Iron studies would be appropriate for diagnosis of hemochromatosis, but patients with that disease do not become symptomatic until late middle age for men and later still for women.

16. The answer is E. Hepatitis A is transmitted mainly by fecal–oral contamination; it generally risks no complications.

17. The answer is A. Hepatitis B is transmitted by body fluids other than gastrointestinal; it carries high risk of chronic hepatitis and sexual transmission.

18. The answer is D. Hepatitis C is transmitted by body fluids other than gastrointestinal; it carries a very high risk of chronic hepatitis; it is prominent in transfusion-induced hepatitis but there is less risk of sexual and accidental needle-stick transmission (4% chance). Approximately 50% of cases progress to chronic hepatitis.

19. The answer is C. Hepatitis D may be transmitted by percutaneous or nonpercutaneous means; it requires presence of hepatitis B in order to procreate.

20. The answer is B. Hepatitis E is transmitted mainly by fecal–oral contamination; it is fraught with no complications except in third-trimester pregnancy.

References

Giboney PT. Mildly elevated liver transaminase levels in the asymptomatic patient. *Am Fam Physician.* 2005; 71:1105–1110.

Lin KW, Kirchner JT. Hepatitis B. *Am Fam Physician.* 2004; 69: 75–82, 86.

Nidiry JJ. Diseases of the liver. In: Rudy DR, Kurowski K, eds. *Family Medicine: House Officer Series.* Baltimore: Williams & Wilkins; 1997:255–268.

Active Drinking = GGT+ c̄ Nl AØ ; Low BUN → 1/3 fatty liver → 15% Cirrhosis

Alcoholic hepatitis = AST:ALT = 2:1

SECTION VI

Problems of the Urinary Tract

chapter 16

Urinary Tract Infection

1 A 35-year-old woman enters your office with complaints of fever, malaise, and vague abdominal discomfort. She denies gastrointestinal symptoms, cough, coryza, and specific areas of pain. A urinalysis reveals positive dip tests for leukocyte esterase, nitrite, and occult blood and a white blood cell (WBC) count of 10 to 15 WBCs/high-power field. She has never had a urinary tract infection (UTI) in the past. Before examining her, you know with 98% certainty that the patient has which of the following diagnoses?

(A) Cystitis

(B) Ureterolithisasis

(C) Bladder cancer

(D) Acute pyelonephritis

(E) Trigonitis

2 The patient in Question 1 most likely has which of the following organisms as the basis of the infection?

(A) *Escherichia coli*

(B) *Staphylococcus saprophyticus*

(C) Proteus organisms

(D) Klebsiella organisms

(E) Enterococci

3 In the case referred to in Question 1, which of the following should be carried out next?

(A) Intravenous urogram

(B) Culture and sensitivity of the urine

(C) Initiation of a course of a fluoroquinolone antibiotic

(D) Computed tomography scan of the kidneys, and upper urinary tracts

(E) Initiation of therapy with double-strength sulfmethoxazole/trimethoprim (e.g., Bactrim)

4 Each of the following would be an indication for hospitalization of this patient, except which one?

(A) Costovertebral angle tenderness

(B) Lack of a responsible other adult in the home

(C) Immunocompromised state (e.g., cancer chemotherapy)

(D) Persistent nausea and vomiting

(E) Discovery of an anatomical basis for the pyelonephritis (e.g., bifid ureter)

5 In which of the following categories of patients is screening for asymptomatic bacteriuria?

(A) Sexually active woman

(B) Sexually active woman with history of recurrent UTIs

(C) Adult man with history of prostatitis

(D) Anyone with a history of pyelonephritis

(E) Pregnant woman

6 You are consulted by a 27-year-old woman who has become sexually active over the past 3 years and had five episodes of cystitis within the last year. She has otherwise been in good health and is not taking medication. Which of the following mechanisms is most likely responsible for the recurrences?

(A) A cystocele

(B) Bifid ureters

(C) A bladder diverticulum

(D) Hydronephrosis

(E) Vaginal seeding by coliform bacteria

7 You are viewing a "KUB" (plain abdominal) x-ray film of a 45-year-old woman who has a history of left bifid ureter and pyelonephritis at least once. You see an opacity that fills and outlines the pelvis of the left kidney. What is the basis and content of this calcification?

(A) Uric acid in hyperuricemia

(B) Calcium oxalate from chronic infection

(C) Calcium oxalate from hypercalciuria

(D) Magnesium ammonium phosphate from urease-producing organisms

(E) Cysteine caused by hypercysteinuria

8 Which of the following bacterial uropathogens is most commonly associated with the stone formation referred to in Question 8?

(A) *E. coli*

(B) *S. saprophyticus*

(C) *Proteus mirabilis*

(D) Enterococci

(E) *Chlamydia trachomatis*

9 A 24-year-old man complains of dysuria and a slight discharge. He was alarmed when he noticed some blood at the beginning of the urinary stream. A urinalysis from split specimens (beginning, middle, and terminal stream) confirms microscopic and chemical evidence of blood in the beginning stream, less in the midstream, and none in the terminal stream. Which of the following is the likely site of the hematuria?

(A) Anterior urethra

(B) Bladder neck

(C) Bladder

(D) Ureter

(E) Kidney

10 A 55-year-old woman who underwent a uterine suspension operation for stress incontinence developed cystitis the day after surgery, having had a Foley catheter inserted the day prior to surgery. Which is the most likely causative organism?

(A) *Pseudomonas aeruginosa*

(B) *S. saprophyticus*

(C) *E. coli*

(D) Enterococci

(E) *Staphylococcus epidermidis*

11 A 49-year-old woman notes bloody urine recurring intermittently during the last several weeks. She denies abdominal pain, dysuria, and frequency. Vital signs are normal, including body temperature. Physical examination is not remarkable and included deep palpation in the abdominal flanks and the suprapubic area. The urinalysis shows only red blood cells with white blood cells in proportion to what one should expect in the peripheral blood. Which of the following is the best working diagnosis?

(A) Ureterolithiasis

(B) Hemorrhagic cystitis

(C) Urinary tract carcinoma

(D) Pyelonephritis

(E) Vaginitis

12 Which of the following is correct regarding the presence of leukocyte esterase in a urinalysis dip test?

(A) Positive test indicates definite presence of leukocytes.

(B) Negative test rules out presence of leukocytes.

(C) Positive test indicates presence of organisms that reduce nitrate to nitrite.

(D) Positive test is suggestive of bacteria.

(E) Positive test indicates presence of blood.

13 You are re-evaluating a 3-year-old girl with cystitis whom you are treating for the second time within 6 months. She has been on amoxicillin for 7 days with complete resolution of her symptoms. Which of the following listed studies would be most likely to demonstrate a most common urinary tract abnormality that is associated with a UTI in this age group?

(A) Radionuclide cystogram

(B) Renal ultrasound

(C) Cystoscopy

(D) Intravenous pyelogram

(E) Urodynamic study

14 Each of the following statements is true regarding UTIs in boys and girls, except for which one?

(A) Girls are more prone to UTIs than boys at all ages.

(B) Girls may be allowed to have one bout of uncomplicated lower UTI without an evaluation for anatomic urinary tract abnormalities.

(C) The onset of sexual activity in females may give rise to UTIs in females aside from sexually transmitted disease.

(D) The first UTI in boy is an indication for evaluation for anatomic abnormalities.

(E) Uncircumcised male infants are prone to UTIs.

15 A 35-year-old woman has required treatment for several UTIs over the last 2 years and she experienced a recurrence last week. Her urinalysis showed WBC counts too numerous to count per high-power field. You diagnosed recurrent cystitis and treated her for 7 days with a combination sulfmethoxazole/trimethoprim preparation. The following weekend you are on call for the group and take a call from this woman. Which of the following should cause concern that she has had subclinical pyelonephritis?

(A) Patient had dysuria for 3 days before seeking treatment.

(B) Patient has gross hematuria developing after 3 days of dysuria and frequency and urgency.

(C) Patient has had four episodes of cystitis in the last year.

(D) Patient developed dysuria and urgency 1 day after intercourse in which a spermocidal jelly was used.

(E) Patient noted recurrence of symptoms 1 day after finishing her 7-day course of antibiotics for cystitis.

Examination Answers

1. The answer is D. A patient with fever, pyuria, and suggestions of systemic illness or symptoms more specific for upper tract involvement has a 98% chance of having pyelonephritis. Chances are quite good, but not certain, that upon examination she will manifest definite costovertebral angle tenderness. Cystitis usually presents with symptoms of frequency and dysuria. Urolithisasis manifests colicky lateralizing pain, at least when the stone is moving. Bladder cancer and hypernephroma (renal cell carcinoma) are notorious for painless hematuria with no particular pyuria. Trigonitis is a syndrome encountered in mature females consisting of irritative bladder symptoms that are out of proportion to clinical findings.

2. The answer is A. *E. coli* is the cause of 88% of cases of uncomplicated pyelonephritis (e.g., cases in nonelderly individuals, nonrecurrent cases, cases with an absence of diabetes mellitus, and cases without known anatomical bases for recurrence, without indwelling catheters, and without clinical sepsis). Diabetics tend to have UTIs caused by Klebsiella, Enterobacter, Clostridium, or Candida organisms. Other complicated cases of pyelonephritis also involve Pseudomonas but usually not Candida organisms. Immunosuppressed patients tend to develop subclinical pyelonephritis caused by nonenteric, aerobic Gram-negative rods and Candida organisms.

3. The answer is B. With the suspicion of pyelonephritis, treatment of this serious infection comes first. Before antibacterial therapy can be started, a culture and sensitivity must be obtained. The fluoroquinolones are a good first choice while one is awaiting the culture results; sulfmethoxazole/trimethoprim, being bacteriostatic as opposed to bacteriocidal, would be a poor choice with suspected pyelonephritis. The diagnostic studies mentioned are important but should take place after therapy is underway and the infection is abating.

4. The answer is A. Costovertebral angle tenderness in an uncomplicated case is not an indication for hospitalization within itself. However, each of the other factors mentioned are such indications. Others are outpatient treatment failure, sepsis or suspected sepsis, age >60 years, inadequate access to follow-up care, and uncertainty of diagnosis.

5. The answer is E. Pregnant women who are between 12 and 16 weeks gestation, if tested by urine culture (rather than urinalysis), will have significantly fewer UTIs, as well as a lower risk of low birth weight babies and of preterm delivery. In no other category is culture of asymptomatic patients supported by evidence at this time.

6. The answer is E. Vaginal lactobacillus has been replaced with rectal coliform bacteria. The coliform bacteria now in the vagina and introitus can easily ascend via the urethra into the bladder. The absence of lactobacillus raises vaginal pH and creates a more favorable vaginal and periurethral environment for these bacteria. Only about 1% of adult women (nongeriatric) with recurrent cystitis have an identifiable anatomic abnormality. The conditions that predispose a woman to this development include sexual activity without voiding both before and afterward; entrapping clothing (more often resulting in Candida infection but leading also to coliform vaginal inoculation); wiping from anus forward after voiding instead of from the vaginal opening backward; voiding without adequately spreading the knees (caused by inadequate lowering of tight underwear); and occasionally changing hormone status, as in inauguration of contraceptive medication. Oral contraceptives, for example, increase vaginal secretions, providing a culture medium for bacteria and contamination of clothing near the anal orifice. All people with recurrent UTIs should take in more water and other fluids than otherwise inclined.

7. The answer is D, magnesium ammonium phosphate from urease-producing organisms. These are called struvite stones, and insofar as they become molded by the calyceal collecting system, they are often referred to as "staghorn" calculi.

8. The answer is C. *P. mirabilis* is associated with struvite stone formation, as are Pseudomonas, Providencia, and, less commonly, Klebsiella, Staphylococcus and Mycoplasma organisms. These organisms commonly produce a urease, which causes the hydrolysis of urea to ammonia and carbon dioxide. The result is an alkaline urine, which is more conducive to struvite stone formation.

9. The answer is A. The anterior urethra of the penis is likely the cause of the hematuria and, in this case, an infection. This could be either gonorrhea or chlamydia. The split specimen results would be similar in the case of urethral trauma as in vigorous sexual activity. Hematuria found through all three specimens, total hematuria, points toward bladder or kidney for the cause. Terminal hematuria suggests bladder neck, prostate, or trigon involvement.

10. The answer is C, *E. coli.* In complicated UTIs (those acquired in anatomically or functionally abnormal tracts or with suspected resistant organisms), the percentage of cases of cystitis caused by *E. coli* drops to about 35%, but it remains the most prevalent responsible organism.

11. The answer is C. Although in a given clinical setting painless hematuria cancer may not pose even a majority probability of cancer, because of the potentially life-threatening nature of the cancers, painless hematuria must be considered to be urinary tract carcinoma until proven otherwise. The cancers are generally transitional cell carcinomas of the bladder or renal cell carcinoma (in the past often called hypernephroma). Occasionally the lesion may be so small as to be missed grossly. Therefore, studies of the urine such as cytology or other chemical evaluation of tumor cell by-products are necessary and must be repeated as long as the cause of painless hematuria, particularly microscopic hematuria, remains unexplained. If hematuria persists and nothing is found grossly, the patient must be monitored every 6 months. Hemorrhagic cystitis is common in women, usually younger than the woman presented in the vignette, and is always characterized by a rapid onset and accompanied by irritative symptoms (frequency and dysuria). Urolithiasis is in the differential diagnosis and must eventually be ruled out but rarely is unaccompanied by lateralized colicky pain. Pyelonephritis rarely occurs without pain or at least flank or costovertebral tenderness (e.g., in chronic cases), and urinalysis would show pyuria rather than microscopic or gross blood.

12. The answer is D. A positive test for leukocyte esterase is suggestive, but not diagnostic, of bacteria. To be sure, the inference is based on the presumed presence of leukocytes (WBCs). Leukocyte esterase is an enzyme elaborated by white blood cells. However, its sensitivity is compromised by the false negatives that can be produced by high specific gravity of the urine, glycosuria, presence of urobilinogen, and medications including rifampin and ascorbic acid. Furthermore, false positives are produced by specimen contamination. There is a separate dip test for organisms that reduce nitrate to nitrite. They include many Gam-negative bacteria but not all. The sensitivity of the nitrite test is only 30%.

13. The answer is A, radionuclide cystogram. Vesicoureteral reflex is the most likely urinary tract abnormality in this age group and setting. A voiding cystourethrogram is the most common initial diagnostic tool but is not used for follow-up because of the radiation exposure. A radionuclide study for reflux involves less radiation exposure and appears to be more sensitive once the fact of reflux is established. Vesicoureteral reflux is most often secondary to UTI in women and as such is reversible with therapy. In both sexes, anatomic abnormalities, such as a short intramural ureteral segment, preclude a functional valve effect. With bladder distention the segment fails to shut off retrograde flow of urine with distention, leading to retrograde spread of infection. Females' incidence and prevalence are significantly greater than males'. However, in males that mechanism accounts for the vast majority of reflux and upper genitourinary tract spread of infection.

14. The answer is A. This statement is wrong. Male infants have a greater incidence of UTIs as a group than female infants do. A significant portion of this excess morbidity, but not enough to account for it alone, is attributed to noncircumcised male infants; thus, Choice E is a correct statement. All other statements are true. Male children over the age of infancy who have a single UTI should be evaluated for anatomic abnormalities. Female children, especially those over the age of 5 years, may be allowed at least one UTI without such evaluation.

15. The answer is E. Risk factors include relapse after recent treatment for cystitis or not seeking treatment after 1 week of cystitis symptoms. Hemorrhagic cystitis and recurrent cystitis are not risk factors.

References

Kurowski K. Urinary tract infections. In: Rudy DR, Kurowski K, eds. *Family Medicine: House Officer Series.* Baltimore: Williams & Wilkins; 1997:269–284.

Ramakrishnan K, Scheid DC. Diagnosis and management of acute pyelonephritis. *Am Fam Physician.* 2005; 71:933–942.

Stoller ML, Carroll PR. Urology. In: Tierney LM, McPhee SJ, Papadakis MA, eds. *Current Medical Diagnosis and Treatment.* 43rd ed. New York: McGraw-Hill/Appleton & Lange; 2004: 899–940.

U.S. Preventive Service Task Force. *Guide to clinical preventive services.* 2nd ed. Washington, DC: Office of Disease Prevention and Health Promotion; 1996.

chapter 17

Nephrology in Primary Care

1 Your 45-year-old type II diabetic weighs 240 lb (108.72 kg) at a height of 5 ft 10 in. (1.77 m). You have treated him with 500 mg of metformin three times daily and 10 mg of glyburide twice daily. His glycohemoglobin this week was measured at 8%. A 24-hour urine specimen reveals 250 mg of albumen. Which of the following is the chief significance of this finding?

(A) It constitutes microalbuminuria.

(B) It is a normal finding.

(C) It indicates nephrotic syndrome.

(D) It is presumptive of pyelonephritis.

(E) It indicates an evaluation for cancer.

2 Regarding Question 1, what are the implications of this finding in the management of the diabetic patient?

(A) It signifies the presence of a lower urinary tract infection.

(B) It signifies the presence of pyelonephritis.

(C) It signifies an early stage of renal insufficiency.

(D) It is of no significance as the amount of albumen in the urine is less than that amount found in nephrotic syndrome.

(E) It signifies the possibility of multiple myeloma.

3 Which of the following pharmaceutical classes protects against decline in renal function in both diabetic and hypertensive individuals, independent of direct effects on either blood sugar or blood pressure (BP) control?

(A) Nonselective beta-adrenergic blocking agents

(B) Beta-2 selective adrenergic blocking agents

(C) Calcium channel blocking agents

(D) Angiotensin-converting enzyme inhibitors (ACEIs)

(E) Alpha-adrenergic blocking agents

4 Which of the following is the mechanism for development of hyperparathyroidism in renal failure?

(A) Failure to retain calcium in the kidneys

(B) Increased catabolism of osteoid matrix in cancellous bone

(C) Failure of absorption of calcium in the gastrointestinal tract

(D) Faulty conversion of 25-hydroxy vitamin D, or 25(OH)D, to vitamin D_3, or 25(OH)2D

(E) Renal retention of phosphates

5 In primary care, part of addressing prevention in addition to treating symptomatic conditions includes alertness to conditions that may initiate or cause or share cause of acceleration of renal disease. Each of the following is listed as such a factor, except which one?

(A) History of congestive heart failure

(B) History of coronary artery disease

(C) History of urinary stones

(D) Atopic disease (eczema, allergic rhinitis, and asthma)

(E) Lower urinary tract obstruction

6 A 45-year-old African American man has been treated by you for cardiomyopathy and has had one significant bout of congestive heart failure. He is 50% overweight. Now he has become diabetic. You find an albumen-to-creatinine ratio of 200 mg of albumen to 1 g of creatinine (normal is <17 mg to 250 mg). Which of the following laboratory studies gives the most accurate measure of renal *function*?

(A) Blood urea nitrogen (BUN)

(B) Serum creatinine

(C) Creatinine clearance

(D) Urinalysis

(E) 24-hour measurement of urinary protein and creatinine

7 Renal failure may be caused by diabetes and hypertension in about two-thirds of the cases. Regardless of causation, as renal failure progresses and BUN and creatinine rise in the blood, anemia develops. Which of the following mechanisms accounts for the anemia associated with chronic renal failure?

(A) Iron deficiency

(B) Hemolysis

(C) Hypovitaminosis B_{12}

(D) Folic acid deficiency

(E) Decreased production of erythropoietin

8 You are considering ancillary imaging studies on your 46-year-old male patient who has had gross and microscopic hematuria over a 1-week period. A helical computed tomography (CT) scan without contrast shows no evidence of stone. Therefore, other causes for hematuria, including cancer, must be considered. Each of the following constitutes a relative or absolute contraindication for repeating the CT scan with contrast, except for which one?

(A) Multiple myeloma

(B) Diabetes with serum creatinine level >2 mg/dL

(C) Chronic renal failure with creatinine level >5 mg/dL

(D) Hypovolemia with BUN level of 45 mg/dl (normal level is 10–20 mg/dL), creatinine level of 1.5 mg/dL (normal level is ≤1.4 mg/dL)

(E) Suspected renal cell carcinoma

9 Regarding the patient in Question 8, if there were a contraindication to the use of contrast materials and a neoplasm were suspected, which of the following would be the most likely choice of ancillary study to rule out neoplasm?

(A) Magnetic resonance imaging

(B) CT scan without contrast

(C) Plain abdominal x-ray

(D) Renal arteriography

(E) Venography

10 Which of the following is the precipitating mechanism of injury that leads to acute renal failure (ARF) after misguided use of a contrast medium in radiographic imaging?

(A) Ischemia

(B) Direct toxicity

(C) Hypoxia

(D) Autoimmunity

(E) Dehydration

11 A 55-year-old white man enters your practice with a complaint of flank pains that have occurred on either side from time to time. He says that he was treated in another city for hypertension over several years. He says he has had positive tests for blood in his urine in the past but that no cause had ever been found. BUN level is elevated at 40 mg/dL (normal is ≤20 mg/dL) and creatinine is 1.8 mg/dL. A complete blood cell (CBC) count is normal. Examination of the abdomen reveals a mass deep in each flank. Which of the following most likely accounts for the clinical picture presented?

(A) Carcinoma of the bladder

(B) Renal cell carcinoma

(C) Pancreatic cysts

(D) Polycystic kidneys

(E) Colorectal cancer

12 A patient who is new to you is a 46-year-old white woman who complains of headaches over the past 3 days and suspects it may be due to her BP. Her BP is 230/120. Each of the following findings constitutes a diagnosis of malignant hypertension, given the BP, except for which one?

(A) Rising BUN and creatinine levels

(B) Onset of dyspnea and orthopnea in the past 1 to 3 days

(C) A finding of papilledema

(D) Systolic BP >220 mm Hg

(E) Mental confusion

13 A 45-year-old white man has type II diabetes and weighs 245 lb (111 kg) at a height of 5 ft 11 in. (1.8 m), despite your efforts to exhort him to lose weight over the previous 2 years. However, for the past 3 months he has complained of low-grade fever, abdominal discomfort, and lack of appetite. During this period he has had a striking weight loss, amounting to 40 lb (18.12 kg). The diabetes has now virtually disappeared so far as clinical evidence exists. However, you cannot explain the weight loss, anorexia, and abdominal pain. Suspecting carcinoma of the pancreas, you ordered a CT scan of the abdomen with and without contrast. The result showed a mass involving the right kidney. Blood studies for liver function, including alkaline phosphatase, and CBC count as well as bone scan reveal no abnormalities. Within 3 weeks after right nephrectomy for renal cell carcinoma, the patient's appetite had returned and he began to gain weight. Which of the following most likely explains the foregoing clinical picture?

(A) Metastases from renal cell carcinoma have caused anorexia and abdominal pain.

(B) The mass was misdiagnosed as cancer, allowing full recovery following surgical removal.

(C) Metastases from renal cell carcinoma have become dormant.

(D) The renal cell carcinoma has entered a remission phase.

(E) The patient had suffered from a paraneoplastic syndrome.

14 A 6-year-old boy is presented to you by his parents with discolored urine, symptoms of an upper respiratory tract infection, including a sore throat, and a rash. All symptoms began on the same day 4 days ago. Other than a dry cough, as expected on the fourth day of a viral upper respiratory tract infection, there are no pulmonary symptoms. There is no facial edema. BP is 126/80. The erythematous rash is mainly on the trunk and blanches with digital pressure. The urine is positive on dip test for blood. Microscopic examination shows misshapen red blood cells and red cell casts and is positive for protein. Which of the following is the best diagnostic impression of this child's condition?

(A) Postinfectious glomerulonephritis

(B) Nephritic syndrome

(C) Immune complex glomerulonephritis

(D) Goodpasture syndrome

(E) Henoch–Schönlein purpura

15 Each of the following drugs may cause nephropathy, except for which one?

(A) Acetaminophen

(B) Aspirin

(C) Phenacetin

(D) Ibuprofen

(E) Naproxen

16 A 58-year-old partly controlled diabetic patient with hypertension has an undiagnosed abdominal pain. In the absence of specific physical examination findings, albeit without elevation of liver enzymes, you fear carcinoma of the pancreas. You decide to order a CT scan of the abdomen with and without contrast. Which of the following laboratory determinations is critical to obtain before contrast material is injected?

(A) CBC count

(B) Serum electrolyte level

(C) Alkaline phosphatase level

(D) Serum creatinine level

(E) Antinuclear antibody level

17 Regarding the patient in Question 16, the serum creatinine level is 1.8 mg/dL. The gastroenterology consultant feels a CT scan with contrast will make the diagnosis the most certain, short of surgical exploration. Which of the following pretreatment medications has been found to reduce the risk of creatinine elevation or renal failure when administered before injection of contrast medium?

(A) Acetylsalicylic acid

(B) Sulfasalazine

(C) Acetylcysteine

(D) Amoxicillin

(E) Furosemide

Examination Answers

1. The answer is A. The 24-hour urine specimen that shows 250 mg of albumen falls within the definition of microalbinuria for a diabetic, which is 30 to 300 mg of albumen in 24 hours. Other, quick methods of detection of microalbuminuria include a urine spot albumen-specific dipstick finding of ≥ 3 mg/dL and spot urine albumen-to-creatinine ratio of 17 to 250 mg of albumen to 1 g of creatinine (men) or 25 to 355 mg of albumen to 1 g creatinine (women). Because small amounts of protein may appear in the urine for brief periods of time, microalbuminuria should be confirmed after a delay of 2 to 3 weeks. If proteinuria persists, the patient should be evaluated for kidney disease, with attention to diabetes, hypertension, and various causes of glomerular disease. Nephrotic syndrome is entirely different, foremost in that the definition of nephrotic syndrome is ≥ 3 g of total protein (both albumen and globulin) per 24-hour period.

2. The answer is C. Microalbuminuria is secondary to glomerulopathy and usually occurs when the creatinine clearance has fallen to near 50 mL/minute/1.73 m^2 (from a normal rate in normal young people of 100 to 110 mL/minute). The development of microalbuminuria and acceleration of renal failure are preventable by control of diabetes mellitus (glycohemoglobin $\leq 6\%$). Microalbuminuria in the presence of hypertension similarly signals acceleration of renal failure and is prevented, along with acceleration of renal failure, if hypertension is controlled to BP $\leq 130/80$. Obviously this patient should have a serum creatinine measurement. Assuming the level is even slightly elevated, metformin must be discontinued on the basis of the guidelines given in the drug literature.

3. The answer is D. ACEIs as well as angiotensin receptor blocking agents (ARBA) protect against renal damage by reducing the glomerular filtration rate per nephron. Glomerular filtration rates per unit number of surviving glomeruli increase as creatinine clearance decreases. An elevated glomerular filtration rate leads to proteinuria. Deterioration of renal function is retarded by control of either BP in hypertensive patients or blood sugar in diabetic patients (see discussion of Question 2). Thus, the other choices, insofar as they are antihypertensive agents, do serve to prevent loss of renal function to the extent that they succeed in control of BP. ACEIs and ARBAs are antihypertensive agents, particularly in patients whose hypertension is driven to a significant degree by the rennin–angiotensin system. Thus, ACEIs and ARBAs protect renal function in hypertensive patients in two ways and in diabetics solely through the effect to reduce the glomerular filtration rate.

4. The answer is E. When creatinine clearance falls to below 60 mL/minute, phosphates are retained and a relative hyperphosphatemia results. The reciprocal relationship between serum phosphates and serum calcium gives rise to hypocalcemia, to which the parathyroid glands respond by increasing the output of parathormone. Negative calcium balance is thus a part of the pathophysiology of chronic renal failure and results in a loss of bone density. Failure of calcium absorption occurs secondary to loss of estrogen support in menopause because of the loss of the parathormone-inhibiting effects of estrogen, relevant in Choices C and D but not in renal failure. The postmenopausal state is associated with hyperparathyroidism for a different reason, which in turn contributes to postmenopausal decrease in postmenopausal bone density.

5. The answer is D. Atopic disease is not listed as a precipitant or aggrevant, and it is not associated with accelerated reduction of renal function. Diabetes and hypertension, as discussed previously, are the most common causes of renal failure, accounting for about two-thirds of cases between them. Any reduction of cardiac output, especially acute or profound congestive heart failure, constitutes a risk to renal function. Coronary artery disease not only risks cardiac output ultimately through the threat of congestive heart failure but also is associated with atherosclerosis that can cause renovascular hypertension. History of urinary stones is a risk factor and may be an initiator of renal disease, probably because of an association with lower urinary obstruction.

6. The answer is C. Creatinine clearance is the measure of renal function. The stages of kidney disease are defined by creatinine clearance. For example, stage 2 is defined as "kidney damage" (e.g., abnormal urinalysis) with creatinine clearance of 60 to 89 mL/minute/1.73 m^2 (somewhat above 50% of normal renal function for a person under 40 years of age). At this stage the parathyroid hormone levels begin to rise because of the renal retention of phosphates (as discussed earlier).

Renal failure, stage 3, is defined as creatinine clearance in the range of 30 to 59 mL/minute/1.73 m^2. It is useful to remember this stage because calcium absorption declines, leading to further secretion of parathormone; lipoprotein activity declines; left ventricular hypertrophy appears; and anemia develops. Stage 4 kidney disease is defined as creatinine clearance in the range of 15 to 29 mL/minute/1.73 m^2; endstage disease shows <15 mL/minute/1.73 m^2. A completely accurate creatinine clearance requires a measurement of both 24-hour urine creatinine and serum creatinine levels. BUN levels are not particularly sensitive to the status of renal function. Serum creatinine is less useful than creatinine clearance because there is such a narrow range of transition from normal to abnormally high levels in the blood, and because by the time serum creatinine begins to rise, renal function has fallen by about 50%. The urinalysis shows evidence of damage to the urinary tract, for example that involving infection or glomerulopathy, but says nothing directly regarding the status of renal function.

7. The answer is E. Decreased production of erythropoietin accounts for the anemia specific to renal failure. Thus, the anemia is normochromic and normocytic. Iron deficiency produces a microcytic, hypochromic anemia whereas both folic acid and B$_{12}$ deficiency cause a macrocytic anemia. The anemia that accompanies renal failure increases the progression of and the ultimate mortality that is due to endstage kidney disease. Therefore, a critical part of the treatment of renal failure is the institution of exogenous erythropoietin. As implied in Question 6, hemoglobin should be followed as creatinine clearance falls below 60 mL/minute/1.73 m^2 and hematocrit falls to less than 30% to 35%, whereupon treatment with erythropoietin is started. Recombinant erythropoietin in the form of epoetin alfa is used clinically.

8. The answer is E. In and of itself, renal cell carcinoma is not a contraindication for contrast media in radiographic studies. In fact, because the contrast medium is filtered by the glomeruli and concentrated in the tables, a CT scan with contrast is an excellent modality for diagnosis of cysts and neoplasms. Serum creatinine >5 mg/dL is a contraindication for contrast media because of the danger of precipitating ARF. In diabetics the tolerance level for serum creatinine is lowered to 2 mg/dL. Even prerenal azotemia (exemplified by the choice showing normal creatinine with elevated BUN) poses a risk for ARF in the presence of contrast medium. Neither glomerular disease nor renal cell carcinoma are contraindications for contrast in the absence of other contraindications.

9. The answer is A. Magnetic resonance imaging is an excellent tool for diagnosing neoplasm when contrast in CT scan or intravenous pyelogram is contraindicated. A CT scan without contrast, as implied in the discussion for Question 8, is not useful in diagnosing neoplasms; certainly, a plain film is not useful either. Although arteriography and venography may be useful in evaluating masses, both require contrast.

10. The answer is B. Direct toxicity by contrast material in radiographic imaging is the proximate cause of ARF in the clinical setting presented. ARF in this case is due to acute tubular necrosis, the cause of 85% of cases of ARF. However, it is not likely to occur unless other causes of renal damage are present. The latter include any cause of ischemia, hypovolemia, or hypoxia. These are dehydration, pre-existing diabetes, hypotension, sepsis, and prolonged anesthesia with vasodilating anesthetic agents. Other causes of direct nephrotoxicity and acute tubular necrosis include the presence of aminoglycosides (gentamicin the most, tobramycin the least potent in that regard); cyclosporine (used to prevent rejection of transplanted organs); various antineoplastic agents (e.g., cisplatin); and organic solvents and heavy metals (e.g., mercury, cadmium, arsenic). Of cases of ARF, 15% of them are caused not by tubular necrosis but by interstitial nephritis. Causes of the latter are generally autoimmune related.

11. The answer is D. Hypertension, history of hematuria, and flank mass together are strongly suggestive of polycystic disease of the kidneys (PCDK). Although any presentation of hematuria of long duration demands evaluation for urinary tract neoplasm, most bladder tumors present with painless intermittent or persistent hematuria, with a small percentage manifesting irritative bladder symptoms (frequency or dysuria). Renal cell carcinoma is notorious for painless hematuria, sometimes over long periods of time before becoming diagnosable. However, neither of the aforementioned cancers present with bilateral masses. Pancreatic cysts may occur in conjunction with PCDK, as may hepatic and splenic cysts. Of patients with PCDK, 50% have hypertension, often preceding the polycystic manifestations; 50% of cases will progress to endstage renal disease by the time the patient reaches the age of 60 years. Despite hematuria that may be significant, anemia is unusual because PCDK is associated with the production of erythropoietin.

12. The answer is D. Although a systolic BP >220, a diastolic BP >125, or both constitute a diagnosis of *accelerated* hypertension, which is an urgent medical state, the diagnosis of malignant hypertension requires these levels of BP in association with any of the other choices presented in the question. Accelerated hypertension is a medical emergency, requiring BP control in order to avoid development of malignant hypertension. Malignant hypertension is a more time-urgent emergency that carries 50% mortality if not treated.

13. The answer is E. The patient had suffered from a paraneoplastic syndrome associated with the renal cell carcinoma, for which the tumor is noted. In cases of paraneoplastic syndromes, the patient becomes ill and manifests symptoms related to a humeral manifestation of the primary tumor that causes systemic symptoms, unrelated to metastases. Renal cell carcinoma may be thus associated with symptoms experienced by the patient in the vignette as well as fever alone, erythrocytosis, thrombocytosis, coagulopathy, and amyloidosis.

14. The answer is B. On the basis of on hematuria and red cell casts, the case can be categorized as a nephritic syndrome (i.e., a glomerulopathy). Each of the other choices is a specific glomerulopathy. However, two can be ruled out based on the history. For the other two choices there is not enough evidence to make a more specific diagnosis without further information. The patient is hypertensive (see the following table, which shows the minimal hypertensive BP levels for four age groups of children). Although Henoch–Schönlein purpura causes a rash, it is indeed purpuric, usually a petechial rash (nonblanching with pressure). Henoch–Schönlein purpura does not cause hypertension. Postinfectious glomerulonephritis (most often caused by group A beta-hemolytic streptococci type 12) does not manifest nephritic signs and symptoms simultaneously with the onset of the upper respiratory tract infection, and the upper respiratory tract infection that precedes the nephritis is a streptococcal infection, not a viral one. Goodpasture syndrome is a progressive glomerulonephritis associated with pulmonary hemorrhage caused by antiglomerular basement membrane antibodies. Among immune complex nephritides, lupus nephritis is representative, along with cryoglobulinemia and subacute bacterial endocarditis. However, one cannot determine the progressivity of the nephritis without following serum creatinine levels over at least many days. In addition, specificity for diagnosis of glomerulopathies requires a kidney biopsy, which in the case of immune complex disease shows crescentic glomerulonephritis with immunofluorescence revealing IgG, IgA, and C3 in the case of lupus nephritis; Goodpasture syndrome shows the same light microscopic findings with IgG but not IgA by immunofluorescence.

Hypertensive BP Levels Among Four Age Groups of Children

Age (y)	Significant Hypertension
3–5	116/76
6–9	122/78
10–12	126/82
13–15	136/86

15. The answer is A. Acetaminophen is the only analgesic among the choices given that does not cause analgesic nephropathy. Aspirin, ibuprofen, and naproxen are all nonsteroidal anti-inflammatory drugs. In all cases, tubulointerstitial inflammation and papillary necrosis are found on pathologic examination.

16. The answer is D. Serum creatinine, if elevated, can result in ARF after injection with contrast medium. Although the other tests are relevant in an investigation of serious possible hepatic or intra-abdominal cancers, they are not necessary before use of contrast medium.

17. The answer is C. Acetylcysteine (Mucomyst), given before radiocontrast media along with infusion of 0.45% saline solution, has been found to result in a relative risk of elevation of creatinine of 0.11 to 0.18 and an absolute risk reduction of 19%. In a control group given 0.45% saline only, creatinine rose 0.5 mg/dL in 9 of 42 control subjects.

References

Johnson CA, Levey AS, Corsh J, et al. Clinical practice guidelines for kidney disease in adults. Part I: Definition, disease stages, evaluation, treatment, and risk factors. *Am Fam Physician.* 2004; 70:869–876.

Johnson CA, Levey AS, Corsh J, et al. Clinical practice guidelines for kidney disease in adults. Part II: Glomerular filtration rate, proteinuria, and other markers. *Am Fam Physician.* 2004; 70:1091–1097.

Neeham ED. Management of acute renal failure. *Am Fam Physician.* 2005; 72:1739–1746.

Snively CS, Gutierez C. Chronic kidney disease: Prevention and treatment of complications. *Am Fam Physician.* 2004; 70: 1921–1930.

Watnick S, Morrison G. Kidney. In: Tierney LM, McPhee SJ, Papadakis MA, eds. *Current Diagnosis and Treatment.* 43rd ed. New York: McGraw-Hill/Appleton & Lange; 2004:863–898.

SECTION **VII**

Problems Unique to Females

chapter 18

Gynecology in Primary Care

Examination questions: *Unless instructed otherwise, choose the ONE lettered answer or completion that is BEST in each case.*

1 A 45-year-old woman complains of increasingly irregular menstrual periods, which are becoming lighter and less frequent, seldom appearing sooner than 35 days after the previous one. She complains also of gaining weight over the last 5 years. During the same period, hair has grown on her upper lip and she has developed acne for the first time in her life. She weighs 165 lb (74.8 kg) at a height of 5 ft 4 in. (1.63 m). Upon examination she manifests central obesity and fading purple striae over the flanks of her abdomen. Which of the following is the best *causal* explanation for these findings?

(A) Type II diabetes mellitus

(B) Hypothyroidism

(C) Metabolic syndrome

(D) Polycystic ovary syndrome (PCOS)

(E) Cushing syndrome

2 Regarding the patient in Question 1, besides an elevation of serum testosterone levels, which of the following laboratory tests, in conjunction with the clinical picture, gives a distinctive pattern for identification of the diagnosis?

(A) White blood cell count

(B) Blood sugar

(C) Serum luteinizing hormone (LH)

(D) Serum electrolytes

(E) Serum creatinine

3 Regarding the patient in Questions 1 and 2, the first treatment option should be which of the following?

(A) Menstrual regulation with cyclic contraceptive hormonal treatment

(B) Increased physical activity and decreased calorie ingestion

(C) Prescription of metformin

(D) Prescription of clomiphene

(E) Epilation and electrolysis

4 Each of the following is a relative contraindication for intrauterine device (IUD) insertion except for which one?

(A) Nulliparity

(B) Active sexually transmitted disease

(C) History of pelvic inflammatory disease

(D) Presence of an intrauterine pregnancy (IUP)

(E) Multiparity

5 A 14-year-old nulliparous girl complains of primary dysmenorrhea. She is overweight and attempting to lose weight. Her parents have recently separated and she has been sporadically involved in drinking fairly heavily and smoking at parties of young people but has not become sexually active. Each of the following aspects of her life situation is a risk factor for dysmenorrhea except for which one?

(A) Drinking alcohol

(B) Smoking

(C) Losing weight

(D) Experiencing family stress

(E) Being nulliparous

6 Which of the following is the only medication approved specifically by the Food and Drug Administration for the treatment of nausea and vomiting of pregnancy?

(A) Prochlorperizine (Compazine)

(B) Promethazine (Phenergan)

(C) Trimethobenzamide (Tigan)

(D) Pyridoxine/doxylamine (Bendectin)

(E) Ondansetron (Zofran)

7 Each of the following conditions occurs at a greater rate than expected in people exposed to diethyl-stilbestrol (DES) in utero except for which one?

(A) Squamous cell carcinoma of the cervix

(B) T-shaped uterus

(C) Clear cell adenocarcinoma of the vagina

(D) Undescended testicle

(E) Hypoplastic uterus

8 A 24-year-old monogamous woman calls from a remote town and complains of a pruritic vaginal discharge. She is unable to see a physician within the next several days and requests prescription for relief of her symptoms. She denies dyspareunia except for slight irritation at the point of entry (i.e., superficial type dyspareunia). She denies urinary symptoms. The discharge is described as white and particulate, like curdled milk. After insisting she seek early medical advice and examination, you decide to treat empirically for the most likely chance of success by phoning in which of the following regimens?

(A) Metronidazole (Flagyl), oral

(B) Podophyllin application

(C) Clindamycin, oral

(D) Fluconazole 150 mg, oral

(E) Amoxicillin course – 10 days of therapy

9 A 21-year-old sexually active woman complains of intense pain in the left vulvar area building over a period of 2 to 3 days. She has not had similar symptoms in the past, and she has not been with her sex partner for several weeks. The pain is of such severity that she has been afraid to attempt intercourse or even to sit down normally. Which of the following is the most likely diagnosis?

(A) Herpes simplex type 2

(B) Craurosis vulvae

(C) Candida vaginitis

(D) Trichomonas vaginitis

(E) Bartholin gland abscess

10 A 65-year-old woman visits you for the first time to complain of vaginal bleeding for the first time since her natural menopause 15 years ago. The bleeding began 2 weeks ago and is mild in flow. Which of the following is the most critical question to be asked in completing the history?

(A) Are there cramps associated with the bleeding?

(B) How many pads per days are needed to keep abreast of the bleeding?

(C) Are you taking hormone therapy of any type?

(D) Have you developed light-headedness upon standing after sitting for prolonged periods of time?

(E) Is there bleeding with intercourse?

11 Regarding the patient in Question 10, you find that she has taken no hormone therapy for the past 10 years but that she was prescribed estrogen replacement therapy for a period of 5 years after the onset of menopause (i.e., until 10 years ago). You note that she has been 25% overweight for most of her adult life and that she has never been pregnant. Which of the following should be the next therapeutic action after doing a routine pelvic examination, performing a Papanicolaou smear, and ordering routine hemographic studies?

(A) Colposcopy

(B) Cervical conization

(C) Await Pap smear and, if negative, repeat in 6 months

(D) Total abdominal hysterectomy

(E) Endometrial biopsy

12 You have diagnosed, on "routine" Pap smear with an enzyme-linked test for sexually transmitted diseases, chlamydia. The woman confessed that she was concerned about the possible infidelity of her husband. Which of the following may be among the aspects of this infection you must explain to this woman?

(A) The course for the infected female is virtually always benign.

(B) Unless successfully treated she will have significantly increased risk of spontaneous abortion and infertility.

(C) The infection responds to amoxicillin.

(D) Macrosomia may occur in newborn babies of mothers infected during pregnancy.

(E) Symptoms, if she notes them, are likely to include a frankly purulent discharge within 48 hours of exposure.

13 A 52-year-old woman, gravida 4, para 4, is diagnosed as having a large uterine "fibroid" (leiomyofibroma).

Although she still has menstrual periods and presumably ovulatory cycles, she does not desire more children. A total abdominal hysterectomy is planned, but because of the size of the fibroid the surgeon requires the patient to receive medical therapy to shrink this benign tumor prior to surgery. Which of the following regimens would be appropriate for that function?

(A) Cycled oral contraceptive medication for 3 months

(B) Intramuscular depot leuprolide, 3.75 mg, monthly for 3 months

(C) Intramuscular depot medroxyprogesterone, monthly for 3 months

(D) Ibuprofen 800 mg, qid for 4 weeks

(E) Oral danazol 400 to 800 mg, daily for 1 month

14 A woman with secondary amenorrhea is given 10 mg of medroxyprogesterone acetate by mouth per day for 5 days and monitored for the onset of bleeding following progesterone withdrawal. Which of the causes for amenorrhea listed here will produce a positive response to this challenge (bleeding upon withdrawal)?

(A) Asherman syndrome

(B) Anovulatory cycle

(C) Gonadal agenesis

(D) Ovarian failure

(E) Menopause

15 You are evaluating a 38-year-old woman who stopped having periods 8 months ago. She has normal secondary sexual development and shows no evidence of virilization. Her pelvic exam shows a normal cervix and fundus and no adnexal masses. Her urine beta-human chorionic gonadotropin (hCG) test is negative. Her thyroid-stimulating hormone and serum prolactin levels are normal. She does not have uterine bleeding during the withdrawal phase of a progestin challenge, but does bleed after being on conjugated estrogen (1.25 mg) for 21 days with a progestin agent added on the last 5 days. Follicle-stimulating hormone (FSH) and LH are both elevated. Which of the following is the most likely diagnosis?

(A) Hypothalamic amenorrhea

(B) Asherman syndrome

(C) Premature ovarian failure

(D) Anovulatory cycle

(E) PCOS

16 A 25-year-old woman who is a ballet dancer has felt the need to lose weight in order to remain competitive. Her height is 5 ft 4 in. (1.63 m) and her weight is 95 lb (43 kg), yet she feels she needs to lose more weight. Her menstrual periods have become scant and infrequent during the past year. Her last menstrual period was more than 3 months ago. You suspect that she has anorexia. Which of the following is a likely finding?

(A) Normal serum estrogen level

(B) Osteoporosis

(C) Sedentary lifestyle

(D) Healthy dentition

(E) Elevated FSH and LH levels

17 A 25-year-old woman who has never been pregnant missed a menstrual period 4 weeks ago, an unusual circumstance for her. She has been using a barrier method of contraception. Until the past week she noticed nausea, but yesterday she passed much blood and now says she feels better, although she is still bleeding. Her beta-hCG level was 2,500 mIU, but the test was repeated 48 hours later and the level found to be 1,000 mIU. Pelvic examination is negative for adnexal mass or tenderness. Transvaginal pelvic ultrasound reveals intrauterine tissue. You diagnose missed spontaneous abortion. The patient's vital signs are normal and her hemoglobin is within normal limits. She is not seriously concerned and in little pain. Which of the following is the best decision for management in the near future?

(A) Expectant observation

(B) Intravaginal misoprostol, 800 µg

(C) Surgical evacuation of the uterus

(D) Naproxen, 500 mg twice daily if needed to control uterine cramps

(E) Initiation of oral contraceptive medication

18 You are seeing an 18-year-old patient with increasingly severe abdominal pain over a span of 4 days. On pelvic examination you find tenderness of the left uterine adnexae. Vaginal ultrasound does not indicate an intrauterine mass, such as an IUP. You order a serum beta-hCG test. Which of the following serum levels signals the threshold above which an ectopic pregnancy should be suspected?

(A) 500 mIU

(B) 1,000 mIU

(C) 1,500 mIU

(D) 3,500 mIU

(E) 10,000 mIU

Examination Answers

1. The answer is D. This patient meets the criteria for the diagnosis of PCOS. The Amsterdam consensus states that a patient must have two of the three following conditions to qualify for the diagnosis: anovulation or oligo-ovulation; chemical or clinical signs of androgenization; and sonographic evidence of polycystic ovaries. Elevated testosterone levels are the common pathway of pathophysiology. Besides the androgenizing effect, this results in lack of a dominant developing follicle during the monthly cycle. Therefore, the ovary fills gradually with uncompleted cystic follicles. Androgenic manifestations that may be found with this condition, besides acne and hirsutism, include male-pattern alopecia. Although metabolic insulin resistance and type II diabetes are part of the syndrome, as is central obesity, they are not necessarily accompanied by androgenizing manifestations. Cushing syndrome manifests purple striae along with its other glucosteroid effects, but not androgenization. Hypothyroidism has nothing in common with the patient in the vignette except for sometimes a mild degree of obesity. In hypothyroidism, menstrual periods are increased in flow and frequency, not decreased.

2. The answer is C. A serum LH that rises to a preovulatory level that is not followed by ovulation within 14 days of the blood drawing is a hallmark of PCOS. The patient with PCOS often goes a long time between periods, 3 months up to a year, so that a random LH level that is elevated to preovulatory levels is suspect immediately. It is as if the hormonal rhythm is "held up" at the preovulatory phase, which is indeed true, caused by androgenic hormone excess. None of the other laboratory tests gives a result distinctive for PCOS. Although blood sugar may be elevated if the patient progresses to diabetes type II, such a finding is not diagnostic of anything except for diabetes. Not listed is serum testosterone, which is typically elevated in PCOS. However, that does not differentiate PCOS from other causes of androgenization, such as adrenal hyperplasia.

3. The answer is B. Increased physical activity and decreased calorie ingestion, that is, weight loss alone, will change the physiology of PCOS in a significant number of patients. Decreased fat stores reduce androgen stores and hence conversion of androgen to estrone, allowing resumption of ovulation. Metformin is an excellent pharmacologic choice as it reduces insulin resistance and aids in weight loss. Metformin is virtually the first choice for drug therapy if weight loss and exercise fail. Menstrual regulation with cyclic contraceptive hormonal treatment is another common approach and may lead to resumption of ovulation. Clomiphene should be used only in women who are anxious to become pregnant in a short time. Epilation and electrolysis are secondary options for treating the hirsutism directly without affecting the underlying pathophysiology at any point.

4. The answer is E. Multiparity is not a contraindication for insertion of an IUD. Nulliparity certainly is a relative contraindication because it may be physically difficult and usually is very painful at the time of insertion and often remains so until it is removed. Having a present or past sexually transmitted disease is a contraindication, unless a matter of 10 or more years has passed. An IUP will likely be aborted by an IUD. Abortions of normal pregnancy constitute malpractice unless the procedure is done specifically for elective abortion. In the latter case, insertion of an IUD is not an approved procedure. Other contraindications include the presence of liver or breast carcinoma or jaundice specific for hormone-containing IUDs; copper allergy or Wilson disease (specific for copper-containing IUDs); known or suspected pelvic malignancy; and immunodeficiency or immunosuppression.

5. The answer is A. Alcohol drinking, though a risk for numerous other health problems, is not statistically a risk factor for dysmenorrhea. Each of the other choices is associated with dysmenorrhea, though none is proven to be a cause thereof. Obesity per se is not associated with dysmenorrhea but attempts to lose weight are so associated, perhaps because of the confounding issue of poor self-image, itself a risk factor. Nulliparity is well known to be associated with primary dysmenorrhea. Primary dysmenorrhea usually begins with the onset of ovulation, 6 months to 2 years after the menarche, and decreases with age after 20 and with parity.

6. The answer is D. Pyridoxine/doxylamine (Bendectin) is known to safely relieve nausea and vomiting of pregnancy and is approved for that usage. In accord with such approval, its Strength of Recommendation Taxonomy

(SORT) classification is A, meaning evidence is case based and adequately studied. Although each of the other drugs mentioned is an antiemetic and utilized for nausea of pregnancy in practice, they are classified as unproven as to safety in pregnancy and not recommended during nursing. Prochlorperizine is classified as SORT C (i.e., usage is based on clinical custom, usual practice, expert opinion, etc.), as are promethazine and trimethobenzamide. Ondansetron is classified SORT B, based on case evidence but not such that rises to statistical significance.

7. The answer is A. Squamous cell carcinoma of the cervix, according to current data, is caused by a papilloma virus. All the other abnormalities, including undescended testicles, are associated with in utero exposure to DES, which was a common practice to prevent miscarriage between 1938 and 1971. In addition to those mentioned in women are other conditions, including cockscomb cervix, cervical collar, cervical pseudopolyp, and vaginal adenosis. Not as well known among clinicians are the abnormalities of male genital development in DES progeny. These include, in addition to undescended testicles, epididymal cysts and sperm and semen abnormalities. There is a resurgence of attention being paid to DES progeny because the female progeny are now postmenopausal and perimenopausal, an epoch of increased susceptibility to the vagaries of hormonal shifts. Both male and female progeny of DES-treated women should be conscientious regarding routine cancer screening for breast, vaginal, and testicular neoplasms.

8. The answer is D. Fluconazole 150 mg is a good one-dose treatment for Candida vaginitis (monilia, thrush), of which the clinical picture is typical, often self-diagnosed. The pruritic discharge is often referred to as "caseous." Candida is a benign infection, when not a complication of an underlying condition, and in the short term may be treated once "empirically." Thus, several treatments are available over the counter. However, Candida vaginitis, especially when recurrent, merits evaluation for underlying causes such as diabetes mellitus, recent or excessive treatment with flora-changing antibiotics, or immunosuppression or immunodeficiency. On occasion it is simply precipitated by the coadministration of contraceptive medication. Metronidazole is the first-line treatment for Trichomonas vaginitis and for bacterial vaginosis; clindamycin is one of the recommended treatments for bacterial vaginosis. Trichomonas organisms cause a thin grayish intensely pruritic vaginitis, caused by a protozoan; bacterial vaginosis is caused most often by Gardnerella organisms and other anaerobic bacteria, resulting in a grayish discharge characterized by a fishy odor (or no symptoms whatever). Podophyllin applications are pre-

scribed specifically for condyloma accuminata (venereal warts). Amoxicillin is seldom used for any vaginitis, with the possible exception being an occasional choice for bacterial vaginosis.

9. The answer is E, Bartholin gland abscess. Herpes simplex produces a sharp, superficial pain aggravated by sheer force contact (i.e., skin or mucosa sliding over the infected area) but not particularly sensitive to pressure. Craurosis vulvae is a premalignant change secondary to long-standing hormonal deficiency (i.e., the postmenopausal state). Candida and Trichomonas vaginitides have been discussed in Question 8; they are both characterized by intense pruritus rather than abscesslike pain, though in severe cases, each may produce a superficial soreness not unlike that associated with herpetic pain. Immediate treatment is incision and drainage, which allows virtually instantaneous relief. To avoid recurrence, definitive treatment requires marsupialization after incision and drainage. Bartholin gland cysts occur without abscess formation and, if asymptomatic, merit no therapeutic measures. The organisms involved are usually not sexually transmitted, but culture should be performed and may yield Gonococcus or Chlamydia organisms. If they are present, these should be treated accordingly.

10. The answer is C. Postmenopausal bleeding must be assumed to be caused by endometrial carcinoma until proven otherwise. If a postmenopausal woman has been on hormone replacement therapy (HRT), three possible answers each determine different pathways investigation. If the patient has been on estrogen cycled with progesterone (HRT), the combination is relatively (but not absolutely) protective against endometrial carcinoma and early in the course of HRT there may be mild breakthrough bleeding. If the patient has been taking estrogen replacement without progesterone and has an intact uterus, the chances of endometrial carcinoma are heightened. Each of the other questions is relevant but only at a secondary level, after an opinion is formed as to what causes the bleeding. Postural light-headedness in the present setting is possibly a symptom of relative hypovolemia and therefore anemia caused by blood loss. In the present vignette that is unlikely, given the history of only recent and modest blood loss. Therefore, also unlikely is the relevance of number of pads required. Having associated cramps generally is related to the volume of flow of vaginal bleeding. Bleeding with intercourse is a nonspecific symptom that could relate to vulvar or uterine causes, including cervicitis.

11. The answer is E, endometrial biopsy. As said in the discussion of Question 10, postmenopausal bleeding is assumed to be due to endometrial carcinoma until proven otherwise. In the present case the risk is compounded by the fact that "unopposed estrogen" (i.e., estrogen prescribed without cycled progesterone when the uterus is intact) constitutes an increased risk of endometrial carcinoma for as along as 10 years after cessation of the medication. Other risk factors for endometrial carcinoma present in the vignette are being nulliparous and being overweight, both of which result in increased lifelong exposure to estrogen. The gold standard for ruling endometrial carcinoma in or out is the endometrial biopsy (short of pathological examination of the organ after hysterectomy or dilatation and curettage). The Pap smear is only 40% sensitive for endometrial carcinoma. Colposcopy and conization are procedural studies specific for the cervix and have no place in investigation of endometrial disease. Total abdominal hysterectomy should generally be performed as a therapeutic, not a diagnostic, procedure.

12. The answer is B. Unless this patient is successfully treated, she will have significantly increased risk of spontaneous abortion and infertility. Women who developed active chlamydial infections during pregnancy are at increased risk for premature rupture of membranes, preterm labor with smaller newborns, spontaneous abortion, and intrauterine deaths. *Chlamydia trachomatis* may cause severe pelvic inflammatory disease, urethritis, and cervicitis, although both women and men with chlamydial infection may be asymptomatic. The infection responds to doxycycline and azithramycin but to none of the penicillins or cephalosporins. The incubation period is between 5 and 21 days.

13. The answer is B. Intramuscular depot leuprolide, 3.75 mg monthly for 3 months, will reversibly cause hypogonadism and reduce the size of leiomyomata. An alternative method is nafarelin 0.2 to 0.4 mg by the intranasal route. Danazol can be used to reduce uterine bleeding and is applicable when fibroids are associated with prolonged heavy menstrual periods, such as when they are submucous in position. Choices A and B, contraceptive regimens, do not reduce the size of fibroids. Ibuprofen, as a prostaglandin inhibitor, may reduce the severity of uterine cramping but does not reduce the size of fibroids.

14. The answer is B, anovulatory cycle. If the patient has no obstruction to the outflow of menstrual blood and if the endometrium has been sufficiently primed with estrogen, the exposure to and withdrawal of progesterone will induce uterine bleeding. This will not occur in primary or secondary ovarian failure that is due to lack of

estrogen priming or if there is an obstruction to uterine outflow such as in Asherman syndrome (uterine obstruction secondary to endometrial scarring, as occurs sometimes after dilatation and curettage). Likewise, gonadal agenesis results in a barren, unprimed endometrium that cannot respond to progesterone withdrawal.

15. The answer is C, premature ovarian failure. The failure to respond to the progestin challenge suggests a problem with estrogen stimulation of the endometrium (either from a pituitary or ovarian problem), or outflow obstruction in the uterus. Because the patient did bleed after reproduction of the estrogen–progestin cycle, outflow obstruction cannot be responsible and the cause must lie in the ovarian or pituitary axis regulating estrogen, with the result being inadequate serum estrogen level. The increase in FSH and LH shows an appropriate pituitary response to these low estrogen levels, and thus the difficulty must be ovarian failure.

16. The answer is B, osteoporosis. This patient exhibits the criteria to diagnose anorexia nervosa: inappropriate voluntary weight loss, distorted body image, and at least 3 months of amenorrhea in a woman not in the perimenopausal age group. The menstrual abnormality is a form of hypothalamic amenorrhea. It is often a response to physical or psychological stress or to excessive exercise or weight loss. It is associated with osteoporosis. Serum estrogen and LH and FSH levels are decreased or normal in hypothalamic amenorrhea. Many anorectics are also bulimic and compensate by purging or inducing vomiting. The latter activity causes severe dental deterioration.

17. The answer is B. Medical management of missed abortion is highly successful when the situation is uncomplicated and ectopic pregnancy is ruled out. Intravaginal misoprostol, a prostaglandin E analog, allows successful evacuation of the uterine contents. Dilatation and curettage is necessary when there is evidence of infection, bleeding is severe, or if the patient is extremely anxious or presses for such intervention. If the uterus is empty on ultrasonic study and expelled products of conception are confirmed and if none of the aforementioned complications are present, expectant observation only is needed. Symptomatic treatment of cramps is inappropriate, as is initiation of contraception at this time.

18. The answer is C. A beta-hCG level of 1,500 to 1,800 mIU is a good starting point for the possible presence of ectopic pregnancy in the absence of evidence of IUP. In any event, the clinical decision to explore further must be based on clinical evidence, such as pain, adnexal mass, fever, or any of the foregoing in the face of hypotension. Beta-hCG levels double every 48 hours in normal IUP. The beta-hCG level should be checked every 48 hours. Falling levels indicate fetal demise, whether intrauterine or ectopic.

References

Bauman KA, Brown DR. Gynecology in primary care. In: Rudy DR, Kurowski K, eds. *Family Medicine: House Officer Series.* Baltimore: Williams & Wilkins; 1997:297–328.

French L. Dysmenorrhea. *Am Fam Physician.* 2005; 71:285–291, 302.

Griebel CP, Halvorsen J, Goleman TB, et al. Management of spontaneous abortion. *Am Fam Physician.* 2005; 72:1243–1250.

Johnson BA. Insertion and removal of intrauterine devices. *Am Fam Physician.* 2005; 71:95–101.

Lozeau A-M. Diagnosis and management of ectopic pregnancy. *Am Fam Physician.* 2005; 72:1707–1714, 1719–1720.

McKay HT. Gynecology. In: Tierney LM, McPhee SJ, Papadakis MA, eds. *Current Medical Diagnosis and Treatment.* 45th ed. New York: McGraw-Hill/Appleton & Lange; 2006:728–762.

Owen MK, Clenney TL. Management of vaginitis. *Am Fam Physician.* 2004; 70:2125–2132, 2139–2140.

Sherif K. Polycystic ovary syndrome in primary care. *Female Patient.* 2005; 70:24–28.

Shrager S, Potter BE. Diethylstilbestrol exposure. *Am Fam Physician.* 2004; 69:2395–2400, 2401–2402.

chapter 19

Problems of the Female Change of Life

Examination questions: Unless instructed otherwise, choose the ONE lettered answer or completion that is BEST in each case.

1 A 48-year-old white woman for whom you have cared for 5 years complains of bouts of depression for the first time in her life. This is the first occasion for her to visit you in the last 6 months. These bouts come on rapidly over periods of less than an hour, last for as long as 12 to 24 hours, and just as rapidly disappear. She denies headaches and difficulty thinking and calculating, although she notes that during the depressive episodes she finds it difficult to concentrate on problems that require focused attention. She denies any relationship between these episodes and the menstrual cycle. Her apical rhythm is regular and the rate is 84. You proceed to entertain a differential diagnosis of this complaint. Which of the following diagnoses is the least likely as a cause of this patient's problem?

(A) Neurotic depression

(B) Thyrotoxicosis

(C) Premenstrual syndrome

(D) Incipient menopause

(E) Hypoglycemic episodes

2 Regarding the patient in Question 1, you notice subtle changes in the patient's complexion and new facial lines that indicate an increased thinness of her skin. She tells of attacks of diaphoresis during which she needs to remove layers of clothing. Specifically there is no sign of acne. The skin is not increased in its oiliness, and to the contrary there is an appearance of increased dryness. Further history reveals that the menses have become irregular and less frequent, with the cycle lengthening to about 35 to 38 days. Which of the following ancillary studies is the most relevant to the developing history and observational findings?

(A) Serum luteinizing hormone level test

(B) Serum adrenocorticotropic hormone (corticotropin) level test

(C) Serum thyrotropic hormone level test

(D) Magnetic resonance image (MRI) of the brain with attention to the hypophysis and anterior pituitary

(E) Follicle-stimulating hormone (FSH) level test

3 Which of the following levels of FSH is confirmatory of ovarian failure or natural or surgical menopause?

(A) 20 IU

(B) 30 IU

(C) 40 IU

(D) 50 IU

(E) 60 IU

4 Regarding the patient in Questions 1 and 2, she asks about hormone therapy. Which of the following is correct regarding hormone replacement therapy (whether estrogen alone, i.e., ERT, or estrogen/progesterone replacement therapy, known as HRT) after menopause?

(A) HRT is protective against cardiovascular atherosclerotic disease.

(B) If progesterone is cycled in an overlapping fashion with estrogen cycling, HRT is protective against breast cancer.

(C) Cycled estrogen with progesterone poses a risk of endometrial carcinoma.

(D) Conjugated equine estrogen (CEE) given daily at 0.625 mg is protective against osteoporosis.

(E) HRT with 0.625 mg of CEE given daily protects against senile dementia.

5 What is the approximate lifetime risk of hip fracture in octogenarian women?

(A) 5%

(B) 10%

(C) 20%

(D) 33%

(E) 50%

6 What dosage of CEE is generally adequate to prevent the acute symptoms of menopause?

(A) 3 mg

(B) 625 mg

(C) 0.3 mg

(D) 0.625 mg

(E) 1.25 mg

7 Of the following categories, which is the most potent in preventing postmenopausal osteoporosis?

(A) Estrogen receptor blocking agents

(B) Bisphosphonates

(C) Estrogen replacement

(D) Oral calcium

(E) Vitamin D

8 Besides suddenness of onset, the way in which surgical menopause is most likely to differ from physiologic menopause is in which of the following characteristics?

(A) Depression is more of a problem in surgical menopause.

(B) Atrophic vaginitis is more severe in surgical menopause.

(C) Osteoporosis is a greater issue in physiologic menopause.

(D) Heart disease is a greater risk after surgical menopause.

(E) Loss of libido is more likely after surgical menopause.

9 A 65-year-old slightly built white woman who is a cigarette smoker is brought to you by her daughter, who is a nurse. The daughter knows that her mother, as a small-boned person, is at high risk for hip fracture, as well as vertebral and radial fractures, as she grows older. The daughter is aware that hip fracture carries a 20% first-year mortality rate and is concerned that if her mother is not placed on hormone replacement therapy then she may suffer that fate. The daughter has learned that HRT has lost favor

and that few physicians are prescribing it as a routine. You attempt to place this information in perspective for the family of this woman. Thus, you point out that the ranking cause of death in postmenopausal females is which of the following?

(A) Coronary artery disease

(B) Endometrial carcinoma

(C) Carcinoma of the breast

(D) Hip fracture mortality in the first year after the occurrence

(E) Stroke

10 Regarding the patient in Question 9, you feel the need to address the smoking issue with the 65-year-old white woman and her daughter the nurse. You explain to her the approximate strength of the risk for osteoporosis from regular smoking as compared with the beneficial effects of natural or replacement estrogen. That is, what proportion of estrogen's benefits is lost by smoking?

(A) Smoking has a detrimental effect 10% as strong as estrogen's beneficial effect.

(B) Smoking has a detrimental effect 25% as strong as estrogen's beneficial effect.

(C) Smoking has a detrimental effect equally as strong as estrogen's beneficial effect.

(D) Smoking is twice as detrimental to bone density as estrogen is beneficial.

(E) Smoking is irrelevant to bone density so long as a postmenopausal patient is given hormone replacement prevention.

11 What is the best course of action to take if (mild) uterine bleeding occurs for longer than 6 months after institution of HRT, whether estrogen and progesterone are cycled with 25 days (estrogen) overlapping with 10 days progesterone or each drug taken daily month around? This assumes that hemoglobin and thyroid function have been evaluated.

(A) Discontinue all hormonal therapy

(B) Double the dosage of estrogen

(C) Adjust the dosage of progesterone

(D) Perform dilatation and curettage

(E) Perform endometrial biopsy

In Questions 12 through 16, match the lettered types of hormone replacement regimens to the numbered candidates for hormone therapy, assuming all candidates should take supplemental calcium as well (1 g of calcium carbonate in addition to dietary intake). A choice may be correct more than once or not at all.

12 A 33-year-old white woman who has undergone subtotal (ovary-sparing) hysterectomy.

13 A 40-year-old woman with early but physiologic menopause. She is of northern European heritage, of lean body habitus, and is a one pack per day smoker.

14 A 55-year-old white woman who has undergone physiologic menopause at the normal age. Hip fractures have been suffered by both her mother and maternal aunt, one of whom died within the first year of the incident.

15 A 40-year-old woman who has undergone total hysterectomy without history of carcinoma of the breast, cervix, or ovary.

16 A 50-year-old woman who is status post total hysterectomy with a history of breast cancer free of evidence of disease 10 years after mastectomy and irradiation therapy. She has suffered two fractures of distal radii and a wedge fracture of the 10th thoracic vertebra.

(A) CEE 0.625 mg and medroxyprogesterone acetate 2.5 mg daily

(B) CEE 0.625 mg daily

(C) Raloxifene 60 mg daily

(D) Observation and periodic measurement of FSH levels

(E) Alendronate 10 mg daily, taken in the morning with significant amounts of water, 30 minutes before eating

Examination Answers

1. The answer is B. Thyrotoxicosis is unlikely in a young person with a normal heart rate. Neurotic depression is always possible with a depressed affect. However, it seldom is expressed in such cataclysmic fashion as occurs in the vignette. Premenstrual syndrome actually fits well with the history, except that women with premenstrual syndrome invariably connect the symptoms with the menstrual cycle. Hypoglycemia, regardless of the root cause, may awaken feelings of failure, guilt, and hence depression. Incipient menopause is certainly possible, given the patient's age.

2. The answer is E. The serum FSH level will be elevated in the menopausal syndrome and after menopause. In the vignette, the skin changes that are apparent to an experienced clinician, the lengthening cycle, and the "hot flashes" point to menopause. The average age of menopause in the United States has passed the age of 50. Thus, many will experience natural menopause as early as the late forties. Thyroid dysfunction is unlikely, as discussed in Question 1, and therefore the thyrotropin level is not likely to be relevant. Luteinizing hormone levels may be elevated in polycystic ovary syndrome, unlikely here because of the lack of androgenizing signs or symptoms. Corticotropin is relevant in investigation of possible adrenal insufficiency or Cushing disease, neither of which is suggested by the present case. MRI of the hypophysis is not indicated unless the studies fail to confirm the most likely cause of the symptoms presented.

3. The answer is C; 40 IU is the level of FSH above which a diagnosis of ovarian failure is secure. Some might choose A, 20 IU, but this cut point is more liberal. The latter would allow a lower threshold for commencing hormone replacement therapy. At younger ages than appropriate, usually arbitrarily taken as <40 years, having menopausal symptoms associated with FSH levels ≥40 IU is referred to as primary ovarian failure.

4. The answer is D. CEE 0.625 mg daily is protective against osteoporosis. Each of the other suggested *benefits* of HRT in the stem question were long considered to be true and valid, but with random prospective studies reported in the last 5 years, they are no longer thought to

be so. The breast cancer risk associated with estrogen and progesterone replacement was acknowledged but felt to be minimal at dosages of HRT being used. Moreover, large prospective controlled trials alluded to, including both the Women's Health Initiative and the Heart and Estrogen/Progestin Replacement Study (HERS), have indicated that cardiovascular brain and heart disease risk appear to be in fact increased with HRT, possibly because of the complication of thromboembolic disease risk. Endometrial carcinoma, although a risk with estrogen replacement unopposed, is, however, relatively prevented by combined estrogen replacement cycled with progesterone. To elaborate, HRT is not cardioprotective, because of the progesterone, and in fact poses an increased risk of atherosclerotic events after 3 to 4 years of HRT.

5. The answer is D. If a woman lives to the age of 80 years, she stands a one in three chance of having a hip fracture. For a man the odds are one in six. In any event, hip fracture is associated with a 20% first-year mortality rate. Therefore, as people live increasingly long after late midlife, the issue of prevention of osteoporosis becomes critical. This is especially so because hormone replacement therapy has been abandoned because of risks of breast cancer and cardiovascular atherosclerosis.

6. The answer is C. CEE 0.3 mg daily will prevent hot flashes in most people during the acute menopause syndrome. This dosage is also safer regarding breast cancer risk. However, 0.3 mg of CEE is not nearly as powerful in preventing osteoporosis as 0.625 mg. The latter dosage is no longer the standard, however, because of the risk of breast cancer.

7. The answer is C. Estrogen replacement is the most potent protector of bone density in the postmenopausal state. Estrogen receptor blockers (e.g., raloxifene, tamoxifen), first used to suppress breast cancers in women with receptor positive tumors, protect against osteoporosis but with not more than about 50% of the potency of estrogens. Bisphosphonates (e.g., etidronate, alendronate) are quite potent but still not to the degree of estrogen. Oral calcium and vitamin D are necessary adjuncts with any of the foregoing therapies, but in themselves they are not adequate to prevent osteoporosis.

8. The answer is E. Loss of libido is more likely after surgical menopause, even with hormone replacement therapy. This is because surgical menopause removes the secondary testosterone source in the case of total hysterectomy, wherein oophorectomy is included. This outcome may occur even after subtotal or ovary-sparing hysterectomy because of the possibility of sacrifice of ovarian blood supply during surgery.

9. The answer is A. Coronary artery disease is the first ranking cause of death in postmenopausal women, whether on hormone replacement or not. Moreover, coronary artery disease deaths are no longer predicted to be reduced (by half) by the application of hormone replacement therapy.

10. The answer is C. Smoking has a detrimental effect equally as strong as estrogen's beneficial effect. Thus, stopping smoking alone will have a huge beneficial effect toward prevention of osteoporosis. Furthermore, the patient's continued smoking increases the risk that the patient will die of coronary heart disease by at least 50%.

11. The answer is E. Perform endometrial biopsy, generally recommended for persistent bleeding beyond 6 months after institution of HRT, or for postmenopausal bleeding of any sort, because of the risk of endometrial carcinoma. In the case of bleeding after HRT (i.e., estrogen and progesterone combined) has been started, this is actually of low urgency because the progesterone in HRT constitutes a negative risk factor for endometrial carcinoma. Bleeding may persist for up to 6 months after HRT is started. ERT (estrogen without accompanying progesterone) in the presence of an intact uterus would increase the risk for endometrial carcinoma. For that reason, ERT is contraindicated in the presence of an intact uterus.

ANSWERS TO MATCHING QUESTIONS

12. The answer is D, observation and periodic measurement of FSH levels. A 33-year-old white woman who has undergone subtotal or ovary-sparing hysterectomy may be presumed to be in an estrogen sufficient state until such time as she undergoes physiologic ovarian involution. In the absence of menstrual periods and assuming no symptoms, humoral menopause can only be diagnosed by a rise in FSH.

13. The answer is A, CEE 0.625 mg and medroxyprogesterone acetate 2.5 mg daily. This is appropriate for the 40-year-old woman with early but physiologic menopause, but for no longer than 3 years, in order to avoid increasing the risk of cardiovascular disease associated with HRT. Smoking cessation is mandatory. All forms of prevention of osteoporosis must be supplemented with oral calcium, at least 1 g per day for women.

14. The answer is A, CEE 0.625 mg and medroxyprogesterone acetate 2.5 mg daily. This is appropriate for the 55-year-old menopausal white woman who is assumed to be at high risk for osteoporosis.

15. The answer is B, CEE 0.625 mg daily. For the 40-year-old woman who has undergone total hysterectomy without history of carcinoma of the breast, cervix, or ovary, the ERT is appropriate. No time limit need be applied to ERT because the increased cardiovascular risk associated with hormone replacement therapy appears to be caused by the progesterone in HRT.

16. The answer is E. Bisphosphonates are recommended for high-risk cases to prevent osteoporosis or as secondary prevention for patients who have already manifested pathologic fractures. Alendronate 10 mg daily, taken in the morning with significant amounts of water, 30 minutes before eating breakfast, is appropriate. As Fosamax, alendronate is also available as 70 mg weekly. A new preparation, ibandronate, as Boniva, is dosed as 2.5 mg daily or 150 mg monthly. This may also be a choice for the 50-year-old woman who is status post total hysterectomy with a history of breast cancer. The history of breast cancer constitutes a contraindication for ERT or HRT. The patient has suffered two fractures of distal radii and a wedge fracture of the 10th thoracic vertebra. Tamoxifen would also be a supplemental agent to consider and, better still, raloxifene. Tamoxifen and the newer agent in the category of estrogen receptor blocking agents, raloxifene, effectively block estrogen receptors in the breast. Still, they retain enough estrogenic properties to retard the progress of osteoporosis. Raloxifene inhibits the progress of atherosclerosis as well. Therefore, given the history of breast cancer, even without evidence of present disease, this class of drugs will be used increasingly to substitute for ERT in patients with a contraindication that is due to a past history of cancer.

References

McKay HT. Gynecology. In: Tierney LM, McPhee SJ, Papadakis MA, eds. *Current Diagnosis and Treatment.* 45th ed. New York: McGraw-Hill/Appleton & Lange; 2006:728–762.

Rudy DR. Problems of the female climacteric. In: Rudy DR, Kurowski K, eds. *Family Medicine: House Officer Series.* Baltimore: Williams & Wilkins; 1997:329–340.

chapter **20**

Diseases of the Breast

Examination questions: *Unless instructed otherwise, choose the ONE lettered answer or completion that is BEST in each case.*

1 Which of the following breast complaints warrants the closest and most persistent evaluation?

(A) Bilateral nipple discharge, milky in appearance

(B) Bilateral tenderness with irregular palpable masses, cyclic in course

(C) Purulent discharge, unilateral, with tenderness

(D) Bilateral nipple irritation during nursing

(E) Unilateral sanguineous discharge

2 A 26-year-old professional woman who is gravida 1, para 1 sees you because she notes bilateral galactorrhea that has not ceased since her baby was born 2 months ago. She had decided against breast feeding her newborn baby. She denies that vigorous sexual stimulation might be a significant factor. She is emotionally well adjusted to the birth and status of parenthood. The breast examination is otherwise within normal limits. Which of the following would be the most appropriate disposition you would make at this time?

(A) Order test for serum prolactin level

(B) Order test for thyroid-stimulating hormone

(C) Order test for growth hormone level

(D) Observe for 4 months before re-evaluating

(E) Order magnetic resonance image (MRI) of the brain

3 Nine months later, the patient referred to in Question 1 returns and says that her galactorrhea has not ceased. A pregnancy test is negative. Without any further information, which of the following is the most common pathological cause of galactorrhea?

(A) Prolactinoma

(B) Gigantism

(C) Thyrotoxicosis

(D) Medication

(E) Breast cancer

4 A 32-year-old woman has bilateral nipple discharge that is found to contain fat globules and not to contain red or white cells and is established to be galactorrhea. She also complains of headaches as well as diminution of her libido and decrease in the flow and frequency of her menses over the last 3 months. Headaches are worse in the mornings. Beta-chorionic gonadotropin level is not elevated and the remainder of the breast examination is negative. The serum prolactin level is elevated at 250 ng/mL. Serum follicle-stimulating hormone and thyroid-stimulating hormone levels are within normal limits. Which of the following is the logical next step?

(A) Prescribe bromocriptine

(B) Refer for surgery

(C) Prescribe cabergoline

(D) Order MRI with contrast

(E) Order plain x-rays of the head

5 A 43-year-old woman seeks your opinion for a breast lump that she discovered the previous week. She has no first- or second-degree family history of breast cancer. She had a negative mammogram 2 years ago. The nodule is 2 to 3 cm in diameter. The remainder of the breast examination is essentially normal, but there is a background of granularity to palpation (like small irregularities in the breast tissue). Which of the following is the best next disposition?

(A) Order a mammogram

(B) Refer for breast biopsy

(C) Draw prolactin levels

(D) Draw serum calcium and alkaline phosphatase levels

(E) Perform aspiration

6 A 28-year-old woman presents with a single breast nodule that is nontender. There is a second-degree family history of breast cancer in that her aunt (mother's sister) had breast cancer at the age of 48. Which of the following is the best diagnostic test at this time?

(A) Mammogram

(B) Excisional biopsy

(C) Aspiration of the nodule

(D) Serum prolactin level test

(E) Ultrasonic study

7 Which of the following diagnostic procedures is the best choice for the least expensive method to differentiate in situ and invasive carcinoma of the breast and to ascertain the status of estrogen receptor presence in the tumor?

(A) Fine-needle aspiration (FNA) biopsy

(B) Core-needle biopsy (CNB)

(C) Excisional biopsy

(D) Lumpectomy

(E) Mammogram

8 A 35-year-old woman comes to an office setting for a routine breast examination (clinical breast examination, or CBE) by the family doctor. Which of the following findings on this CBE least suggests the possibility of breast cancer in a palpable nodule?

(A) Lack of liquid retrieval on aspiration

(B) Location in the superior-lateral quadrant

(C) Fixation to underlying tissues

(D) Hardness measured at 60 durometers

(E) Irregular shape

9 You decide the patient in Question 8 has a nodule that you judge to be suggestive of malignancy. You perform FNA and encounter a solid lesion. Cytology is negative. Which of the following studies should be ordered next?

(A) Mammogram

(B) Breast ultrasound

(C) Open biopsy

(D) Radical mastectomy

(E) Repeat CBE after the next menstrual period

10 The test you ordered in Question 9 is interpreted as suggestive of malignancy. The combination of three particular tests, that is, the CBE, tissue sample, and imaging, has been called The Triple Test (TTS). What is the score of TTS in this case?

(A) 1

(B) 2

(C) 3

(D) 5

(E) 7

11 On the basis of the results of TTS in Question 10, what is the most probable next disposition?

(A) Order a CNB

(B) Repeat the examination(s)

(C) Perform excisional biopsy

(D) Order a mammogram

(E) Evaluate for oncological treatment

12 Of the following age groups, in which does the largest proportion of breast cancers occur?

(A) Menarche to 25 years

(B) 20 to 40 years

(C) <50 years of age

(D) 50 to 65 years

(E) >65 years

13 A 26-year-woman presents herself to you with a complaint of a breast lump. Upon examination, the nodule is found to be apparently 1 cm in diameter and tender. It is more tender this week than it was last week, but it has been like this several times for a week or so over the last 3 months. What is the best course of action at this time?

(A) Order mammography this week

(B) Refer for breast biopsy

(C) Observe for 3 months, examining the patient monthly during that time

(D) Perform needle aspiration

(E) Reassure the patient that she is not in the age group to fear cancer of the breast

14 Assume a patient presents with the same complaint as in Question 13, except instead of having the lump for several weeks, she has known of it for only 2 weeks. She gives a history not of cyclic pain and swelling but of trauma to the area about 2 weeks ago. Now what is the best action at the present time?

(A) Order mammography this week

(B) Refer for breast biopsy

(C) Observe for 3 months, examining the patient monthly during that time

(D) Perform needle aspiration

(E) Reassure the patient that she is not in the age group to fear cancer of the breast

15 Each of the following may be complications of breast implantations except which one?

(A) Capsule contraction and scarring around the implant

(B) Firmness and distortion of the breast

(C) Rupture of the implant

(D) "Bleeding" of silicone gel through the implant capsule

(E) Precipitation of autoimmune diseases in the recipient

16 In performing a CBE, which of the following is most appropriate in advising your patient regarding this examination?

(A) The sensitivity of the CBE is 90% in the hands of a professional.

(B) Specificity of the CBE is virtually 100%.

(C) If a patient avails herself of the CBE then she needn't perform breast self-examination.

(D) When performed optimally, the CBE is about 70% sensitive.

(E) The patient should make a decision to undergo either CBE or mammography starting at age 40 years.

Examination Answers

1. The answer is E. Unilateral sanguineous discharge warrants the closest and most persistent evaluation because it is the most likely to be a sign of cancer, most types of which begin as intraductal carcinomas. The chances that bloody nipple discharge is caused by cancer are 1:3. Bilateral nipple discharge, milky in appearance, is galactorrhea, associated with a variety of causes, including pregnancy, mechanical stimulation, pituitary adenoma (prolactinoma), hypothyroidism, and Cushing disease, as well as chronic renal failure. Bilateral tenderness with irregular palpable masses, cyclic in course, is caused by fibrocystic disease and is seen commonly in primary care practice. Purulent discharge with tenderness represents infection, often in a lactating woman.

2. The answer is A, order growth hormone level testing. Galactorrhea may continue normally for 6 months after parturition. Neurogenic factors, such as sexual stimulation, may cause galactorrhea through the inhibition of hypothalamic prolactin inhibitory factor.

3. The answer is D. Drugs are the most common pathologic cause of galactorrhea. Galactorrhea may be normal for a brief time in newborns, postpartum women, and pregnant women. The most common drugs associated with galactorrhea are categorized as follows, with certain examples given. First, there are dopamine receptor blocking agents: butyrophenones, metoclopramide, phenothiazines, selective serotonin re-uptake inhibitors, tricyclic antidepressants, and thioxanthenes. Second, there are dopamine-depleting agents, such as methyldopa and reserpine. Third, there are inhibitors of dopamine release: codeine, heroin, and morphine. Fourth, there are histamine receptor blocking agents. Fifth, there are lactotroph-stimulating agents: oral contraceptives and verapamil. Each of the other options may be associated with galactorrhea, but all are unusual except for prolactinoma.

4. The answer is D. Prolactin levels above 200 ng/mL should be considered to be caused by prolactinoma until proven otherwise. However, the size of this slowly growing benign tumor and the patient's total symptomatology and attitude toward fertility together determine the therapeutic approach. The best modality for confirming the tumor's size and presence is the MRI, preferably enhanced by gadolinium. Microadenomas may be treated with dopaminergic agents such as bromocriptine. Cabergoline is a longer-acting and thus more convenient drug, but it is more expensive. Macroadenomas, especially if suprasellar, may warrant surgical removal, particularly so if fertility is a critical issue.

5. The answer is E. Performing aspiration before otherwise legitimate options makes sense in this woman, who is over the age of 40 and not with epidemiologic evidence of high risk. Fluid-filled cysts are most likely to occur in women over the age of 40. If aspiration results in fluid with the disappearance of most of the nodule, the likelihood of cancer as a basis for the mass is very low. To be sure, the patient should be followed for several weeks afterward and a mammogram should be done early, if only as a recommended routine for all women over the age of 40. Nodules in women younger than 40 years of age are more likely to be fibroadenomas and other benign solid tumors. Breast biopsy need not be rushed into in this circumstance, although it should never be withheld unnecessarily. Prolactin levels are reserved for nipple discharge. Calcium and alkaline phosphatase are indicated when metastatic disease is suspected.

6. The answer is E. An ultrasonic study of the breast tissue is appropriate in a young woman, even with a second-degree family history of breast cancer. Sonography is 89% sensitive for breast abnormalities in symptomatic women. Women younger than the midthirties are likely to have dense breast tissue that renders mammography less accurate (less sensitive and less specific). Aspiration is less likely to be fruitful, as fluid-filled cysts are more common in women who are older than 40 years of age. Prolactin levels are indicated in galactorrhea or other bilateral nipple discharge. Excisional biopsy should be delayed, pending the results of the noninvasive studies. FNA biopsy may be considered and the revelation of fluid would rule out cancer, making the FNA a fluid aspiration procedure, with the same limitations already mentioned.

7. The answer is B. The CNB, done with 14- to 18-gauge needle, is as much as 99% sensitive in palpable lesions and 93% sensitive in nonpalpable nodules for diagnosing breast cancer. A minimum of four cores is required to gain these statistics, which include a higher predictive value than found in FNA. Excisional biopsy is the gold standard but is obviously more expensive and more traumatic than the CNB. Lumpectomy is a therapeutic technique, designed to cure a known cancer under favorable circumstances.

8. The answer is B. Although the so-called upper-outer quadrant will contain the most breast cancers, so is that location the quadrant that contains the most breast tissue. Lack of an aspirant retrieval by tap does not signal breast cancer, but appearance of fluid aspirant in that situation rules strongly against cancer. The durometer is a measure of hardness; 20 durometers is comparable to a soft to medium grape and 60 durometers approaches the hardness of calcified bone, a sign suggestive of cancer. Irregular shape, as opposed to well-circumscribed roundness, is suggestive of cancer as well.

9. The answer is B. Breast ultrasound is the most appropriate imaging study for the woman under the age of 40 in the present circumstance. This is so for two reasons. First, women younger than 40 years of age are more likely to have dense breast tissue that is more difficult for mammographic interpretation. Second, ultrasonography is better than mammography in differentiating between benign and malignant solid masses.

10. The answer is D. The TTS scores 1 point for an interpretation of benign, 2 for suggestive, and 3 for an adjudgement of malignancy in each of the three categories of CBE, tissue sampling, and imaging. Thus, all three tests being evaluated as malignant would render a score for TTS of 9. Tissue sampling for this purpose may be CNB instead of FNA. In the vignette, the TTS score in the present case is 5.

11. The answer is C. A TTS score of 5 or more is an indication for surgical intervention. (A score of 3 obviates further intervention.) A CNB may have already been accomplished but a TTS score of 5 dictates the more certain obtainment of histological diagnosis. Mammography is a form of imaging and the ultrasonography has already placed the patient in the suggestive category for imaging. A TTS score of 4 may legitimately justify repeating the examination. Oncology consultation is inappropriate in virtually all cases until tissue diagnosis is made definitively.

12. The answer is E. Nearly 50% of breast cancers in women in the United States occur in women older than 65 years of age. About one-quarter occur in the age group of 50 to 65 years, leaving about one-quarter for the under 50 age group. The latter, as was implied earlier, tend to contract more aggressive cancers, giving rise to a changing view of screening that calls for more frequent routine mammography (i.e., yearly) in the age group of 40 through 49 years of age. This point is not heavily emphasized in the chapter by Bowman and Szewczyk (1997), but a telling report on the subject was freshly published as that manuscript was being processed.

13. The answer is D. Needle aspiration is the first step choice for a 26-year-old woman with a cyclically tender breast lump. All other choices given in the vignette have relevance at certain times and under certain circumstances. However, the clinical picture is that of fibrocystic disease. If the nodule disappears as fluid is yielded in the procedure in the given setting, cancer can virtually be ruled out, assuming the fluid is clear. Disappearance is defined as nonrecurrence of the cystic nodule after a period of several monthly cycles. If the fluid is bloody, cytological examination of the fluid should be routine in that circumstance. Any other result requires, at the least, an imaging study and the invoking of the TTS as outlined in Questions 10 and 11.

14. The answer is C. Observing for 3 months is acceptable, given the history of trauma, because hematomas can persist for 6 weeks or longer before resolving. A mammogram may be obtained, though inaccuracies are attendant to the patient's age; thus, an ultrasound would be preferable. On the basis of the aforementioned information, the breast biopsy can wait. Needle aspiration is acceptable but need not be done on this visit because hematoma is a logical diagnosis.

15. The answer is E. Although there was a flurry of medicolegal litigation during the early 1990s surrounding the claim of autoimmune disease associated with breast implants, there was never, either at the time or since, even purported incidence or prevalence attached to that alleged association; there were only patients (deluded or self-serving) and eager lawyers driving the claims through courts and too often succeeding, which gave birth to that wave of economic waste. All the other complications do occur. Capsule contraction and scarring occur in 15% to 25% of cases of silicone implants; implant rupture occurs in 5%.

16. The answer is D. Several points are relevant here. Perhaps the most important is that the doctor should explain both the strengths and weaknesses of any test to which he or she requests the patient submit. This is foremost so as to arm the patient with the best data by which to guide her or his health care in concert with the doctors, but in addition to avoid placing the physician in a defensive medicolegal position. Thus, the patient in this case is informed that a negative CBE is not a guarantee against breast cancer in the near future. Further, in the present example, there is an approximately 30% chance that the CBE may miss diagnosing a cancer (i.e., 70% sensitivity). It follows that patient and doctor must avail themselves of other reasonable means of screening for breast cancer, such as mammography yearly beginning at the age of 40 years, after a baseline study at the age of 35 (for women of average expected lifetime risk). Mammography itself has been estimated to be only 70% sensitive. Presumably, the cancers missed are most likely to be the smallest nodules by both methods. Although sensitivity is questionable, breast self-examination appears to confer additional advantages only if performed monthly or more often, even by an initially insecure and unpracticed woman.

Specificity of all three methods is obviously imperfect and negative breast biopsies will necessarily occur.

References

Barton MB, Harris R, Fletcher SW. Does this patient have breast cancer? The screening breast examination: Should it be done? How? *JAMA*. 1999; 282:1270–1280.

Bowman MA, Szewczyk MB. Diseases of the breast. In: Rudy DR, Kurowski K, eds. *Family Medicine: House Officer Series*. Baltimore: Williams & Wilkins; 1997:341–350.

Kerlikowske K, Grady D, Barclay J, et al. Effect of age, breast density, and family history on the sensitivity of first screening mammography. *JAMA*. 1996; 276:33–38.

Klein S. Evaluation of palpable breast masses. *Am Fam Physician*. 2005; 71:1731–1738.

Leung AKC, Pacaud D. Diagnosis and management of galactorrhea. *Am Fam Physician*. 2004; 70:543–550, 553–554.

Lucas JH, Cone DL. Breast cyst aspiration. *Am Fam Physician*. 2003; 68:1983–1986, 1989.

SECTION **VIII**

Problems Unique to Males

chapter 21

Genitourinary Problems of the Male

Examination questions: *Unless instructed otherwise, choose the ONE lettered answer or completion that is BEST in each case.*

1 A 14-year-old boy has the rapid onset (<2 hours ago) of severe right testicular pain associated with right flank pain and nausea and vomiting. Upon examination the right testicle is riding higher than the left and is markedly tender within an edematous scrotum. Each of the following may be reasonably included in the differential diagnosis of this case, except for which one?

(A) Epididymitis

(B) Testicular trauma

(C) Torsion of the testicle

(D) Varicocele

(E) Testicular cancer

2 Regarding the patient in Question 1, which of the following may yield the quickest office diagnosis?

(A) Urinalysis

(B) Complete blood count (include white blood cell count and differential)

(C) Doppler stethoscope

(D) Testicular technetium scan

(E) Intravenous pyelogram

3 Which of the following dispositions is most appropriate for the patient in Question 1?

(A) Intramuscular ceftriaxone 250 mg followed by 100 mg of oral doxycycline bid for 10 days

(B) Elective exploration of the scrotum to obtain gross and microscopic evidence to rule out a malignancy

(C) Emergency exploration to perform bilateral orchiopexy

(D) Sulfamethoxazole/trimethoprim given twice daily for 7 days

(E) Elective general surgery for repair of hernial defect

4 An 80-year-old gentleman complains of testicular pain that had its onset 3 days ago and has built since to prevent sleep the night before this visit. On examination the testicle seems on palpation to be irregular in shape and quite tender. The scrotal contents are difficult to differentiate. The patient's temperature is 100.8°F. The urinalysis demonstrates 20 to 30 white blood cells/high-power field. Which of the following is the most likely diagnosis?

(A) Epididymitis

(B) Testicular trauma

(C) Torsion of the testicle

(D) Orchitis

(E) Testicular cancer

5 A 34-year-old factory worker whose daily activity involves heavy lifting seeks advice for a growing groin mass. He first noted the swelling about 2 months ago after lifting a 75-lb (34-kg) packet of steel rods, and now it has become apparent to him during dressing and undressing. You examine him and find a scrotal mass that transilluminates well. You diagnose an inguinal hernia. Which of the following additional findings renders this clinical situation an emergency?

(A) Inability to reduce the hernia

(B) Finding a direct rather than an indirect inguinal hernia

169

(C) Associated testicular pain

(D) Tenderness of the hernial sac

(E) History of urinary tract infection

6 A 25-year-old man develops an inflammatory arthritis in his left knee that has been present for 1 week. Upon questioning, he avers that he has had bloody diarrhea that nevertheless had abated by the time of onset of his knee pain, and he complains of blurred vision in the right eye. He denies any history of trauma and any previous history of joint pain or swelling and there is no family history of connective tissue disease. On examination he exhibits some redness of the right eye and the pupil is smaller than that of the left eye. Which of the following is the most likely etiology for this problem?

(A) Rheumatoid arthritis

(B) Osteoarthritis

(C) Reflux sympathetic dystrophy

(D) Reactive arthritis

(E) Systemic lupus erythematosus

7 You examine a 35-year-old man who presents with a painless enlarged testicle noticed by him over the last 3 months. On examination the testicle is irregular in shape and does not transilluminate. Alpha-fetoprotein (AFP) and human chorionic gonadotropin levels are within normal limits (i.e., barely perceptible), as is the lactic dehydrogenase level. You also note developing gynecomastia. You diagnose a testicular tumor. Which of the following types is it *most* likely to be?

(A) Seminoma

(B) Embryonal cell carcinoma

(C) Teratocarcinoma

(D) Choriocarcinoma

(E) Leydig cell carcinoma

8 A 25-year-old man and his 22-year-old wife are seeking consultation in order to find out why they have been unable to achieve fertility in the marriage after trying for pregnancy for more than 3 years. The wife's pelvic examination showed normal anatomy. The couple has confirmed and timed her ovulations by a temperature graph over the past year and attempted impregnation during the period surrounding ovulation, with no success. You initiate an evaluation to investigate the problem. Which of the following is the most logical first step?

(A) Hysterosalpingogram on the wife

(B) Computed tomography scan of the brain to investigate for pituitary adenoma

(C) Pelvic ultrasound to rule out polycystic ovary syndrome in the wife

(D) Sperm count on the husband

(E) 24-hour urine collection for 5-OH ketosteroids

9 Regarding the case in Question 8, which of the following is the most common cause of male infertility?

(A) Malnutrition

(B) History of undescended testicle

(C) Varicocele

(D) Adrenal hyperplasia

(E) Klinefelter syndrome

10 A 55-year-old male patient complains of gradually increasing prostatism over the last 6 months. This has taken the form of increasing difficulty in initiating the urinary stream (hesitancy), decreasing size of the stream, and increasing nocturia. There have been times when his symptoms were worse than others. Each of the following statements are correct regarding these developments except for which one?

(A) One cause may be prostatic cancer.

(B) The differential diagnosis includes benign prostatic hyperplasia (BPH).

(C) The symptoms may be caused by epididymitis.

(D) The symptoms may be aggravated by ingestion of drugs with anticholinergic side effects.

(E) Prostatitis may be a cause of the symptoms.

11 Each of the following has been proven to reduce symptoms of BPH except which one?

(A) Transurethral resection

(B) Transurethral microwave thermotherapy

(C) Alpha-1 adrenergic blocking agents

(D) 5-alpha reductase inhibiting agents

(E) *Pygeum africanum*

12 Regarding the patient in Question 10, as a matter of course the patient underwent a transrectal needle biopsy that returned a histopathologic diagnosis of prostate cancer, with a Gleason score of 3. Which of the following statements is true regarding the Gleason score and this patient in the context of that score?

(A) The probability of this patient dying of prostate cancer over the next 15 years is greater than 50%.

(B) The Gleason score is a scale of values directly related to the degree of differentiation of the tumor.

(C) This patient is less likely to have an increase in quality-adjusted life years (QALYs) as a result of treatment than he would have if his Gleason score were 8.

(D) The Gleason score renders surgical staging an outmoded concept.

(E) This patient has a small chance of dying of something other than prostate cancer.

13 A 65-year-old man inquires regarding the use of sildenafil or related drugs for his self-perceived relative erectile dysfunction. Which of the following statements regarding that class of drugs, phosphodiesterase type 5 inhibitors (PDE-5s), is correct?

(A) The drugs have caused a significant number of deaths in hypertensive patients.

(B) Headache is the most common side effect.

(C) Color vision changes are equally incident in all the PDE-5 drugs with tadalafil.

(D) Men with coronary artery disease are at increased risk of coronary events after taking this medication.

(E) There is no risk in taking PDE-5 drugs along with any other medication.

14 Regarding the patient in Question 13, before prescribing for the man with erectile dysfunction, you decide to survey the man's medications for possible causes of impotence. Which of the following medications would be *least* likely to cause erectile dysfunction?

(A) Chlorthiazide diuretics

(B) Cimetidine

(C) Albuterol

(D) Propranolol

(E) Finasteride 4

15 A 52-year-old African American man makes an appointment to inquire about the risks of prostate cancer. He has heard that the risk is higher in African Americans than in other racial groups. Following guidelines from The American Cancer Society, at what age and by what method(s) do you recommend that he begin submitting to screening for prostatic carcinoma?

(A) Age 30 years – digital rectal examination (DRE)

(B) Age 40 and every 5 years – DRE and blood prostate-specific antigen (PSA)

(C) Age 40 and yearly – DRE and PSA

(D) Age 50 years and yearly – DRE

(E) Age 50 – DRE and PSA

16 Regarding the PSA, each of the following statements is true except for which one?

(A) The normal limit of 4 ng/mL is a hard-and-fast rule.

(B) A level of 3 ng/mL in a 35-year-old man may be a cause for concern (i.e., without symptoms and a normal DRE).

(C) A PSA level of 6.5 ng/mL in a 75-year-old man need not be further evaluated.

(D) A minimum proportion of the total PSA should be in the free as opposed to the bound form.

(E) The yearly rate of rise in PSA levels, regardless of their absolute values, should not exceed 0.7 ng/mL.

Examination Answers

1. The answer is D. A varicocele is the one choice listed that is not painful. Epididymitis is a well-known cause of acute testicular pain that typically has a slower onset than that portrayed in the vignette. Epididymitis virtually always is associated with pyuria. Trauma should be obvious in the history unless it was associated with head trauma and amnesia for the event. Cancer is typically painless but may be acutely painful and acutely swollen if there occurs hemorrhage into the tumor. The story fits that of testicular torsion in that it occurred in an intra-adolescent boy, and none of the other possibilities has as rapid an onset as torsion. Abdominal pain, nausea, and vomiting are often found in torsion. Thus, although varicocele is ruled out by history and the other choices figure in the differential diagnosis, the most likely diagnosis is torsion of the testicle.

2. The answer is C. A Doppler stethoscope test may be the most readily available test. In torsion it will demonstrate the audible bruit of arterial blood in the uninvolved side but not on the affected side, except in rare cases. The technetium scan is helpful in confirming the diagnosis and should be the next test to be performed. Complete blood cell count and urinalysis are unremarkable in torsion. The intravenous pyelogram has no application in the diagnosis of any of the choices in the differential diagnosis.

3. The answer is C. Torsion of the testicle must be relieved in order to restore arterial circulation to the testicle within 6 hours. Otherwise, the testicle is functionally (and cosmetically) lost. Doxycycline is indicated for expectant treatment of infection by *Neisseria gonorrhoeae* and Chlamydia organisms, both of which are frequently implicated in epididymitis. Elective exploration is appropriate for cancer and elective repair for varicocele. Sulfamethoxazole/trimethoprim (Bactrim) is a typical regimen for cystitis and some cases of prostatitis.

4. The answer is A. Epididymitis is well described in the vignette. Although the testicular anatomy may be difficult to differentiate, careful examination usually allows the physician to identify the epididymis and the testicle proper as ovoid and not deformed. Torsion was described and is best identified by the methods alluded to in Questions 1 and 2. However, in torsion, despite confounding edema, one should appreciate that the testicle itself is the source of tenderness and that the epididymis is normal in size and not tender. Orchitis manifests tenderness of the testicle and, in most cases, enlargement but no change in the basic shape of the organ. The signs of ischemia and lack of evidence of obstructed arterial flow usually allow torsion to be ruled out. Testicular cancer manifests an irregular shape of the testicle proper and nearly always is nontender. The exception is the rapidly growing tumor into which occurs hemorrhage.

5. The answer is D. Tenderness of the hernia sac indicates the complication of strangulation of an incarcerated hernia. This surgical emergency requires timely correction to prevent ischemic death of the tissues involved in the hernia, usually a loop of bowel. In the latter case the specter of bowel obstruction adds a further threat. Inability to reduce the hernia confers urgency and is the precursor of strangulation. Direct inguinal hernias are less likely to become incarcerated than indirect hernias. The latter herniate down the inguinal canal, a defined tight tunnel.

6. The answer is D. Reactive arthritis (formerly called Reiter syndrome in the context of the vignette) is the most common etiology for an acute inflammatory arthritis in a young adult. When following exposure to Yersinia or Shigella organisms, the incidence is equal in male and female patients. When following a sexually transmitted disease, the incidence in men is nine times that in women. The joint fluid is sterile by definition (as opposed to that in septic arthritis). Other components of the classic tetrology of urethritis, conjunctivitis, arthritis, and dermatitis may be present or absent.

7. The answer is E, Leydig cell carcinoma. Leydig cells produce testosterone. Because of the dedifferentiation of these cells and the lack of circulating testosterone, 30% of patients with Leydig cell tumors exhibit gynecomastia. All the remaining tumors mentioned in the choices are germ cell tumors. Although 97% of testicular cancers are germ cell tumors and 5% of them manifest gynecomastia, all except seminomas among them are characterized by elevations of alpha-fetoprotein or human chorionic gonadotropin; 60% manifest elevated lactic dehydrogenase as well.

8. The answer is D. Performing a sperm count on the husband is the most logical initial step after a thorough history and physical examination, the latter including pelvic examination to rule out anatomic causes of female infertility. Forty percent of cases of infertility are male related. Polycystic ovary syndrome is unlikely because is appears to be established that the patient is ovulating so that pelvic ultrasound is unnecessary. The other studies are quite expensive compared with the cost of the sperm count.

9. The answer is C. Varicocele is the most common cause of male infertility, accounting for 30% of cases.

10. The answer is C. Prostatism may be caused by or aggravated by all the choices given, except for epididymitis. Epididymitis, though not a cause, may be associated chronologically with prostatitis.

11. The answer is E. *P. africanum*, an herb, has not been proven by random controlled trials to reduce symptoms of BPH. However, there have been some reports from systematic reviews that urinary residual volume and peak urine flow were improved after the use of the herb for 6 weeks. Similar reports come from systematic reviews of rye grass pollen extract. Saw palmeto plant extracts have, in fact, been found to improve symptom scores comparably to the alpha-blocker tamsulosin and the 5-alpha reductase inhibitor finasteride.

Alpha-adrenergic receptor blocking agents that are specific for alpha-1A receptors (relevant in 85% of BPH cases) and for alpha-1D (15% of cases) are quite effective in reducing symptoms of BPH, as are 5-alpha reductase inhibitors. Examples of the former are terazosin (Hytrin) and doxazosin (Cardura), first brought out as antihypertensive agents. Newer versions are tamsulosin and alfulosin. The 5-alpha reductase inhibitors are effective, the most well known of which is finasteride (Proscar). Drugs in this class are inhibitors of dihydroxytestosterone. It is known that BPH is dependent on androgenic stimulation and that dihydroxytestosterone is more potent in that regard than testosterone.

Transurethral resection is a time-honored surgical method of treatment of BPH. Transurethral microwave thermotherapy is new. Studies appear to be limited to fairly short periods of follow-up of <2 years, which indeed do show beneficial effects over 1 to 2 years.

12. The answer is C. This patient is less likely to have an increase in QALYs as a result of treatment than he would have if his Gleason score were 8. The Gleason score is a scale from 1 to 10 *inversely* related to the degree of differentiation (directly related to aggresivity). Therefore, it

may seem ironic that the patient with the lower score will gain fewer (or even lose) QALYs. However, the point to be made is that curative treatments are fraught with side effects of varying severity, depending on the individual patient. On balance the patients with the least aggressive tumors may suffer a net loss of QALYs by aggressive treatment. Those patients with advanced disease gain the most in QALYs, at least for the near future. Given the foregoing definition of the Gleason score, it follows that those with the smallest score are least likely to die of the disease and the most likely to die of an unrelated cause. However, the Gleason score has not replaced surgical staging in rendering a prognosis.

13. The answer is B. Headache is the most common side effect of PDE-5s. Contrary to early hysterical reports regarding precipitation of heart attacks and hypotensive crises, the only firm contraindication to prescription of PDE-5s is the concurrent treatment with nitrates. In that case, clinically critical hypotensive crisis may be precipitated. Color vision changes have been reported during the action of PDE-5s, apparently reversible after the medication wears off. However, this side effect is much less frequent with tadalafil (Cialis).

14. The answer is C. Among the drugs mentioned, literature for albuterol does not list impotence or erectile dysfunction. As this drug is a beta-2 agonist, some patients will complain of heart pounding if use of the drug is excessive. Such adrenergic effects may interfere with sexual function because of the effect of preoccupation. However, the other medications are well known to cause impotence to varying degrees at therapeutic levels. It behooves physicians to inquire directly of people who take those medications (and many others) about that problem, even if the chief complaint is not related to the symptoms of sexual dysfunction.

15. The answer is C, age 40 and yearly. Employing DRE and PSA is the American Cancer Society (ACS) recommendation for screening African American men. Arbitrary as this question may seem, there are a few messages that the student or resident should keep well in mind. First, African Americans have an earlier onset and higher case mortality than whites and Asians do. Second, all other groups should, according to the ACS, be screened exactly the same way except that the screening need not begin until the age of 50, unless there is a family history of prostate carcinoma. Third, although the ACS recommends the foregoing, the conservative U.S. Preventive Services Task Force is neither for nor against prostate screening by PSA. That is because the PSA, although it has good sensitivity, is not as specific as, for example, the

Pap smear, so that positive PSA screening leads to a high rate of negative biopsies and much worry on the part of the patient.

16. The answer is A. The incorrect statement is that the upper limit of normal in PSA level is 4 ng/mL in all circumstances. This can be inferred from the other choices (i.e., that the upper limit of normal rises with age and levels <4 can be an indication of cancer in younger men). From the other correct statements can be inferred that the free as opposed to bound form of PSA should be present at a minimum of 27% of the total. Less than that is a criterion for biopsy and is used in cases of marginal PSA levels for age. Finally, the yearly rate of rise in PSA levels, regardless of their absolute values, should not exceed 0.7 ng/mL. If it does, further investigation is critical so as not to miss the opportunity for early diagnosis of prostate carcinoma.

References

Hellmann DB, Stone JH. Arthritis and musculoskeletal disorders. In: Tierney LM, McPhee SJ, Papadakis MA, eds. *Current Medical Diagnosis and Treatment*. 45th ed. New York: McGraw-Hill/Appleton & Lange; 2006:807–864.

Strode SW. Genitourinary problems of the male. In: Rudy DR, Kurowski K, eds. *Family Medicine: House Officer Series*. Baltimore: Williams & Wilkins; 1997:351–369.

Swebber R. Clinical evidence concise (a publication of the British Medical Journal). Reprinted in *Am Fam Physician*. 2004; 70:1325–1326.

Tunnila J, Lassen P. Testicular masses. *Am Fam Physician*. 1998; 57:685–692.

SECTION **IX**

Musculoskeletal and Connective Tissue Problems

chapter 22

Musculoskeletal Problems of the Neck and Back

Examination questions: Unless instructed otherwise, choose the ONE lettered answer or completion that is BEST in each case.

1 A 25-year-old woman comes to you for neck pain that had its onset 6 hours after she was "rear ended" in her automobile. In addition to her pain, she complains that her head feels "heavy" on her shoulders. She denies radiation of the pain into her arms. She was seen at an emergency room soon after the accident because of the insistence of the emergency medical technicians, and x-rays of the cervical spine were negative for fracture and dislocation. Besides the finding of normal strength and deep tendon reflexes of the upper extremities, you find you can elicit tactile crepitus when you move the larynx against the cervical vertebral column. Which of the following expresses best the significance of the last finding in this situation?

(A) It rules out fracture of a vertebral body.

(B) It assures you that there is no retrolaryngeal neoplasm.

(C) It assures you that there is no Ludwig angina.

(D) This finding raises the likelihood of a laryngeal fracture.

(E) It rules against the presence of a hematoma between the larynx and the cervical vertebrae.

2 A 65-year-old man complains that he has deep hip and buttock pain on both sides, worse the longer he walks and when dorsiflexing the spine. The pain is immediately alleviated when he sits down. Deep tendon reflexes of the lower extremities and straight-leg raising (SLR) tests are normal and symmetrical. Which is the most likely diagnosis?

(A) Herniated disc at L5, S1

(B) Lumbosacral strain

(C) Cauda equina syndrome

(D) Lumbar spinal stenosis

(E) Prostatitis

3 A 35-year-old woman complains of tingling and numbness of the little finger on the left hand. On examination you corroborate hypesthesia of the fifth finger and also all of the ring finger, and you find also left-side weakness of flexion of fingers and wrist. The patient is able to spread the fingers adequately. Which of the following diagnoses is likely to account for these symptoms?

(A) Ulnar nerve injury

(B) Carpal tunnel syndrome

(C) C6 nerve root compression

(D) C7 nerve root compression

(E) C8 nerve root compression

4 A 19-year-old patient who is obese had a fall on the ice last week and since then has had pain radiating down both posterior thighs. Three days later, the pain was of such severity as to require hospitalization. In the hospital his family noticed that the young man said he was having trouble making it to the bathroom for voiding without losing some urine, as well as once for defecation of formed stool. The physician in charge noted that the patient had normal ability to sense position in space with eyes closed and heels together, albeit exhibiting pain, and that he has "urinary and fecal urgency." The physician orders urinary culture and sensitivity. Which of the following is the cause of the foregoing findings?

(A) Perineal contusion incurred in the fall

(B) Acute cystitis

(C) Diabetes insipidus caused by brain injury

(D) Central disc herniation

(E) Ataxia caused by posterior column injury

5 You have a 38-year-old female patient who complains of lower back pain with no radiation with its onset 2 days ago after she did some heavy lifting. She is afebrile. There is some limitation to full flexion and rotation. There is no spinal or paravertebral tenderness. Motor and sensory examinations of her legs are normal. On the SLR test you can raise each of her legs (with her knees in extension) 80 degrees off the table without any radicular pain. Her pain is made worse when she bends forward at the waist or twists at the waist. The patellar and Achilles deep tendon reflexes are 2+ and symmetrical bilaterally. When she arises from the examining table she turns onto one side, throws her legs over the table side, and arises from her flank down position with the help of her arms. Which of the following therapies or evaluations would you recommend?

(A) Order a magnetic resonance image (MRI) of her lumbar spine after plain x-rays of the lumbar spine

(B) Complete the physical examination and then order strict bed rest at home for 1 week

(C) Order a nerve conduction velocity (NCV) test, electromyogram (EMG), and alkaline phosphatase isoenzyme testing (hepatic vs. bone origin)

(D) Order physical therapy sessions consisting of traction, massage, and diathermy three times per week for 2 weeks

(E) Prescribe nonsteroidal anti-inflammatory drugs (NSAIDs) for 5 to 7 days

6 A patient comes to you with the exact same story as the one in Question 5 except for two differences. Instead of 38 years old she is 55 years old, and the pain, instead of starting at a definite known time 2 days before she consulted you, has been present for several weeks. She is unable to tell you what day or even what week the pain began. What she says is that the pain had been bothering her mostly at night for a number of weeks during which she had difficulty finding a position comfortable for sleeping. For the last 2 to 3 weeks, she notices the pain by daytime as well. Her pain is not influenced by position and she can bend forward at the waist and twist at the waist without aggravating the pain. Her SLR test is negative, and the knee jerks and ankle jerks are 2+ and symmetrical bilaterally. Which of the following therapies or evaluations would you recommend first?

(A) Complete the physical examination, order an MRI of her lumbar spine, and draw alkaline phosphatase isoenzymes

(B) Complete the physical examination and then order strict bed rest at home for 1 week

(C) Order NCV test and EMG

(D) Order physical therapy sessions consisting of traction, massage, and diathermy three times per week for 2 weeks

(E) Prescribe NSAIDs for 5 to 7 days

7 The car driven by a 35-year-old woman was struck from behind. She notes the onset of pain several hours later and by morning has significant neck pain with movement in any direction. Which of the following mechanisms is most likely the cause of her symptoms?

(A) Hyperextension of neck

(B) Subluxation of the body of C3 on C4

(C) Contusion to the neck

(D) Extreme rotation of the cervical spine

(E) Fracture of a cervical vertebra

8 You suspect a 55-year-old man has cervical radiculopathy. On examination you note that there is diminished sensation over the right radial aspects of the thumb and index finger. The triceps reflex is normal and compares with the left triceps, but the biceps reflex is diminished as are the strengths of right elbow flexion and supination, as compared with the left side. The patient is right handed. Which of the following listed cervical roots do you believe is most affected in this patient's radiculopathy?

(A) C4

(B) C5

(C) C6

(D) C7

(E) T1

9 Regarding the patient in Question 8, he reports 1 week later that his pain is no better after heat, massage, NSAIDs, and cervical traction. You consider seeking the opinion of a neurosurgeon. Which of the following studies would be the most helpful to provide the specialist with a useful database before he or she sees the patient?

(A) Plain x-rays of the cervical spine

(B) EMG of the upper extremities

(C) NCV test of the upper extremities

(D) MRI of the cervical spine

(E) Erythrocyte sedimentation rate

10 A 60-year-old man is referred back to you from your hospital's emergency department (ED), which he visited 2 nights ago for increasingly severe back pain. The pain is located in the midline at about the 11th thoracic vertebral spinous process. The patient has no radicular symptoms or signs (neither sensory involvement nor complaint of weakness, and he does not show reflex changes or positive SLR test). In reviewing the ED report, you notice a white blood cell count of 19,000 and a temperature of 100.8°F recorded in the ED. You are reminded that you have recently diagnosed him with type 2 diabetes mellitus. What should be your next step?

(A) Stat MRI of the thoracolumbar spine

(B) Stat lumbar puncture

(C) Prescribe amoxicillin at a dosage of 875 mg twice daily for 10 days

(D) Order plain x-rays of the thoracolumbar spine

(E) Order EMG and NCV test of the lower extremities

11 A 24-year-old man has complained of back pain and stiffness sometimes radiating into his right groin for the past 4 years. In the last 2 months, he has noticed limitation of motion of twisting. There has been no trauma. He was treated for iritis by you 3 years ago and again in another city while on vacation last year. The back pain increases with spine rotation. On physical examination he is afebrile with tenderness of the right sacroiliac joint and with loss of lumbar lordosis and a slight increase in the thoracic kyphosis. A sedimentation rate is 50 mm/hour and a test for rheumatoid factor is negative. You find on routine examination aphthous buccal ulcerations, whereupon the patient is reminded of this annoyance that has been present for several weeks. Which of the following is correct in the diagnosis, treatment, and prognosis of this condition?

(A) Of afflicted patients, 85% are positive for human leukocyte antigen (HLA) B-27.

(B) The majority of patients with this condition are female.

(C) Most patients experience resolution of their pain within 4 to 6 weeks.

(D) Proximal interphalangeal and metacarpophalangeal joints are involved with morning stiffness and afternoon gelling.

(E) Radiographs of the peripheral joints will show symmetrical involvement manifesting erosions and demineralization.

12 A 45-year-old male patient complains of low back pain for the last 2 days after doing heavy lifting of furniture. He denies radiation of pain into the lower extremities. He is afebrile. There is significant limitation to full flexion and rotation that is due to pain.

There is no spinal or paravertebral tenderness. Motor and sensory examinations of his legs are normal. The SLR test elicits low back pain at 5 to 10 degrees of hip flexion on both sides. Which of the following therapies or evaluations would you recommend?

(A) An MRI of the lumbar spine

(B) Strict bed rest at home for 1 week

(C) Urgent consultation of a neurosurgeon for presumptive cauda equina syndrome

(D) Physical therapy sessions consisting of traction, massage, and diathermy three times per week for 2 weeks

(E) Use of NSAIDs for 5 to 7 days

13 A 54-year-old man complains of neck, shoulder, and left arm pains that are aggravated by certain neck movements. You suspect herniated nucleus pulposus of a cervical disc. Which of the following is the most appropriate regarding such cervical radiculopathy?

(A) Hand and arm muscle atrophy can be observed in chronic cases.

(B) Acutely, an EMG will show signs of denervation.

(C) There is usually a history of recent blunt neck trauma.

(D) Numbness of the fifth finger and the medial aspect of the adjacent ("ring") finger are typical symptoms.

(E) The Spurling test is highly sensitive and specific in confirming the diagnosis.

14 You are asked to be a consultant for a company that is employed in manufacturing small parts for the automotive industry. The chief of human resources is concerned about the rate of disability among both floor workers and office staff, as defined by days of absence from the job because of health reasons. Without knowing anything specific about the types of illness reported by the employees, which of the following is most likely the leading cause of disability in the employees under the age of 50?

(A) Upper respiratory tract infections

(B) Depression

(C) HIV infection

(D) Heart disease

(E) Lower back pain

15 A 45-year-old woman, otherwise healthy, complains of pain in the left hip area (located in a diffuse area inferior to the iliac crest), present for the last 3 weeks.

The pain radiates down the left anterior thigh. She complains of pain while walking with an extended stride. You examine her and find you can evert the left hip without inducing aggravation of the pain. Deep tendon reflexes are symmetrical at about 2+ in the lower extremities, in both the Achilles and the patellar tendons. The SLR test is negative bilaterally. You find tenderness to fairly firm palpation with two fingers distal to the iliac crest over the prominence of the "hip bone." Which of the following is the likely diagnosis?

(A) Hip fracture

(B) Aseptic necrosis of the left femur

(C) Trochanteric bursitis

(D) Herniated nucleus pulpous at the L3-L4 level

(E) Colon diverticulitis

16 Regarding the patient in Question 15, which of the following is the most logical diagnostic or therapeutic approach?

(A) Order 25 to 35 lb (11.3 to 16 kg) of pelvic traction for 30 minutes, repeated every 3 hours, daily

(B) Order 5 days of modified bed rest in the supine Williams position

(C) Order an MRI of the lumbosacral spine

(D) Make a paralesional injection of a glucocorticoid and a local anesthetic agent

(E) Refer the patient for a neurosurgical opinion

Examination Answers

1. The answer is E. The presence of retrolaryngeal crepitus against the vertebral column is a normal finding. In this situation it rules against a hematoma resulting from the cervical ligament strain, from which this patient suffers. "Whiplash" by auto accident through rear-ending is the most common cause of neck pain in young people. The best way of ruling out vertebral body fracture is, of course, by x-ray. Although retrolaryngeal crepitus disappears in the presence of a neoplasm in that space, it is not the reason for effecting the maneuver in this circumstance. Ludwig angina is cellulitis of the submaxillary and hence sublingual and submandibular spaces. It does not occur on the retrolaryngeal space. This maneuver is not needed to rule against a laryngeal fracture. The latter would be manifested by crepitation and tenderness in the thyroid cartilage.

2. The answer is D. This story is typical of spinal stenosis. The majority of patients are over 60 years of age, though there are uncommon congenital versions. The cause is any combination of degenerative changes about the lumbar spinal cord: Osteophytic spurs, herniated disc(s), or hypertrophied ligamentum flavum. This syndrome may lead to weakness of the proximal lower extremities. Only 25% of patients with this syndrome exhibit decreased deep tendon reflexes, and 10% have positive SLR tests. Eighty percent of cases will respond to laminectomy, at least for an indefinite period of time.

3. The answer is E. Sensory deficit of the fourth and fifth finger is typical of a C8 root syndrome, as are weakness of flexion of the fingers and wrist. The fact that the hypesthesia involves all of the ring finger as opposed to only the ulnar half favors C8 rather than ulnar nerve compression, as does the intact lumbrical and interosseous muscle function. Carpal tunnel syndrome causes median nerve symptomatology, that is, sensory deficit of the palmar aspects of the thumb and fingers through the radial half of the ring finger, as well as dorsal aspects of those fingers distal to the proximal interphalangeal joints. Carpal tunnel syndrome also causes a motor deficit consisting of weakness of thumb–finger apposition. The C6 syndrome is associated with hypesthesia and anesthesia of the palmar and dorsal aspects of the thumb and pointing finger; C7 lesions cause sensory involvement of the middle finger and the narrow corresponding aspects of the distal ventral forearm and a longer streak of the dorsal forearm.

4. The answer is D. The 19-year-old obese man has cauda equina syndrome. It occurs with central intervertebral disc herniation. The significant clue to the correct diagnosis is the history of bilateral radiation of pain into both legs. The patient does not have urinary urgency but rather urinary and fecal incontinence. If examined correctly, the patient may manifest bilateral positive SLR tests and perineal hypesthesia or anesthesia as well as bilateral deep tendon reflex depression and hypotonia of the rectal sphincter. Neurosurgical consultation is indicated on an urgent basis. If intervention does not occur within 2 to 4 days, the patient may suffer permanent problems with control of urine or stool and possibly neurological deficit in the lower extremities.

For there to be a perineal contusion, the patient would have had to land astride something akin to a fence rail. And his chief complaint would likely have been perineal pain and perhaps blood in the urine. Cystitis would cause urinary urgency, not incontinence, and would have had to be coincidental to the fall, which is unlikely. Diabetes insidious (from a head injury) would cause polyuria, not incontinence. Incontinence could conceivably result from a back injury, but the patient's gait would have been wide based and his proprioception defective when he stood with eyes closed.

5. The answer is E. Without more chronicity than is found in this case and in the absence of radicular symptoms and signs, one should treat the case as lumbosacral strain, with NSAIDs given for a period of about 1 week. Bed rest in a case such as this is to be recommended only until the patient feels she can begin to move and is not to be overemphasized. There is no hurry for x-rays and certainly no hurry for an MRI. It takes 3 or 4 weeks for the NCV test and EMG to show denervation changes in acute compression radiculopathies, even when there are positive symptoms and signs of radiculopathy such as sensory or motor changes (e.g., changes in deep tendon reflexes, dermotomal numbness, and weakness of heel or toe walking). Physical therapy modalities would be employed only after more conservative measures fail over a period of at least 2 weeks.

6. The answer is A. This patient is in the age group for breast cancer; there are no symptoms or signs of radiculopathy, and there are no signs of any musculoskeletal condition whatever. Completion of the physical examination is, in this case, for the specific purpose of searching for a breast lesion (after review of her family history for breast cancer and inquiry as to whether she has had timely mammograms as recommended for the patient 40 years of age and older). Although the MRI could await the results of the plain x-rays, it might as well be ordered immediately, along with alkaline phosphatase testing. The latter is sensitive for bone metastases. Electrical studies are not indicated in the absence of suggestions of radiculopathy. NSAIDs may be helpful but are not relevant to the main thrust of ruling out cancer.

7. The answer is A, hyperextension of neck, commonly referred to as whiplash injury. The hyperextension is most typically produced by the victim's being in a motor vehicle that is rear ended by another vehicle. Cervical vertebral body subluxation or fracture would cause most certainly neurological symptoms. The greatest risk for either of these injuries would be a sharp hyperextension such as occurs with a sharp blow to the head from the front as opposed to the hyperextension that occurs with the whiplash mechanism. Extreme rotation of the neck also is fraught with serious sequelae but does not commonly occur in the whiplash mechanism. Contusion of the neck itself requires a direct blow to the soft tissues of the neck, something that would not occur in a rear-end strike unless there were objects loose in the cab of the car. In this and any of the alternative examples given, the pain would not be expected to be delayed as it is in the cervical ligament strain employed in the whiplash mechanism.

8. The answer is C; that is, the affected cervical nerve root is C6. This is a result of a herniation of C6 to C7 or, less often and certainly more possible in a person over the age of 50 years, an osteophytic spur. The classic picture of a C6 lesion shows sensory symptoms of the radial forearm, the index finger, and thumb, and motor involvement of the biceps and wrist extension. Patients are treated conservatively at first, by NSAIDs, warm applications, massage, physical therapy, and possibly cervical traction with 5 to 15 lb (2.3 to 6.8 kg).

9. The answer is D. An MRI is useful as a diagnostic tool for herniated discs but should rarely be used for neck (or back) pain in the absence of radicular symptoms because the test is too sensitive. The more sensitive a test's criteria for positivity, the less specific. Many patients will have positive findings of intervertebral discs showing discernible degrees of herniation that will never become surgical cases. Thus, consulting a neurosurgeon implies not only radicular symptoms (radiation of pain in the distribution of the involved root, sensory symptoms in the appropriate dermatomes, motor symptoms appropriate

to the foregoing findings, or any combination thereof) but also the possibility of the case becoming appropriate for surgical correction. Electrical studies are helpful for pinpointing symptoms but do not generally become positive until the symptoms have been present for 3 weeks. Plain films, though included virtually always in evaluation of neck pain, tend to be too sensitive and not specific enough. Sedimentation rate is useful in evaluating a patient for inflammatory arthritis, which would not be considered in this case because of the rapidity of onset and the precipitating activity.

10. The answer is A. The most serious possible diagnosis to explain the symptoms in the presence of a leukocytosis and fever is that of spinal epidural abscess. In that case the patient is at risk for the rapid onset of a spinal cord transection syndrome (paraplegia if at the level described in the vignette) that can set on within 72 hours to as long as 5 days. While the MRI is being obtained, a neurosurgeon must be consulted for the possibility of emergency decompression of the abscess encroaching on the spinal cord at the T7-9 level. Risk factors for this condition include recent lumbar puncture and diabetes. Lumbar puncture has no place in this case acutely because there are no signs suggestive of meningitis. Amoxicillin prescribed orally would be an inadequate treatment, though there are case reports of patients treated successfully by intravenous antibiotics. Plain films would not show the abscess. Electrical studies would not be helpful because there is no evidence of radiculopathy.

11. The answer is A. This is an example of ankylosing spondylitis. These patients are HLA B-27 positive in 85% of cases. Men are affected more often, more severely, and earlier than women. Peripheral joint involvement occurs transiently in about 50% of cases, and hips, shoulders, and knees permanently in about 25%. Involvement is not symmetrical and does not manifest erosion and demineralization as occurs in rheumatoid arthritis.

12. The answer is E. At this point, NSAIDs for 5 to 7 days is all that is needed. This patient's presentation is consistent with lower back strain. The SLR test is not positive, as it did not elicit radiating pain typical of radiculopathy. Such a pseudopositive SLR is common when the patient has not been coached as to what to expect when he is in significant pain caused by back strain. With full explanation that the patient is to remain only passive (i.e., without guarding of the postural muscles), the same patient can often be straight-leg-raised to 70 to 80 degrees without radiation of pain. If the SLR were indeed positive bilaterally, cauda equina must be considered and the patient evaluated further for saddle-area hypesthesia and bowel or bladder incontinence. Prolonged bed rest was not shown to be beneficial for back strain in one recent study. There are no controlled double-blind studies that demonstrate the effectiveness of physical therapy in this situation either. Muscle relaxers are indicated only if the patient is believed to be experiencing paravertebral muscle spasms.

13. The answer is A. Hand and arm atrophy are common advanced signs of herniated nuclear pulposus of a cervical disc. It takes 3 or 4 weeks for the EMG to show denervation changes in acute compression radiculopathies. The Spurling test is positive when there is aggravation of the patient's radicular pain or sensory changes when the neck is rotated toward the side of the pain (while in extension) with pressure applied to the head. Although this test is highly specific, it is poorly sensitive. Patients do not usually report a history of recent blunt trauma to the neck, but they may report noticing their symptoms after activities that stress the cervical musculature, including sneezing or violent maneuvers of snuffling during upper respiratory infections. Numbness of the fifth and the medial half of the ring finger are typical symptoms of ulnar nerve dysfunction. Although radiculopathy involving C8 causes hypesthesia of the fourth and fifth fingers, the syndrome is dermotomal and does not spare the lateral half of the ring finger.

14. The answer is E, lower back pain. Even in patients older than 50 years of age, it ranks second only to heart disease as cause of disability. Although upper respiratory tract infection competes with all other causes of disability in incidence of illness, the number of days of absence caused by back pain in the under-50 age group exceeds that caused by upper respiratory tract infection and, certainly, HIV infection.

15. The answer is C. The pain in the lateral hip area, radiation down the ipsilateral thigh, and tenderness over the greater trochanter are typical. Aseptic necrosis of the femoral head and fracture both would have been very painful upon eversion of the hip. Colon diverticulitis most often occurs in the sigmoid colon and results in deep tenderness in the left lower quadrant of the abdomen. Hip fracture would prevent the patient from walking into the office; a herniated disc would have resulted in a positive SLR test.

16. The answer is D. Injection of a glucocorticoid mixed with a local anesthetic agent into the area of tenderness would be appropriate and effective in the great majority of cases. Such injections are best directed to within a centimeter of, but not into, the most tender point. Pelvic traction was in the past employed in lumbar disc herniation but never had a place in the management of this condition. MRI of the lumbar spine would, at some point, be appropriate in lumbar disc disease, not in trochanteric bursitis. Neurosurgical opinion would not be sought in trochanteric bursitis.

References

Boyd, RJ. Evaluation of neck pain. In: Coroll AH, May LA, Mulley AG, eds. *Primary Care Medicine*. Philadelphia: JB Lippincott Co; 1995.

Hellmann DB, Stone JH. Arthritis and musculoskeletal disorders. In: Tierney LM, McPhee SJ, Papadakis MA, eds. *Current Medical Diagnosis and Treatment*. 43rd ed. New York: McGraw-Hill/Appleton & Lange; 2004:778–832.

Maropis CG. Musculoskeletal problems of the neck and back. In: Rudy DR, Kurowski K, eds. *Family Medicine: House Officer Series*. Baltimore: Williams & Wilkins; 1997:371–382.

chapter 23

Common Problems of the Upper Extremities

Examination questions: *Unless instructed otherwise, choose the ONE lettered answer or completion that is BEST in each case.*

1 A 45-year-old man has had intermittent numbness in his (dominant) right hand palmar index and middle fingers for 2 years, particularly in the night. Since experiencing prolonged use of a handheld posthole digging tool a year ago, he has found that the numbness has persisted even by day and involves the thumb and part of the ring finger. He complains also of midventral forearm pain and shoulder pain on the right. He exhibits weakness of thumb opposition with all four fingers but denies and exhibits no hypesthesia of the dorsal aspects of any of the fingers of the right hand. He denies triggering of the digits with flexion of the fingers. Which of the following is the most likely cause of his symptoms?

(A) Median nerve compression

(B) Cervical disc herniation involving C5, C6, and C7

(C) Scalene anticus syndrome

(D) Herpes zoster

(E) Ulnar nerve compression

2 Regarding the patient in Question 1, you perform and find positive the Phalen and Tinel tests. These are increased numbness in the median nerve distribution within 30 seconds of 90-degree flexion of the wrist (Phalen test) and numbness and paresthesia in the median nerve distribution when tapping with the percussive finger the ventral wrist in the position of the median nerve (Tinel test). You consider conservative management consisting of wrist splinting in the neutral position, to prevent repetitive gripping and wrist flexion, glucocorticoid injection into the carpal tunnel space, or both. What are the chances of alleviation for an indefinite or permanent period?

(A) Excellent

(B) Good

(C) Not good

(D) Poor

(E) Nil

3 A 28-year-old male patient slips and falls onto his outstretched left hand during a winter ice storm. He is complaining of wrist pain and you examine him. You conclude that the distal radius is neither tender to direct pressure nor painful with application of longitudinal or torque stress to the distal radius. An x-ray is negative for fracture of the distal radius or distal ulna. You apply a wrist brace and ask the patient to return in 1 week. However, 3 days later the patient is still complaining of wrist pain. Upon re-examination you note tenderness at the base of the left thumb metacarpal. The patient complains that the persistent pain is made worse by clenching his fist. Which of the following is the likely diagnosis?

(A) Fracture of the thumb metacarpal

(B) Colles fracture of the wrist

(C) Soft tissue sprain of the wrist

(D) Carpal navicular fracture

(E) Rupture of the flexor carpi radialis tendon

4 Regarding the patient in Question 3, x-rays of the left wrist performed on the third day are normal. Which of the following is the best choice for disposition today?

(A) Reassure the patient and a request a return visit in 1 week

(B) Prescribe ibuprofen 400 mg q6h prn for pain

(C) Apply a short-arm thumb spica and bring the patient back for re-examination and repeat x-ray in 2 weeks

(D) Place the patient in an arm sling for 2 weeks and order a return visit for re-examination and x-ray

(E) Prescribe active range of motion exercises for the left wrist and recheck in 3 weeks

5 An 18-year-old high school student got into a fist fight after school and is brought to you the next morning complaining of pain in the right hand where he had struck his adversary with his doubled fist. He has swelling of the hand seen prominently on the dorsal aspect. There is a break in the skin over the dorsal aspect of the fourth metacarpophalangeal joint. You assume this skin break was incurred by the teeth of the opponent. Sensation of the fingers is intact, as is the radial pulse. Which of the following would be your mainstay of therapy?

(A) Warm soaks, nonsteroidal anti-inflammatory drugs (NSAIDs), and return in 2 days; tetanus, toxoid booster injection if indicated

(B) Tetanus toxoid injection and reassurance

(C) Antibiotic coverage for gram-positive cocci plus Choice A here

(D) First-generation cephalosporin antibiotic coverage and Choice A here

(E) Surgical consultation to prevent hand compartment syndrome

6 Regarding the patient in Question 5, after deciding for the medical coverage to treat and prevent critical infection of the hand, you notice that when you ask the patient to flex the fingers of the right hand the distal fifth finger points ulnad rather than lying parallel to the other three digits. Which of the following accounts for this finding?

(A) The patient has a congenital anomaly.

(B) This is a normal variant.

(C) The patient has incurred a fracture of the fifth matacarpal.

(D) The patient has a fracture of the fifth middle phalanx.

(E) The patient has a fracture of the fifth distal phalanx.

7 A 35-year-old house painter who was a catcher in baseball on his high school and industrial league teams complains of right shoulder pain that has become increasingly annoying over the past 3 weeks. His pain interferes with his work because it is engendered by the motion of abduction and by forward placement of his dominant right arm. Which of the

following maneuvers would be useful in determining whether this man has the impingement syndrome?

(A) Testing the proximal biceps insertion for tenderness

(B) Testing the biceps for flexion strength of the arm

(C) Active forward flexion of the shoulder while pressing downward over the acromion

(D) Testing for pain with active extension of the elbow against resistance

(E) Observe patient's performance of digit-to-thumb apposition

8 A 35-year-old man, while playing touch football at a family reunion, fell on his abducted right shoulder with his right arm in abduction behind his back. He heard a "pop." The patient is fully alert but in pain, holding his right arm with his left; the arm is held in slight abduction and external rotation. On examination his right acromion is prominent, a depression is noted in the superior portion of the deltoid, and his right humeral head is palpated anterior to the acromion. Which of the following fractures is commonly associated with this dislocation?

(A) Fracture of distal third of clavicle

(B) Posterolateral humeral head

(C) Posterior rim of glenoid

(D) Transverse fracture of upper third of humerus

(E) Coracoid process fracture

9 If the patient in Question 8 had not sustained a fracture, you would be preparing to reduce the dislocation. Assuming the ABCs of trauma triage have been accomplished and are negative, which of the following is most crucial to perform before effecting a Kocher maneuver?

(A) Press with an examining finger deep into the lateral popliteal fossa for radial head intactness

(B) Examine the distal radius to rule out a Colles fracture

(C) Check for pulsus paradoxicus to rule out pericardial tamponade

(D) Examine for papilledema

(E) Check the radial and ulnar pulses

10 A 21-year-old wide receiver on a prominent college football team, in catching a pass, makes a twisting leap and lands directly on his right shoulder. Immediately he is in pain, holding his right arm with his left hand. There is no glenohumeral tenderness and there is full range of motion. The right acromion manifests prominence that is reduced by downward pressure on the clavicle. There is tenderness and ecchymosis around the acromioclavicular (AC) joint. Distal motion, pulses, and sensory examinations are normal. Which of the following examinations or ancillary studies would you obtain?

(A) Anteroposterior (AP) and lateral and modified axillary view of left shoulder

(B) Magnetic resonance image (MRI) of the left shoulder

(C) AP views of both AC joints with the patient holding 10-lb (4.5-kg) weights in each hand

(D) Right clavicle x-ray

(E) Arthrogram of left AC joint

11 A 35-year-old male mechanic sustained a small puncture wound on the volar surface his left index finger while working on an engine. Three days later he complains of increasing pain in the digit. You find the finger to be swollen to about half above its normal diameter and being held in a semi-flexed position. There is pain with passive extension of the finger and the hand otherwise presents no remarkable change. Active flexion and extension are intact though painful. Which of the following is the most likely diagnosis?

(A) Cellulitis of the hand

(B) Palmar space infection

(C) Flexor tendon rupture of the index finger

(D) Tenosynovitis of the flexor tendon

(E) Stoving injury involving the joint capsule of the proximal interphalangeal (PIP) joint

12 A 32-year-old former competitive athlete complains of 3 weeks of right elbow pain, coming on 2 weeks after he had decided to take up tennis. There has been no trauma to the elbow. He first noted his pain when performing his backhand stroke on the tennis court. Later he began to complain of pain upon shaking hands, turning a screwdriver, and now even when he turns a doorknob. He denies any other musculoskeletal symptoms. He is afebrile and there is no elbow joint swelling or discoloration. There is tenderness over the lateral epicondyle of the proximal forearm. Each of the following therapeutic approaches would be appropriate except which one?

(A) Addressing the ball with increased wrist and elbow extension during the backhand stroke

(B) Hand grip exercises with a rubber ball

(C) Forearm splinting

(D) Paralesional injection of a glucocorticoid solution

(E) Cold applications to the elbow

13 A 35-year-old woman has an accident in the kitchen with a paring knife. As she is brought to your office, you note a laceration of the skin across the dorsum of the PIP joint of the middle finger of the left hand. You note also that the PIP joint is in partial flexion while the distal interphalangeal (DIP) joint is in extension. Which of the following injuries causes this result?

(A) Collateral ligament injury

(B) Transection of the flexor tendon of the middle finger

(C) Laceration of the central slip of the extensor tendon

(D) PIP dislocation

(E) Stoving injury to the end of the middle finger

14 A 16-year-old male catcher on the high school baseball team had a foul tip strike his left (nongloved) hand and arrives with pain the next day to your office. There is tenderness and ecchymosis over the dorsal aspect of the DIP joint of the thumb. The patient can fully flex the joint, but he has lost 20 degrees of extension, compared with the normal hyperextension seen in the thumb. No fracture is revealed on x-rays. What is the most likely treatment of the patient?

(A) Surgical repair of injured extensor mechanism

(B) Continuous splinting in extension for 6 weeks

(C) Continuous splinting in 20 degrees of flexion for 6 weeks

(D) Arthrodesis (fixation of the joint) in hyperextension of the thumb PIP joint

(E) Only NSAIDs because the x-ray shows no fracture

15 A patient has incurred a fracture of the middle phalanx of left ring finger that extends into the DIP joint, involving 50% of the articular surface. Which of the following treatment plans is most appropriate?

(A) Use open reduction and internal fixation

(B) Splint the finger in 25 degrees of flexion for 6 weeks

(C) Buddy tape the finger to the adjacent middle finger

(D) Use immobilization for 2 weeks followed by active range of motion

Examination Answers

1. The answer is A. This patient has, of course, classic carpal tunnel syndrome, compression of the median nerve, secondary to relative contraction of the flexor retinaculum of the wrist that contains the tendons, blood supply, and median nerve. It occurs commonly and is aggravated by repetitive hand gripping. Involvement of three cervical disc levels is unlikely. More important, however, is that this patient does not exhibit dermatomal distribution of the sensory symptoms, because the dorsa of the thumb, index, middle, and (half) the ring fingers are not involved proximal to the PIP joints. The scalene anticus syndrome is a variant of thoracic outlet syndrome wherein the scalene anticus muscle in the thoracic outlet contracts and causes compression of the peripheral roots of C7, C8, or both, thus involving a distribution that approximates the ulnar nerve (sensation to the ring and fifth fingers). Herpes zoster, or "shingles," causes mostly superficial pain rather than hypesthesia and is associated with a painful varicelloid rash in a dermatomal distribution. Ulnar nerve lesions cause fourth (ulnar half) and fifth finger sensory involvement and weakness of lumbrical and interosseous musculature of the hand (abduction or spreading) of the fingers, not opposition movements.

2. The answer is D. The chance of indefinite alleviation with conservative management is 6.8%. See the table that follows here.

Predicting the Outcome of Conservative Treatment for Carpal Tunnel Syndrome

1. Have symptoms been present for more than 10 months?	Yes___	No___
2. Does the patient have constant paresthesias?	Yes___	No___
3. Does the patient have tenosynovitis (triggering of the digits)?	Yes___	No___
4. Is the Phalen maneuver positive within less than 30 seconds?	Yes___	No___
5. Is the patient older than 50 years of age?	Yes___	No___

Used with permission from Viera (2003).

Score 1 point for each yes answer and zero for each no answer. The scoring key for success rate is as follows: 0 points, 65%; 1 point, 41.4%; 2 points, 16.7%; 3 points, 6.8%; 4 or 5 points, 0%.

3. The answer is D. Fracture of the carpal navicular (also called the scaphoid) occurs with falls onto an outstretched hand, acutely showing tenderness in the "anatomic snuffbox," which is that space between the extensor tendons of the thumb at the base of the metacarpal. Tenderness at this locus is 90% sensitive for scaphoid fracture but only 40% specific. Thus, diagnosis must be confirmed by x-ray with specific focus for the scaphoid bone. Chronically, failure to diagnose may lead to aseptic necrosis and osteoarthritis. Missing this fracture has been the subject of litigation for failure to diagnose.

4. The answer is C. If the initial x-ray is negative, a fracture may show 2 weeks later. Immobilization from early on should prevent aseptic necrosis. If the fracture is confirmed, then the immobilization must continue for the standard length of time for fracture healing, which is 6 weeks. An alternative to the preliminary 2-week immobilization and follow-up x-ray is an MRI of the wrist. Sensitivity and specificity of the MRI are superior to the x-ray.

5. The answer is D. This patient must be treated as if he incurred a human bite and, given the critical sequelae of infection of the hand, antibiotic coverage should be instituted immediately and should cover the gram-negative as well as gram-positive bacterial spectrum. The former includes especially *Pasteurella multoceda* and *Eikenella corrodens*. For the latter two organisms, amoxicillin/clavulanate would be appropriate as well. The compartment syndrome of the hand is a critical development and a surgical emergency. In this case, given that the circulation and sensory functions are intact and that the edema involves only the dorsal rather than the palmar aspect of the hand, the patient does not exhibit evidence of the compartment syndrome.

6. The answer is C. This patient has, in addition to the "fight bite" injury described in Question 5, a fracture of the fifth metacarpal. This is called a boxer's fracture, though a professional boxer would be less likely to incur this injury than would an amateur. Typically the punch was not landed squarely and strikes laterally, loading excessively on the fifth metacarpal, a smaller and weaker bone than the midmetacarpal and fourth metacarpal. The significance of this injury is that the distal fragment of the fracture rotates readily and results in a rotational deformity if not diagnosed and corrected at the time of the reduction of the fracture.

7. The answer is C. Active forward flexion of the shoulder while pressing downward over the acromion, called the impingement maneuver, causes pain in the deltoid area in a positive test for impingement syndrome. Pain of the impingement syndrome is also particularly increased by active abduction at the shoulder. Radiographs are usually normal, but the MRI will reveal any swollen tendon producing impingement and can identify tears in the rotator cuff. The pain of rotator cuff tendonitis usually has an insidious onset and is poorly localized. Tenderness in the proximal insertion of the biceps is found in biceps tendonitis. Neither biceps nor elbow extensor strength is an issue in impingement syndrome because abduction of the shoulder is involved. Thumb–finger apposition tests the motor function of the median nerve, as commonly done in probing for carpal tunnel syndrome.

8. The answer is B. A right anterior glenohumeral dislocation is associated posterolateral humeral head fracture. The dislocation tends to occur anteriorly, and it is the anterior rim of the glenoid that may take off the posterolateral part of the humeral head.

9. The answer is E. Before and after reducing a shoulder dislocation, the peripheral pulses and the peripheral nerve function of the extremity must be affirmed. This is because the brachial neurovascular structures can be caught between the humeral head and the glenoid fossa. A radial head fracture is not incurred by the dynamics given in the vignette. Pulsus paradoxicus, a diminished pulse with inspiration, the opposite of the physiologic state, is found in hemopericardium and constrictive pericarditis. In the absence of a history of falling on the outstretched hand and absence of pain in the wrist, there is no reason beyond standard trauma audit to check the distal radius (Colles) fracture. In the absence of head trauma, and because acute trauma triage in this instance was negative, there is no reason to expect papilledema.

10. The answer is C, AP views of both AC joints with the patient holding 10-lb (4.5-kg) weights in each hand. Clinically the case seems to involve a grade III or IV sprain of the right AC joint (suggested by the high-riding right clavicle). Hanging weights bring out the separation between the clavicle and acromion if the joint capsule is torn and comparison with the contralateral side is made. MRI or arthrogram could also show the capsule tears, but they are more expensive and unnecessary in deciding treatment. For this purpose the right clavicle will be adequately viewed on the AC joint films.

11. The answer is D. Tenosynovitis of the hand is a surgical urgency calling for interruption and control of the infection and surgical drainage and decompression when indicated in order to save function of the affected digit. Cellulitis of the hand produces diffuse swelling of the whole hand; palmar space infection causes swelling of either the thenar or midpalmar space. Flexor tendon rupture, assuming no infectious involvement, is not noted for the degree of swelling found in the vignette and active flexion would not be demonstrable at all. A stoving injury of the PIP joint is caused by a blow to the end of an extended finger wherein the impact is transmitted axially to the joint capsule of, usually, the PIP joint. It produces fusiform swelling centered on the joint itself, not the whole finger.

12. The answer is C. Hand grip exercise would aggravate the problem, which is a type of overuse syndrome, lateral epicondylitis. It is commonly called tennis elbow; lateral epicondylitis is caused in tennis by an amateurish tendency to stroke the backhand with the heavy tennis racquet as if it were a table tennis paddle. However, it may develop through any repetitive supination or gripping action (handgrip calls upon the wrist extensors to stabilize the wrist against flexion in doubling the fist as well). The brachioradialis muscle attaching to the epicondyle operates at a great mechanical disadvantage. Forearm splinting prevents the wrist extension and supination. A glucocorticoid mixed with a local anesthetic injected into the region of the epicondyle, but not directly into it, may give dramatic relief. Relief may be lasting, provided the underlying mechanical cause is dealt with. Cold applications may give relief during the acute phase.

13. The answer is C, laceration of the central slip of the extensor tendon. The configuration of the boutonniere deformity is flexion of the PIP and extension of the DIP joint. The DIP attachment of the extensor tendon is a convergence of two lateral slips that course to the two sides of the PIP and thus are spared in an injury to the dorsal midline of the proximal phalanx and the PIP joint. However, the central slip is involved by that injury. Activation of the extensor tendon apparatus without the functional presence of the central slip allows the lateral strands of the tendon to slip sideways and relatively ventrally, allowing their action to take a "shortcut" to the DIP, resulting in paradoxical flexion of the PIP while extending the DIP.

14. The answer is B, continuous splinting in extension for 6 weeks. This is an example of a partial avulsion of the extensor tendon, in this case brought about by the careening baseball's striking the patient's flexed thumb and violently stressing the PIP into hyperflexion. In a similar case involving one of the fingers, the result is referred to as a mallet finger. Prolonged splinting (6 to 8 weeks) in extension is necessary for the extensor mechanism to heal. Delayed treatment can result in the situation in which the patient is unable to extend the finger at DIP joint without surgical intervention. Surgical repair has not produced satisfactory results; splinting in flexion is counterproductive; arthrodesis is virtually never resorted to; and NSAIDs as a sole treatment is inadequate.

15. The answer is A, open reduction and internal fixation of the fracture. Closed treatment in a fracture involving more than 30% of the articular surface is highly likely to develop degenerative arthritic change. All the other choices offer less aggressive treatment than either open reduction or 6 weeks of splinting.

References

Daniels JM, Zook EG, Lynch JM. Hand and wrist injuries: Part I. Emergent evaluation. *Am Fam Physician.* 2004; 69:1941–1948.

Daniels JM, Zook EG, Lynch JM. Hand and wrist injuries: Part II. Non-emergent evaluation. *Am Fam Physician.* 2004; 69: 1949–1956.

Myers A. Common problems of the upper extremities. In: Rudy DR, Kurowski K, eds. *Family Medicine: House Officer Series.* Baltimore: Williams & Wilkins; 1997:383–398.

Phillips TG, Reibach AM, Slomiany WP. Diagnosis and management of scaphoid fractures. *Am Fam Physician.* 2004; 70: 879–884.

Viera AJ. Management of carpal tunnel syndrome. *Am Fam Physician.* 2003; 68:265–272.

chapter 24

Mechanical Problems of the Lower Extremities

Examination questions: *Unless instructed otherwise, choose the ONE lettered answer or completion that is BEST in each case.*

1 A 24-year-old male graduate student and committed amateur athlete comes to see you one day after suffering an inversion injury (ankle turned violently inwardly) of the left ankle in pick-up basketball. He was able to bear weight painfully and applied ice last evening with a resultant reduction of moderate swelling. On examination the patient has a "goose egg" type of swelling just inferior to the lateral malleolus, with a negative anterior drawer test; passive inversion of the ankle allows 10 degrees as it does on the right (noninjured) side. There is no tenderness of the tip or posterior edge of the left lateral malleolus and no tenderness of the posterior edge of the medial malleolus. Which of the following initial dispositions is the most logical?

(A) Use supportive dressing (e.g., double layers of sheet wadding or similar material before applying two 4-in. or 10-cm elastic support bandages) followed by a magnetic resonance image (MRI) of the left ankle.

(B) Order stat x-rays of the left ankle and same-day referral to an orthopedic surgeon.

(C) Order stat x-rays, as well as crutches for ambulation for 3 weeks.

(D) Use supportive dressing or an air cast, order crutches until weight bearing takes place without pain, and suggest continued ice application for 1 day more. Have the patient return for follow-up in 1 week.

(E) Encourage immediate weight bearing by the patient and have him return if not improved in 3 days.

2 The patient in the previous question did well on your management but returns to you 1 year later after another inversion injury of the left ankle. On this occasion he was unable to bear weight at the site of the accident. Examination within the first 2 hours showed a large fusiform swelling centered anteriorly on the lateral malleolus. When you grasp the ankle and pull the foot forward, there is definite forward motion compared with the response to the same maneuver on the right. Which of the following dispositions constitutes the wisest course?

(A) Use supportive dressing (e.g., double layers of sheet wadding or similar material before applying two 4-in. or 10-cm elastic support bandages) followed by MRI of the left ankle.

(B) Order stat x-rays of the left ankle, supportive dressing, crutches, and referral to an orthopedic surgeon.

(C) Order stat x-rays, as well as crutches for ambulation for 3 weeks.

(D) Use supportive dressing or an air cast, order crutches until weight bearing takes place without pain, and suggest continued ice application for 1 day more. Have the patient return for follow-up in 1 week.

(E) Encourage immediate weight bearing by the patient and have him return if not improved in 3 days.

3 A 35-year-old woman comes to you with the complaint of left heel pain, which had its onset over several days with no history of trauma. It is worst during the woman's first steps in the morning or after she has been sitting for prolonged periods or standing for significant periods of time. You ask her to walk without shoes in the back hallway of your office suite. You note that she exhibits valgus deformities at both ankles when walking slowly or standing. The os calcis is tender to compression but exhibits no erythema. There is neither hypesthesia of the overlying skin of the heel nor the medial tract from the heel to the proximal sole. Which of the following is the most likely cause of this patient's complaint?

(A) Achilles tendonitis

(B) Retroachilles bursitis

(C) Tarsal tunnel syndrome

(D) Plantar fasciitis

(E) Osteomyelitis

4 An 18-year-old high school football player complains of left hip pain after being tackled. The pain increases with rotation and lateral bending of the trunk. He denies radiation of the pain into the lower extremities. He bears weight well and examination finds increased pain neither with eversion of the left hip nor with active flexion at the waist. Which of the following is the probable diagnosis?

(A) Contusion of the iliac crest

(B) Inflammation of the greater trochanter of the hip

(C) Inflammation of the lesser trochanter of the hip

(D) Fracture of the left hip

(E) Contusion of the pubic ramus

5 A 19-year-old male high school football player is brought to you 2 hours after the sudden onset of severe right anterior thigh pain during an explosive sprint in an early-season practice game. From a sitting position on the examining table, he is able to extend the knee painfully. He exhibits visible swelling of the thigh with ecchymosis but no depression or unnatural concavity of the thigh contour. Which of the following is the least appropriate in the initial management of a grade II muscle strain of the quadriceps?

(A) Stretching of the affected muscles to decrease shortening

(B) Resistance training to rebuild muscle strength

(C) Ice and compression with an elastic wrap

(D) Crutch walking until patient can ambulate without limping

(E) Avoidance of strenuous physical activity

6 A 20-year-old female college student who is an athletics enthusiast complains of intermittent bilateral knee pain, worse after family reunion volleyball. She denies any trauma or twisting injury to her knees. She notices increased knee pain when sitting with her knees flexed at study in the campus library. She

weighs 135 lb (61 kg) at a height of 5 ft, 4 in. (16.3 m). There are no visible or palpable effusions above or subcutaneously in the anterior aspect of the knee and no joint line or other local tenderness except for discernible lateral subpatellar tenderness. Which of the following diagnoses is most strongly suggested by these findings?

(A) Osgood–Schlätter disease

(B) Patellofemoral instability

(C) Prepatellar bursitis

(D) Patellar tendonitis

(E) Medial collateral ligament strain

7 An 18-year-old high school football player was tackled from the right side by a linebacker who hit low with his shoulder thrusting against the lateral aspect of the knee. This occurred just as your patient was planting his right foot to pivot for turning left. The event occurred 8 days earlier, and he has been trying to walk on the leg despite pain and swelling. Which of the following would you expect to find on examination (assume swelling has decreased enough to allow adequate examination), in addition to a positive anterior drawer test, if your patient tore his anterior cruciate ligament 8 days earlier?

(A) Prepatellar swelling

(B) Abnormal degree of varus deformity with varus pressure on the leg below the knee

(C) Tenderness of the patella

(D) Tenderness over the anterior aspect of the knee

(E) An abnormal valgus deformity with valgus pressure applied below the knee

8 In the case of the running back in Question 7, if the same pivotal motion while being tackled from the side had resulted in a torn medial cartilage, which of the following symptoms or signs would be among those characteristic of that knee injury?

(A) Positive posterior drawer sign

(B) Immediate intense pain

(C) A knee-locking sensation

(D) Pain and tenderness in the patella

(E) A palpable spongy sensation overlying the patella

9 A 17-year-old boy has grown from 66 in. (1.68 m) to 71 in. (1.8 m) within the past 18 months. He now complains of pain in the posteromedial aspect of the distal one third of his right tibia since initiation of track training in the past 7 days. On examination he exhibits pes planus and tenderness in the area of described pain. The 128-Hz tuning fork applied to his medial malleolus gives a normal result. Which of the following is the most likely diagnosis of this condition?

(A) Tibial stress syndrome

(B) Stress fracture of the tibia

(C) Fracture of the fibula

(D) Grade 3 anterior ankle sprain

(E) Venous insufficiency of the long saphenous system

10 A 30-year-old athlete develops pain in the proximal posterior medial aspect of the right calf after long-distance running earlier that day. He is afebrile. He limps on his right leg. There is swelling and ecchymosis and tenderness in an area approximately 5 cm in diameter in the proximal posterior medial aspect of the calf as well as ecchymosis in the lower leg and heel. He cannot stand on his toes on the right. Which of the following diagnoses is most likely?

(A) Achilles tendonitis

(B) Achilles tendon rupture

(C) Shin splints

(D) Tibial stress fracture

(E) Gastrocnemius tear

11 A 40-year-old former athlete had been playing football during the annual family reunion. He noted sudden pain in the left lower calf area and is brought to you complaining of posterior distal leg pain. With the patient supine and with his knee flexed, you squeeze the midportion of his calf and do not observe any plantar flexion of the foot. Which of the following diagnoses is most strongly suggested by these findings?

(A) Shin splints

(B) Ruptured Baker cyst

(C) Deep venous thrombosis

(D) Tibial stress fracture

(E) Achilles tendon rupture

12 A 35-year-old male former athlete suffered a severe right lateral ankle sprain in an inversion injury. The injury occurred when he landed after jumping to catch a rebound in "alley" basketball. You suspect instability and perform an anterior drawer test. In that test, where do you look for displacement, assessing stability of a lateral ankle sprain?

(A) The talus on the navicular

(B) The fibula on the talus

(C) The talus on the tibia

(D) The talus on the calcaneus

(E) The navicular on the talus

13 A teenaged boy attended a rock concert in an outdoor theater with standing room only. In the crush of the crowd, he is pushed down to his right by a heavy person who has fallen against his left knee. You note a 10-mm opening when you apply valgus stress with the knee in 20 degrees of flexion and an 8-mm opening when the knee is fully extended. There is no knee effusion appreciated, but there is tenderness along the medial joint line. The Lachman test is negative. Which of the following lesions do you expect to find?

(A) Anterior cruciate along with medial collateral ligament sprain

(B) Lateral collateral ligament sprain

(C) Patellofemoral instability

(D) Posterior cruciate ligament tear

(E) Medial collateral ligament with posterior capsule tears

14 An 18-year-old white female collegiate track competitor has complained of pain in the left midportion of the tibia over the last 2 weeks during her training, increasingly severe and longer lasting after running sessions. In evaluation of this condition you utilize the test of the vibrating 128-Hz tuning fork, for sensation when the stem is placed upon the ipsilateral medial malleolus. The patient complains of pain in the area of complaint. Which of the following is true regarding the condition from which this patient suffers?

(A) Normal x-rays rule out stress fractures as a potential cause of a patient's symptoms.

(B) Some limited running or jumping is permitted after 2 weeks of treatment.

(C) This is the most common of stress fractures.

(D) It is caused by a blow to the lower leg.

(E) Swimming is forbidden for the first 4 weeks of treatment.

15 A 35-year-old male army infantry reservist returns from 2 weeks of annual field training that consisted of daily marches increasing in distance from 5 miles (8 km) the first day to 40 miles (64 km) the last day. He complains of pain in the left foot that began 3 days before the end of the tour and increased in severity with the distance walked. The pain lasted longer each evening. Which of the following parts of the bony anatomy of the foot deserves special attention on the plain x-ray?

(A) First metatarsal

(B) Talus

(C) Navicular

(D) Calcaneus

(E) Fifth metatarsal

16 A running back on a high school football team falls backward while being tackled. He lands with one defender on his chest and another on his right foot, which is thus subjected to forced plantar flexion. As team physician you examine the player in the locker room in the supine position and perform the "bounce test," pressing downward on the forefoot. The patient reacts with pain. If the player has a fracture, which of the following sites for it is most likely?

(A) Navicular

(B) Fibula avulsion

(C) Talus

(D) Calcaneus

(E) First metatarsal

17 For several years, your 65-year-old male patient has complained of deep pelvic area pain following strenuous physical activity. Lately he finds this pain comes on whenever he walks any distance beyond 1 mile (1.6 km). If he stops and sits down for as little as 1 minute, the pain subsides and he can resume walking for another 10 minutes or so. The pain tends to radiate into both posterior proximal thighs, not reaching below the knees. He denies bowel or bladder symptoms of dysfunction. Occasionally he notices weakness and tends to buckle in the left leg before getting relief from sitting and resting. Deep tendon reflexes, results of the straight-leg raising test, and pulses of the lower extremities are all within normal limits. Which of the following is the most logical diagnosis to explain this patient's symptoms?

(A) Lumbar spinal stenosis

(B) Herniated nucleus pulposus at the L5 to S1 level

(C) Osteoarthritis of the lumbar spine

(D) Prostatitis

(E) Lumbosacral strain

Examination Answers

1. The answer is D. On the basis of the moderate swelling and lack of evidence of grade III sprain, this patient had a grade II inversion ankle sprain. This patient has no indications for a plain x-ray, not to mention an MRI. This is based on the patient's ability to bear weight immediately, a negative anterior drawer test, and a negative inversion test; both tests, if positive, would not allow weight bearing according to most experts. Weight bearing in this scenario does not mean the ability to push off normally on the toes in walking but to stand on the axis of the ankle. Indications for plain x-rays of the ankle, in the interest of cost effectiveness, are based on the Ottawa rules: tenderness of the posterior edge of the lateral malleolus (in an inversion injury or medial malleolus in an eversion injury), or inability to bear weight immediately, or in the emergency care situation. To send the patient out bearing full weight would be foolhardy, risky (because of the possibility of aggravating an unappreciated grade III sprain or a fracture), and probably unenforceable. The use of supportive dressing or an air cast can never go wrong. Grade I or II sprains should be 90% well in 10 days and completely well and ready for full athletic activity in 3 weeks.

2. The answer is B. This patient has a grade III sprain, based on the positive anterior drawer test, and thus a complete rupture of the talotibial ligament. Therefore, as a devoted athlete under the age of 40, he becomes a surgical candidate. Stat x-rays are indicated based on the Ottawa criteria that include inability to bear weight, virtually always present in the case of grade III sprains. Failure to appreciate the extent of this injury results in sending the patient forth with an unstable ankle. The latter may lead to further injury. That said, however, the outcomes of repair in the acute phase are very little different from those of repair of chronic ankle instability.

3. The answer is D, plantar fasciitis. This patient, by her ankle valgus deformity (eversion), shows that she has pes planus. That condition is one of the causes of plantar fasciitis through the process of increasing tension on the plantar fascia. Others are pes cavus, decreased subtalar joint mobility, and tight Achilles tendon. The other choices are possible causes of heel pain as well. Retroachilles bursitis is caused by a loose-fitting shoe band at the heel that allows repetitive motion of the skin

overlying the bursa. (Quick relief is achieved by cutting a slit in the shoe at the area of friction.) Achilles tendonitis is made worse by running, jumping, and quick turning on the ball of the foot and is aggravated by dorsiflexion. Tarsal tunnel syndrome causes numbness or pain of the heel radiating medially into the sole of the foot. Osteomyelitis would be apparent by the signs of inflammation and infection.

4. The answer is A. The patient has a contusion of the iliac crest, commonly referred to as a "hip pointer." These are usually produced by a direct blow to the iliac crest, such as by a football helmet as the patient is being tackled. Seldom does the player lose playing time beyond a few minutes or a quarter, after cold applications and increased local padding. Hip fracture is ruled out by failure of eversion to elicit the pain. Trochanteric bursitis pain radiates anteriorly down the ipsilateral thigh and is characterized by local tenderness at the greater trochanter. The lesser trochanter is "not in play" for injury except in the presence of a hip fracture, in which case one of the two common types is the intertrochanteric fracture. The patient would neither be bearing weight with hip fracture nor would he painlessly do so in the face of a pubic ramus fracture.

5. The answer is B. The patient has a grade 2 strain of the quadriceps. Resistance training to rebuild muscle strength should not be initiated until swelling and pain have resolved and full range of motion has been restored, usually within about 10 to 14 days. Grade 1 strains show no specific physical findings and little functional impairment. Grade 3 strains involve a complete tear of any of the quadriceps muscles and require ice and compression initially followed by crutch assistance for ambulation until the patient can walk limp free. This would not occur for at least 6 weeks.

6. The answer is B, patellofemoral instability. This condition occurs in patients with genu valgus ("knock knees") wherein the quadriceps tendon tends to draw the patella across the lateral ridge of the patellar groove, taking a "shortcut" between the insertion at the anterior tibial tuberosity and the belly of the quadriceps muscle in the anterior thigh. Patients with patellofemoral instability experience a lot of pain with jumping during basketball, as well as bike riding and running whereupon the knee is flexed during exercise. The pain of patellofemoral instability will usually be felt diffusely behind the patella, whereas all the other listed entities will have the pain localized to the anatomic site that is inflamed. Patellar tendonitis pain is located in the tendon inferior to the patella; prepatellar bursitis is "housemaid's knee" and exhibits effusion in the prepatellar bursa; medial collateral ligament injury causes pain in the medial joint space and instability with valgus stress upon examination; Osgood–Schlätter disease manifests anterior tibial tuberosity tenderness and enlargement.

7. The answer is E. Valgus deformity with pressure applied is indicative of an associated torn medial collateral ligament, an injury that often accompanies an anterior cruciate ligament tear.

These patients may have medial or lateral joint line tenderness secondary to menisci or collateral ligament injury, but no anterior aspect tenderness. The Lachman test is a variant of the anterior drawer test, which is the confirming test for anterior cruciate tear, and as such would be positive. These injuries usually produce a large knee effusion. The effusion would have decreased in size by 8 days later, but it would still be present.

8. The answer is C. As an acute change, a locking sensation is fairly specific for a ruptured meniscus. Of interest is that immediate pain is not characteristic of meniscal tear. A posterior drawer sign is diagnostic of a posterior cruciate ligament tear. Patellar pain occurs with direct injury to the patella, either a contusion or a fracture from a direct blow. Anterior knee sponginess is a description of prepatellar effusion, found in prepatellar bursitis (housemaid's knee).

9. The answer is A. The patient has tibial stress syndrome, also known as shin splints. Although precipitated by running exercise, patients who have pes planus or have recently come through rapid growth are more susceptible. Stress fractures may have a similar history (without the association with the foregoing risk factors). If followed for longer periods, unlike with medial tibial stress syndrome, tibial stress fractures result in increasing pain precipitated by decreasingly strenuous activity. Testing for vibration sense upon the tibia results in pain in the case of tibial stress fracture. Neither fibula fractures nor anterior ankle sprain would manifest tibial tenderness and pain. Long saphenous venous insufficiency could cause soft tissue congestion with visible venous ectasia or soft tissue tenderness.

10. The answer is E, torn medial head of the gastrocnemius. The tenderness and swelling are proximal in gastrocnemius tears, whereas in Achilles tendon injuries the pain and tenderness are distal. Swelling and ecchymosis are not typical of shin splints or stress fractures. Ecchymosis distal to the injury site is typical of gastrocnemius tears and actually nonspecific for any injury in a dependent portion of a limb that results in internal bleeding, such as any sprain or other soft tissue renting.

11. The answer is E. The question describes the Thompson test. If the Achilles tendon were intact, squeezing the calf between the examining thumb and fingers would produce plantar flexion. Often, with this injury one can appreciate a notch or depression in a segment of the Achilles tendon. The Homan test (poorly sensitive for deep venous thrombosis) involves forced dorsiflexion of the foot with a positive test elicited if the patient complains of calf pain. See the explanation for Question 9 for a discussion of shin splints and tibial stress fracture. A Baker cyst is a popliteal extension of the joint capsule of the knee. When this cyst ruptures, diffuse calf swelling ensues. However, it is not characterized by focal tenderness, and extravasation of blood is not of defining significance.

12. The answer is C, the talus on the tibia. The tibia is stabilized and the calcaneus is pulled forward. Anterior displacement of the talus on the tibia signifies a positive test. By definition this injury constitutes a grade III sprain. The patient under 40 years of age may be a candidate for surgical correction. For patients over 40 years of age, conservative management would be tried first.

13. The answer is E, medial collateral ligament with posterior capsule tears. Even with collateral ligament tear, if the knee is in full extension, components of the posterior capsule stabilize the knee during valgus and varus stress, so opening even with full knee extension indicates a posterior capsule tear also.

14. The answer is C. Tibial stress fracture is the most common of stress fractures, except in the military population, in whom metatarsal ("march") fracture has the highest incidence of stress fracture. Tibial stress fracture occurs most commonly in white female athletes. This is directly related to associated amenorrhea in female track athletes and baseline bone density in white as compared with black athletes. Plain x-rays do not always rule out stress fractures, and bone scans may be necessary. There is no one blow that causes stress fracture; it is the results of cyclic repetitive axial impact. Cortical thickening on x-ray may be seen in advanced stages of stress fractures. Running and jumping are forbidden for at least 6 weeks but swimming is allowed as early as tolerated.

15. The answer is E, fifth metatarsal. Metatarsal stress fractures are the most common stress fracture among military personnel. Metaphyseal fifth metacarpal stress fractures carry a higher risk of conversion to a complete fracture and nonunion. For that reason, unlike with other metatarsal fractures, a fifth metatarsal fracture has to be managed more aggressively, including short-leg-cast application, complete non-weight-bearing status, or open reduction and internal fixation.

16. The answer is C, posterior process of the talus. Rapid plantar flexion of the ankle (the bounce test), reproducing the original mechanism of injury, will produce pain in the posterior talus.

17. The answer is A. This is a story typical of lumbar spinal stenosis: lumbosacral and deep pelvic pain, more often than not symmetrical, coming on during walking upright and relived by the sedentary position. It occurs most often in a person's seventh decade and later. The cause tends to be a mixture of osteophytic spur formation and varying degrees of herniated discs (nuclei pulposi), effectively narrowing the spinal canal. Claudication is often suspected but palpability of the pulses rules it out. Although a herniated disc can contribute to the syndrome, it seldom occurs with this presentation; knee buckling, as mentioned in the vignette, implies the L4 to L5 root, not the L5 to S1. Prostatitis should be considered in the differential diagnosis of deep pelvic pain, but back pain referral in that situation is sacral and the pain of prostatitis has no relationship to posture or activity. Lumbosacral strain does not radiate from the low back.

References

Aldridge T. Diagnosing heel pain in adults. *Am Fam Physician.* 2004; 70:332–338.

Sickles RT. Mechanical problems of the lower extremities. In: Rudy DR, Kurowski K, eds. *Family Medicine: House Officer Series.* Baltimore: Williams & Wilkins; 1997:399–412.

Terrell TR, Leski MJ. Sports medicine. In: Rakel RE, ed. *Textbook of Family Practice.* 6th ed. Philadelphia: WB Saunders; 2002:845–890.

Wexler RW. The injured ankle. *Am Fam Physician.* 1998; 57: 474–480.

chapter 25

Approach to the Patient with Rheumatic Disease

Examination questions: *Unless instructed otherwise, choose the ONE lettered answer or completion that is BEST in each case.*

1 A 35-year-old woman consults you for pain in the left knee region that appears to be associated with an effusion. No other musculoskeletal pain is present and there is no history of trauma. Each of the following is among the first group of measures to take in diagnosing this patient, except which one?

(A) Take a complete history and perform a relevant physical examination

(B) Determine whether the pain emanates from the knee joint

(C) Obtain plain x-ray films of the joint

(D) Perform arthrocentesis

(E) Order a magnetic resonance image of the knee

2 Regarding the patient in Question 1, you determine that she has an effusion in the left knee joint, which is warm to the touch. The pain had its onset only over the last 3 weeks. The bouts of this pain have had no relationship to atmospheric changes. There has been no history of trauma, whether acute or chronic. Which of the following is the most likely cause of the monoarthritis in this patient?

(A) Rheumatoid arthritis

(B) Gout

(C) Staphylococcal septic arthritis

(D) Gonococcal arthritis

(E) Osteoarthritis

3 Regarding the patient in Questions 1 and 2, aspiration yields no crystals and shows a white blood cell (WBC) count of 35,000/mm³. To your surprise, a culture of the joint fluid yields growth of Gram-negative rods. Which of the following items might explain this departure from the flora expected in this situation?

(A) Positive human immunodeficiency virus (HIV) titer

(B) Positive antinuclear antibody

(C) A uric acid level of 11 mg/mL

(D) A transferrin saturation level of 60%

(E) A re-examination shows erythema migrans

4 A 25-year-old woman complains of pain in the wrists, index, and middle metacarpophalangeal (MCP) joints on both sides as well as morning stiffness, lasting 45 minutes more or less. Which of the following findings is most likely to be present as well?

(A) Elevated uric acid level

(B) Radiographic evidence of erosion or loss of density of bone adjacent to affected joints

(C) WBC in involved joint fluid of 45,000/mL³

(D) Presence of rheumatoid nodules

(E) Elevated serum alkaline phosphatase level

5 Regarding the patient in Question 4, you consider starting her on a disease-modifying antirheumatic drug (DMARD), based on the belief that the early use of DMARDs results in delayed progression of bone erosion, compared with delayed treatment. Each of the following is an example of a DMARD, except which one?

(A) Methotrexate

(B) An antimalarial drug

(C) Intramuscular gold

(D) A COX-2 inhibiting nonsteroidal anti-inflammatory drug (NSAID)

(E) A tumor necrosis factor antagonist

6 A 45-year-old man complains of low back pain, worse in the morning and occasionally during the nights, which has gradually increased over the last 3 months. Three days ago he began to have discomfort in the left eye, which, as the patient enters the office, appears red; the patient is squinting in the lights of the examining room. There are neither gastrointestinal complaints nor skin lesions. Stain of the cornea with fluorescein is negative for disruption of the epithelium. The pupil in the left (affected) eye is smaller than that of the right. You draw blood tests and find that the patient's human leukocyte antigen is type HLA-B27. Which of the following tests or signs is likely to be positive or present?

(A) Plantar reflex

(B) Murphy sign

(C) Schirmer test

(D) Rovsig sign

(E) Schober test

7 Regarding the patient in Question 6, while awaiting tests ordered during the first visit, he now complains of foot pain on the left. In what part of the foot is the most likely locale for this pain to appear?

(A) Retrocalcaneal

(B) First metatarsal

(C) Between the first and second metararsals

(D) Across the dorsum of the forefoot

(E) Supracalcaneal

8 A 65-year-old man complains of pain and stiffness of the right shoulder, both hips, and low back. Muscle strength is normal in all extremities. Radial, femoral, and dorsalis pedis pulses are easily palpable. A complete blood count shows a normal WBC count and normochromic normocytic anemia (hemoglobin of 9 g/dL); the erythrocyte sedimentation rate is elevated at 50 mm/hour. No other joints are involved. The patient denies headaches and difficulty chewing. He denies sensory or motor symptoms and radiating pain into either the arms or the legs. His pain and stiffness have gone on for several months at the time he makes his consultation. Which of the following is the most likely diagnosis?

(A) Gout

(B) Rheumatoid arthritis

(C) Ankylosing spondylitis

(D) Polymyalgia rheumatica

(E) Polymyositis

9 You are examining a 12-year-old male patient with a history of arthralgias. Upon examination you note that the skin is easily stretched and has a dry, rubbery feel. The patient's mother asks him to demonstrate that he can place his hand flat on the examining table, then lift it and rotate it painlessly 360 degrees and place it back flat on the table. Which of the following is the most likely diagnosis?

(A) Congenital dislocation of the shoulder

(B) Ehlers–Danlos syndrome

(C) Polymyositis

(D) Fibromyalgia

(E) Rheumatoid arthritis

10 A 45-year-old white woman complains of pain on the sole of the foot. It has been present for several weeks, is worse in the mornings for several minutes, and tends to subside when the patient walks significant distances; it is aggravated by walking upstairs. Which of the following is the likely diagnosis?

(A) Calcaneal epiphysitis

(B) Lumbar radiculopathy

(C) Osteomalacia

(D) Claudication of the foot

(E) Plantar fasciitis

11 Which of the following statements regarding fibromyalgia (fibrositis) is correct?

(A) In its pure form, NSAIDs are often of benefit.

(B) Affected patients usually have decreased delta-wave sleep on sleep studies.

(C) Affected patients have evidence of neuropathy on nerve conduction studies that is consistent with the paresthesias they report.

(D) Sedimentation rates and C-reactive protein levels are elevated.

(E) Patients demonstrate diffuse joint effusion.

12 A 60-year-old man complains of right hip pain, which has progressed over the last 5 years. There have been no recent falls or trauma. He used to play halfback in football during his high school and college days. He is afebrile and has no visible joint deformities on examination. You note poor right hip abduction and slight pain to palpation. You believe he may have osteoarthritis of his right hip. Which of the following statements regarding osteoarthritis is correct?

(A) Women tend to have fewer joints involved than men.

(B) Patients typically complain of 1 to 2 hours of morning stiffness.

(C) It is more likely to be seen if significant trauma has occurred to the affected joint.

(D) There is usually pain only on active range of motion of the involved joint.

(E) It is always symptomatic with pain, crepitus, and stiffness.

13 You are evaluating the hand and knee x-rays of a 50-year-old woman who complains of pains in these joints. Which of the following x-ray changes would be most consistent with osteoarthritis?

(A) Joint erosions

(B) Osteoporosis of articulating bone

(C) Asymmetrical joint space narrowing

(D) Subperiosteal bone resorption

(E) Calcifications of the hyaline and fibrous cartilage

14 After being started on hydrochlorthiazide, a 60-year-old man complains of bouts of intense pain at the great toe metatarsophalangeal (MTP) joint, and you suspect gout. Which of the following would have to be true in order for you to confirm this diagnosis with certainty?

(A) The pain is located in the first MTP joint.

(B) The patient has an elevated serum uric acid level.

(C) The patient has an erythematous, painful joint associated with a fever and serum leukocytosis.

(D) A 24-hour urine uric acid level is <800 mg/dL.

(E) Aspirated joint fluid shows negatively birefringent, needle-shaped crystals within WBCs when viewed with a polarizing microscope.

15 Which of the following is correct with respect to calcium pyrophosphate deposition disease (CPDD, also known as pseudogout)?

(A) Its incidence is increased with advanced patient age.

(B) The crystals are easier to detect in this disease than in gout.

(C) It may be associated with hypoparathyroidism.

(D) It typically affects only the weight-bearing joints.

(E) Attacks are always monoarticular.

For Questions 16 through 20, match the numbered soft tissue causes of heel pain with the lettered descriptions of clinical presentations.

16 Fat pad atrophy

17 Heel contusion

18 Plantar fascia rupture

19 Posterior tibial tendonitis

20 Retrocalcaneal bursitis

(A) Pain is retrocalcaneal.

(B) Pain is in the inside of the foot and ankle.

(C) There is an intense tearing sensation on the bottom of the foot.

(D) There is a history of trauma.

(E) Pain is in the area of a thinned plantar aspect of the heel.

Examination Answers

1. The answer is E. At the point at which this patient enters the system, the patient presents with a monoarthralgia that may or may not be a monoarthritis. Monoarthritis is defined as arthritis existing in one joint for more than a few days. The first priorities are to obtain a complete history and physical examination in order to ascertain that the pain indeed originates in the (knee) joint. If a determination is made that monoarthritis exists, then plain x-rays and joint aspiration should be obtained, along with basic laboratory studies (complete blood cell count, sedimentation rate, and uric acid level), before a magnetic resonance image study is ordered. Many patients complain of pain in the *regions* of joints whose pains are not truly arthralgias.

2. The answer is D. Gonococcal arthritis is the most common form of nontraumatic monoarthritis. It is three times as common in women as in men. Rheumatoid arthritis may pass briefly through a monoarticular phase but generally affects joints in a symmetrical fashion. Nongonococcal arthritis is most often caused by *Staphylococcus aureus* and is much more destructive to the joint than is gonococcal arthritis. It is also monoarticular in 80% of cases and most often affects the knee. Osteoarthritis of severity to produce an effusion would be unusual in a young woman without significant history of trauma.

3. The answer is A. Monoarticular *septic* arthritis (as opposed to traumatic arthritis or gout, among others) in which Gram-negative or anaerobic bacteria, Lyme disease, or tuberculosis organisms grow from joint fluid, must be investigated for the possibility of immunodeficiency.

4. The answer is B. Radiographic evidence of erosions adjacent to affected joints is present in about 80% of cases of rheumatoid arthritis (RA). The case in this vignette is quite representative of RA in that there is symmetry of involvement of three or more typical joints and morning stiffness (wrists; proximal interphalangeal, MCP, and MTP joints; elbows; knees; ankles) occurring in a female (RA affects females more than twice as frequently as males). Rheumatoid nodules are present in about 50% of cases of rheumatoid arthritis. Uric acid is usually elevated in gout (but not always). There is no association between either uric acid elevation or clinical gout and RA. A WBC count >25,000 in joint fluid is said to be septic arthritis until proven otherwise. Alkaline phosphatase is elevated in the presence of destructive bone lesions; this is not so in RA.

5. The answer is D. COX-2 NSAIDs are not disease modifying, although they are anti-inflammatory as well as analgesic. Each of the other drugs or categories is disease modifying. Other DMARDs besides those mentioned include auranofin, leflunomide, azathioprine, penicillamine, and sulfasalazine.

6. The answer is E, the Schober test. This is a test of mobility of the spine, performed by marking the spinous process of L5 and marking at a point 10 cm above the L5 spine. The patient is directed to bend forward, and the two marks should be observed to move apart by 5 cm or more. Although the test is nonspecific, when back pain exists in the presence of spine immobility and extra-articular manifestations, the Schober test may clinch the diagnosis of ankylosing spondylitis. The differential diagnosis includes, besides ankylosing spondylitis, reactive arthritis (Reiter syndrome), as well as psoriatic arthritis and spondyloarthropathy related to inflammatory bowel disease. Each of the alternate diagnoses mentioned manifests skin findings (circinate balanitis, psoriatic plaques, and erythema nodosum or hypodermal gangrenous, respectively), but skin changes are not found in ankylosing spondylitis. The eponym *Schober test* in this case is more convenient than a descriptive term; therefore, the student will expect to hear mention of the Schober test in practice and training. Spastic paresis or paralysis may result in immobility of the spine, and hence an upper motor neuron sign such as Babinski response to the plantar reflex stimulus. However, this is hardly likely in the vignette presented. The Murphy and Rovsig signs are relevant in the surgical diagnosis of abdominal pain, and the Schirmer test is for adequacy of lacrimal response in the eye (see chapter 27).

7. The answer is A. The retrocalcaneal would be the location of pain in the foot area associated with ankylosing spondylitis. Two common sites of inflammation of the attachment of tendon to bone (enthesitis) in ankylosing spondylitis are the Achilles tendon at the calcaneus and plantar fascia at the calcaneus. Enthesitis occurs also with Reiter syndrome and psoriatic arthritis, but not with sponyloarthropathy related to inflammatory bowel disease.

8. The answer is D. Polymyalgia rheumatica exhibits stiffness in the shoulders or pelvic girdle, fever, normochromic anemia, normal WBC count, and elevated sedimentation rate. The age range of older than 60 years is also typical. RA is within the differential diagnosis but usually occurs in younger people, women more than men. Ankylosing spondylitis is not high on the list of possibilities at this time, as there is no axial involvement. Polymyositis affects the proximal muscle groups and is distinguished by its marked muscle weakness. Gout, of course, is highly improbable with the presentation in the vignette.

9. The answer is B. To test for Ehlers–Danlos syndrome, one should assess for passive hyperextension at the knee, elbow, and MCP joints. There are no characteristic joint deformities or effusions in patients with Ehlers–Danlos syndrome, although many affected patients can develop a secondary osteoarthritis. In fact, the greatest morbidity over time is osteoarthritis.

10. The answer is E. Plantar fasciitis is well described in this vignette. Ten percent of the U.S. population suffers from this malady at some time in their lives. Calcaneal epiphysitis causes heel pain in adolescents but no plantar pain. Lumbar radiculopathy causes referred pain that radiates from the lumbar area to the foot when it is referred to that extent. Referred pain is not aggravated by local factors. Osteomalacia is a systemic disease that causes bone pain in multiple sites and total body weakness. The pain of claudication is made worse by exercise and, when involving the lower extremities, generally is felt in the calf, more than the foot proper. Plantar fasciitis is worst after inactivity, usually improving with usage.

11. The answer is B. Fibromyalgia is a diagnosis of exclusion. The two themes that appear consistently are multiple musculoskeletal pains without weakness and sleep dysfunction. Patients affected with fibromyalgia usually have decreased delta-wave sleep on sleep studies. There is no physical or laboratory evidence of joint inflammation in these patients and no documentable neuropathies, even though patients frequently complain of paresthesias. NSAIDs are only useful if the patient has some superimposed osteoarthritis or other NSAID-responsive condition.

12. The answer is C. Osteoarthritis is more likely to be seen if significant trauma has occurred to the affected joint. Osteoarthritis is frequently asymptomatic for years. The typical stiffness of osteoarthritis lasts less than 5 minutes. Women are more likely to have more severe disease than men, with increased numbness of joints involved and deformities. Both passive and active range of motion produces pain in the involved joint. Osteoarthritis may exist without symptoms. However, such cases have a way of popping into view with precipitating trauma, which may be relatively mild in and of itself. An example might be a man who, in his late fifties, makes a sudden initial movement in a family reunion football game and falls to the ground in pain as a result of osteoarthritis in a knee of which he was previously unaware.

13. The answer is C. Asymmetrical joint space narrowing is a typical x-ray finding of osteoarthritis. Joint erosions are found in RA. Chondrocalcinosis (Choice E) is typical of calcium pyrophosphate deposition disease. Subperiosteal bone resorption is typical of hyperparathyroidism. Bone spurs, joint space narrowing (from loss of articular cartilage) and subchondral new bone formation are also typical of osteoarthritis.

14. The answer is E. In gout aspirated joint fluid shows negatively birefringent, needle shaped crystals within WBCs when viewed with a polarizing microscope. It is true that the vast majority of patients who present with isolated acute first MTP joint pain will have gout. However, such a description of pain is not 100% specific for gout. Many patients have hyperuricemia (from overproduction or underexcretion), and yet never have attacks of gouty arthritis. Septic joints are also erythematous with fever and serum leukocytosis.

15. The answer is A. Its incidence is increased with advanced patient age. CPDD, especially in its idiopathic form, is seen more with increasing age. CPDD is also associated with hyperparathyroidism, gout, hypothyroidism, and hemochromatosis. It is more likely to be polyarticular than gout is, and it does not have a predilection for the weight-bearing joints.

MATCHING THE NUMBERED CAUSES WITH THE LETTERED DESCRIPTIONS

16. Fat pad atrophy: **The answer is E,** pain in the area of a thinned plantar aspect of the heel.

17. Heel contusion: **The answer is D,** history of trauma.

18. Plantar fascia rupture: **The answer is C,** intense tearing sensation on the bottom of the foot.

19. Posterior tibial tendonitis: **The answer is B,** pain in the inside of the foot and ankle.

20. Retrocalcaneal bursitis: **The answer is A,** the pain is retrocalcaneal.

References

Chokkalingam S, Velasquez C, Mody A, et al. Diagnosing monoarthritis in adults: A practical approach for the family physician. *Am Fam Physician.* 2003; 68:83–90.

Cole C, Seto C, Gazewood J. Plantar fasciitis: Evidence based review of diagnosis and therapy. *Am Fam Physician.* 2005; 72: 2237–2242, 2247–2248.

Derk CT, Vivino FB. A primary care approach to Sjogren's syndrome. *Postgrad Med.* 2004; 116:48–65.

Emery Susarez-Almazor ME. Rheumatoid arthritis. *Am Fam Physician.* 2003; 68:1821–1823.

Seigel LB, Gall EP. Approach to the patient with rheumatic disease. In: Rudy DR, Kurowski K, eds. *Family Medicine: House Officer Series.* Baltimore: Williams & Wilkins; 1997: 413–438.

chapter 26

Musculoskeletal Problems in Children

Examination questions: Unless instructed otherwise, choose the ONE lettered answer or completion that is BEST in each case.

1 A 7-year-old boy is brought to your office by his parents with complaint of pain in the right knee whose onset was gradual over the last 3 weeks. It is worsened by athletic play and by kneeling on a hard surface. Upon examination, there is seen to be a tender swelling inferior to the patella. Which of the following statements is true regarding this condition?

(A) Quadriceps exercises are a mainstay of treatment during the acute phase.

(B) There usually is associated knee joint effusion.

(C) This condition is an expression of juvenile rheumatoid arthritis (JRA).

(D) The condition usually remits after fusion of the tibial tubercle with the diaphysis.

(E) The condition is caused by premature closure of the tibial tuberosity with the diaphysis.

2 A 6-year-old boy has developed a limp over a period of 5 days. He appears to be ill and has had a fever with temperatures rising to 102°F. During examination, eversion of the left hip elicits pain. Which of the following is the least logical next step in the disposition in this case?

(A) Open surgical exploration

(B) Determination of complete blood cell (CBC) count and sedimentation rate

(C) Needle aspiration of the left hip joint

(D) Plain x-rays of the left hip

(E) Arthroscopy

3 A 7-year-old boy began limping after exercise several months ago. The parents questioned him at first and he denied pain. Later the boy began complaining of pain in the right hip, and at times the right thigh and knee. Over the past week the pain has been disabling. Vital signs are normal; on examination, the boy is unable to actively abduct and internally rotate as a result of muscle spasm. A CBC count is normal. A plain x-ray shows a "moth eaten" appearance of the femoral epiphysis, flattening of the head, and irregular contours of the acetabulum. Which of the following is the likely diagnosis?

(A) Slipped femoral capital epiphysis

(B) Legg–Calvé–Perthes disease

(C) Septic arthritis of the right hip

(D) Toxic synovitis

(E) Osteomyelitis of the right femur

4 A 4-year-old girl complains of pain in the left hip and is limping as the parents bring her into your office. While you are obtaining further history, the parents mention that the girl is in the second week of a viral upper respiratory tract infection whose onset was about a week before the appearance of the hip pain. There is fever with a temperature of 100.8°F at the time of this appointment (10 AM). The CBC count is entirely within normal limits. Which of the following is the correct diagnosis?

(A) Slipped femoral capital epiphysis

(B) Legg–Calvé–Perthes disease

(C) Septic arthritis of the right hip

(D) Toxic synovitis

(E) Osteomyelitis of the right femur

5 A 14-year-old boy, who is in the early stages of sexual development, complains of left knee pain, developing over a course of 2 weeks. He walks with a limp. On examination his weight is 184 lb (83.4 kg) at a height of 5 ft, 5 in. (1.65 m). He holds his left hip in about 5 degrees of flexion and is unable to fully extend the hip to 180 degrees. He has no constitutional symptoms or signs. The result of a CBC count is unremarkable. A plain posteroanterior x-ray film of the left hip is unremarkable. Which of the following is the most logical next step in obtaining a diagnosis?

(A) Order a lateral view x-ray of the left hip

(B) Order serum level tests of calcium and alkaline phosphatase

(C) Perform left hip joint aspiration

(D) Order a magnetic resonance image of the left hip

(E) Consult a surgeon for arthroscopic exploration of the left hip

6 While examining a female newborn, you perform a Barlow maneuver (attempting to dislocate the newborn's femoral heads interiorly from the acetabulum with your forefinger, while grasping the thigh with your thumb placed on the medial proximal thigh). You sense a clear movement interiorly of the femoral head on the baby's left hip. Each of the following statements is true regarding the condition in the patient in the vignette except for which one?

(A) Female infants are affected more than male infants.

(B) For optimal outcome the condition must be diagnosed and treated before the child reaches the age of 6 months.

(C) There may be a history of this condition in the baby's family.

(D) If the baby is not diagnosed before the age of walking, the baby's gait becomes waddling and the perineum broadened.

(E) The presence of intoeing effectively rules out developmental dislocation of the hip.

7 A 5-year-old girl has complained for 5 months of pain in her left wrist and right second and third metacarpophalangeal joints. This week she complains of photophobia in the left eye. Examination shows the left pupil to be constricted, compared with the right eye. An antinuclear antibody level is elevated. Which of the following is the most likely and most precise diagnosis, given the clinical picture?

(A) Rheumatic fever

(B) JRA, or Still disease

(C) Reiter syndrome

(D) Pauciarticular JRA

(E) Rheumatoid arthritis

8 A young mother brings to you her second child, a male infant of 3 months of age. She is concerned that the baby is consistently found with the head turned to the left and tilted to the right. Upon examination, which of the following is a likely finding?

(A) Passive limitation of motion of flexion and extension of the neck

(B) Limitation of passive motion of turning the head to either side

(C) Upper motor signs in the upper extremities

(D) Palpable mass on the left side of the neck

(E) Palpable mass on the right side of the neck

9 Parents frequently are concerned with "intoeing" in infants. It may be safe to say that parents bring it to their doctors' attention more than the other way around. Being armed with data regarding this complaint makes it much quicker and easier for physicians to manage the families as well as the patients. Which of the following is not true in regard to intoeing?

(A) Metatarsus adductus may be the cause.

(B) Internal tibial torsion may be the cause.

(C) Excessive femoral anteversion may be the cause.

(D) Developmental hip dislocation may be associated with it.

(E) The majority of cases require surgical correction if they have not resolved by the time the child reaches the age of 8 years.

10 A father brings to you a 6-year-old boy who fell onto his outstretched hand while playing at recess in grade school. The boy complains of pain and the extremity manifests swelling in an area just proximal to the wrist. An x-ray done stat in the office building comes back to reveal a buckling of the distal radius, visible in both anteroposterior and lateral views. Which of the following is the best treatment strategy?

(A) Open reduction

(B) Short-arm cast for 6 weeks

(C) Closed reduction followed by casting for 3 weeks

(D) Long-arm cast for 3 weeks

(E) Observation only

Examination Answers

1. The answer is D. The condition is called Osgood-Schlatter's disease and is caused by traction apophysitis of the tibial tubercle. The tibial tubercle becomes enlarged (the apophysis) in a preadolescent boy (more often than a girl) and the unclosed connection to the diaphysis becomes inflamed as a result of microtrauma and traction on the tubercle by the quadriceps apparatus at its attachment; thus, the condition is called a "traction" apophysitis. Quadriceps exercises would likely aggravate the condition in the acute phase, but activity level in general is guided by the symptoms associated; that is, activity is curtailed when it aggravates symptoms. The condition usually remits when the tubercle fuses with the diaphysis, when the child is between the ages of 9 and 15 years. The knee joint is not involved; therefore there is no joint effusion. Osgood-Schlatter's disease is not related to JRA. Because the disease is a result of trauma to an unclosed ossification system, it cannot be a sequela of a lack of closure of tubercle with diaphysis.

2. The answer is A. Open exploration of the hip joint need not be the first move. The differential diagnosis of acute hip pain in a child includes septic arthritis and toxic synovitis, as well as Legg–Calvé–Perthes disease. The most critical in terms of early diagnosis in order to prevent joint destruction is septic arthritis of the hip. All three would present with pain upon hip eversion. The patient with septic arthritis is ill. The first step is aspiration of the joint along with a determination of CBC count and sedimentation rate. The joint fluid is cultured and examined for white blood cells and glucose. In septic arthritis, but not toxic synovitis, there is a leukocytosis and neutrophilia with a left shift. The most common organism involved is *Staphylococcus aureus*. Plain x-rays will pick up osteomyelitis, Legg–Calvé–Perthes disease, and slipped femoral capital epiphysis. While culture and sensitivity are awaited, an empiric choice of antibiotic is started. Only if there is no response within 48 hours need there be an arthroscopic approach to the joint. Open exploration appears to be increasingly less frequently employed.

3. The answer is B. Legg–Calvé–Perthes disease is avascular necrosis of the femoral head. It occurs more often in boys than girls at a ratio of 5:1. Early referral for orthopedic correction is crucial.

4. The answer is D. Toxic synovitis is a self-limited syndrome that often follows an identifiable upper respiratory tract infection. If the course and pain are apparently severe, joint aspiration is indicated but will show only yellow fluid without white blood cells. The peripheral CBC count is within normal limits or presumably may show a relative lymphocytosis as a reflection of the viral infection. Although toxic synovitis occurs more frequently in male patients, it may be found in female patients as well.

5. The answer is A. This boy's hip pain fits the clinical setting of slipped femoral capital epiphysis; he is an obese adolescent boy with late and underdeveloped sexual maturation. The posteroanterior view of the hip may fail to show the displacement of the femoral head posteriorly with respect to the femoral neck. Thus, a lateral view x-ray of the left hip would pick up that abnormality. Calcium and alkaline phosphatase levels are of value in investigating possibilities of destructive lesions of the bone, among other things, but they are not relevant in slipped femoral capital epiphysis. Joint aspiration would not be justified as an early diagnostic step, in the absence of constitutional symptoms and signs. A magnetic resonance image would make the diagnosis but is unnecessarily expensive. Although the problem is treated surgically, an early exploration is not necessary to achieve diagnosis.

6. The answer is E. The described maneuver, the Barlow maneuver, has elicited the diagnosis of congenital hip dysplasia or hip dislocation. The opposite maneuver, that of reduction of the hip dislocation, is called the Ortolani maneuver. If the hip joint is dislocated at the initial examination, the Ortolani maneuver may provide the primary diagnostic sign. Examination for asymmetry of skin folds in the thighs posteriorly was taught on pediatric rotations of old. However, such asymmetry is present in 40% of all (i.e., normal) newborns and thus is not helpful. The congenital hip dislocation may be a cause of intoeing. Female patients are affected more than male patients by a ratio of 6:1. The left hip is affected alone 60% of the time, and in 20% of cases the affliction is bilateral. A positive family history exists in 20% and this serves as a guiding principle for sonographic screening, when present. The sooner the diagnosis is made, the better the ultimate outcome after correction, the best results occurring if the diagnosis is made no later than 6 weeks after the infant's birth.

The waddling gait seen in uncorrected cases is associated with a broadened perineum because of the lateral displacement of the femoral head(s).

7. The answer is D. The onset of fewer than four joints involved in arthritis, within the first 6 months of arthritic pain, is called pauciarticular JRA and carries an increased risk for iritis. A positive antinuclear antibody titer increases the risk. These patients are rheumatoid factor negative. This type of pauciarticular JRA is the foremost cause of blindness in children. These patients need periodic slit-lamp examination by an ophthalmologist. A second type of pauciarticular JRA affects boys between the ages of 8 and 10 years. These boys are antinuclear antibody and rheumatoid factor negative but manifest a high prevalence of human leukocyte antigen, type HLA-B27.

8. The answer is E. A palpable mass will likely be found on the right side of the neck. The mass is a fibrotic area of infiltration in a zone of chronic spasm. The baby has torticollis, caused by spasm of the right sternocleidomastoid muscle, a muscle that causes the head to turn to the opposite side and the neck to abduct to the ipsilateral side. According to pediatric texts, this may be caused by birth injury or cervical spine abnormalities. The course is benign in the vast majority of cases, but if the problem is not treated by stretching exercises or (rarely) surgery, the long-term result may be asymmetry of the face.

9. The answer is E. The statement that "the majority of cases require surgical correction if not resolved by time the child reaches the age of 8 years" is not true in regard to intoeing, though it is relevant that 95% of intoeing cases resolve spontaneously by the time the child reaches the age of 8 years. The most common cause of intoeing is excessive femoral anteversion and it has its onset between the ages of 2 and 3 years. It causes cosmetic and sometimes functional gait changes and may lead to osteoarthritis. As its name would indicate, the intoeing that is due to femoral anteversion is associated with a turning in of the patellae as well as the feet, because the problem exists at the hips. Although most cases will have resolved by the time the child reaches the age of 8, those that do not are best accepted in accommodation, unless the affectation is severe. Osteotomy, the only treatment available, is fraught with complications and thus is extended to only a minority of cases that have persisted to that point. Although three other conditions listed may be causes of intoeing and each has its own pathophysiology and therapeutic approach, each seldom requires surgery. Rarely, cases of developmental hip dislocation occur in association with metatarsus adductus and chances of surgery would depend on timeliness of diagnosis. Metatarsus adductus virtually always resolves by the age of 1 year or later in childhood, and internal tibial torsion responds poorly to any surgical approach. Tibial torsion has usually ceased to be noticeable by the time the child reaches the age of 16 months. If it has not, it may be ameliorated by mechanical devices.

10. The answer is D, long-arm cast for 3 weeks. The fracture described is a torus or "green stick" fracture, seen in preadolescent children. It is well named and refers to the fact that the bone is soft, not brittle, at these ages. Virtually by definition, reduction of any type is unnecessary because there is no separation of fragments and seldom angulation. The immobilization should be standard for the fracture, generally following the rule to include a joint both proximal and distal to the fracture within the cast. However, this immobilization need be only for 3 weeks instead of the usual 6 weeks for most fractures.

References

Eilert RE. Orthopedics. In: Hay WW, Levin MJ, Sondheimer JM, et al. eds. *Current Pediatric Diagnosis and Treatment.* 17th ed. New York: McGraw-Hill; 2005:810–828.

Wenacur R, Tucker JB. Musculoskeletal problems in children. In: Rudy DR, Kurowski K, eds. *Family Medicine: House Officer Series.* Baltimore: Williams & Wilkins; 1997:439–446.

chapter 27

Connective Tissue Diseases

Examination questions: Unless instructed otherwise, choose the ONE lettered answer or completion that is BEST in each case.

1 A 45-year-old woman who has been diagnosed with conjunctivitis twice over the past year and has been frequently complaining of pruritus now complains of a foreign-body sensation in the left eye. Examination discloses corneal ulceration. Her office record also shows that she has complained of various muscular pains over the past year. Which of the following is the most logical first test you might order?

(A) Schirmer test

(B) Antinuclear antibody (ANA) test

(C) Complete blood cell (CBC) count

(D) Serum uric acid

(E) Slit-lamp examination

2 A 25-year-old African American woman living in the Midwest complains of fever, fatigue, malaise, and weight loss over the last 3 months. Lately she has started to have a dry cough. She has never smoked cigarettes. A CBC is unremarkable. A chest x-ray shows bilateral lymphadenopathy and two noncavitating nodules. Which of the following is least likely in the differential diagnosis?

(A) Pulmonary tuberculosis

(B) Histoplasmosis

(C) Hypersensitivity pneumonitis

(D) Pneumococcal pneumonia

(E) Sarcoidosis

3 The patient in Question 2 began to feel significantly better and has been followed for several more weeks. A tuberculosis skin test, repeated after 2 weeks, was negative. The serum calcium is elevated slightly, and in a bronchial lavage specimen the ratio of CD4 to CD8 lymphocytes is 4.0. Now she complains of painful red nodules on her lower legs. Which of the following is the most likely diagnosis?

(A) Pulmonary tuberculosis

(B) Histoplasmosis

(C) Hypersensitivity pneumonitis

(D) Acquired immunodeficiency syndrome (AIDS)

(E) Sarcoidosis

4 A 35-year-old African American woman has complained of weight loss and fatigue for several weeks. In advising her on the phone as to measures to take before her appointment with you the following week, you asked her to keep a record of her temperature four times per day. She arrives for the appointment with the record. She also notes loss of hair and you note her diffusely thinning hair. The temperature graph shows that her temperature has sometimes been as high as 101°F. However, the high points of the daily graphs appear at various times in the early hours of the morning or late mornings, not in the afternoons or evenings. She complains also of arthralgia involving her metacarpophalangeal joints of the first and second fingers bilaterally, with 30 to 60 minutes of stiffness in the morning. A urinalysis yields microscopic hematuria and red cell casts. Which of the following diagnoses is most likely, given the combination of clinical findings?

(A) Chronic glomerulonephritis

(B) Alopecia areata

(C) Lupus erythematosus

(D) Chromic pyelonephritis

(E) Pulmonary tuberculosis

5 Which of the following clinical constellations would make the diagnosis of the case in Question 4?

(A) Elevated sedimentation rate and leukopenia

(B) Hemolytic anemia and positive ANA

(C) Positive lupus erythematosus preparation and false-positive serologic test for syphilis

(D) Positive antibody to double-stranded DNA and positive ANA

(E) Oral ulcers and photosensitivity

6 In lieu of the foregoing, one basis of the diagnosis of systemic lupus erythematosus (SLE) requires the presence of 4 of 11 clinical criteria. Among those are four dermatologic conditions. Each of following is one of the dermatologic criteria, except which one?

(A) Urticaria

(B) Malar rash

(C) Discoid rash

(D) Photosensitivity

(E) Oral ulceration

7 A 35-year-old white woman has had two bouts of pleurisy and a bout of pericarditis, none associated with infection, within 3 months. In addition she manifests a hemolytic anemia with reticulocytosis and leukopenia (3,500 white blood cells/mm^3) on two occasions. You suspect a connective tissue disease and order an ANA test. The result is positive for the homogeneous pattern. Which of the following is the best conclusion to draw from that result?

(A) The patient has SLE.

(B) The patient could have a connective tissue disease or drug-induced SLE.

(C) The patient has had undiagnosed pneumonia.

(D) The patient should be evaluated for mesothelioma.

(E) The patient has a blood dyscrasia.

8 Regarding the patient in Question 7, if the ANA titer were positive with the rim pattern, which of the following conclusions would be the most valid?

(A) The patient has SLE.

(B) The patient could have a connective tissue disease or drug-induced SLE.

(C) The patient has had undiagnosed pneumonia.

(D) The patient should be evaluated for mesothelioma.

(E) The patient has a blood dyscrasia.

9 Each of the following is characteristic of scleroderma, except for which one?

(A) Polyarthralgia

(B) Raynaud phenomenon

(C) Intestinal malabsorption

(D) Positive test for Sm antibodies

(E) Pulmonary hypertension

10 A 33-year-old woman complains of the gradual hardening of her skin, as well as its waxy appearance and feel. She complains also of dysphagia, consisting of a "sticking" sensation in the lower portion of the chest during swallowing, and color changes to her index and middle fingers that manifest, especially during exposure to cold, damp weather, definite lines of demarcation at the proximal interphalangeal joints. First, the color changes to white, then purple, followed by recovery of normal coloration when the extremities are warmed. The hardness involves only the skin of the face and hands. She denies tendon friction rubs. You ordered an anticentromere antibody level that is returned with a positive result. Which of the following is the most likely diagnosis of her condition?

(A) SLE

(B) Diffuse scleroderma (systemic sclerosis)

(C) CREST syndrome (limited scleroderma)

(D) Dermatomyositis

(E) Rheumatoid arthritis

11 A 45-year-old woman complains of difficulty initiating swallowing and increasingly early onset of fatigue of her legs as she climbs stairs and in her arms as she lifts baskets of laundry. She notices skin changes that you see consist of violaceous coloration about the eyes and in the periungual areas that also are manifested over the shoulders and anterior chest. You notice also clubbing of her nails and that she has a cough that she relates to her smoking. Which of the following accounts for her systemic symptoms and rash?

(A) Photosensitivity eruption

(B) Contact dermatitis

(C) Polymyositis

(D) Dermatomyositis

(E) SLE

12 Regarding the patient in Question 11, which of the following most likely accounts for the nail clubbing?

(A) Chronic obstructive pulmonary disease

(B) Reversal of left-to-right shunt through an interventricular septal defect (the Eisenmenger syndrome)

(C) Hepatic cirrhosis

(D) Congenital variant

(E) Lung cancer

13 A 25-year-old man complains of prolonged upper respiratory congestion. You have treated him for sinusitis twice and for otitis media over the past year, although these are the first such occasions he has had these problems in his adult life. This week he complains of redness of the eyes with vascular ectasia that does not move over the sclera the way one notes the conjunctival movement with changes in gaze. Blood pressure levels are normal. You consult by telephone your favorite rheumatologist, who suggests ordering a number of antibody levels. Their results are as follows: ANA, anti-Sm, SS-A, SS-B, and anticentromere, all negative; rheumatoid factor and ANCA (antineutrophil cytoplasmic antibody) positive. Which of the following is the most likely condition to account for the symptomatology?

(A) Wegener granulomatosis

(B) SLE

(C) Dermatomyositis

(D) Systemic sclerosis

(E) Rheumatoid arthritis

For Questions 14 through 18, match the numbered clinical characteristics with the lettered diseases.

14 Formation of sialoliths (salivary duct stones)

15 Nephrocalcinosis

16 Proximal muscle weakness and difficulty in initiation of swallowing

17 Pleural and pericardial effusions

18 Heliotrope rash about the eyes

(A) Sarcoidosis

(B) Sjogren syndrome

(C) Polymyositis

(D) SLE

(E) Dermatomyositis

Examination Answers

1. The answer is A. This patient may well have sicca syndrome and Sjogren syndrome. Her myositis could be one of the many extraglandular manifestations of Sjogren syndrome. It is commonly known by physicians that patients with this syndrome complain of dryness of the eyes, mouth, and other mucosae (sicca syndrome). Dryness of the eye also makes the patient more susceptible to corneal ulcerations and bacterial conjunctivitis. The Schirmer test is simple and available to any primary care office. It consists of laying fluorescein-impregnated filter paper on the lower lid to measure how much the migration of the wetness caused by tears advances in a given time period. Each of the other choices has a place in the evaluation of autoimmune diseases or eye problems but involves expense and, in the case of slit-lamp examination, consultation with an ophthalmologist.

2. The answer is D. Pneumococcal pneumonia is the least likely in a patient with a subacute course such as that presented in the vignette. Each of the other choices is reasonable to consider. Depending on the clinical setting, in addition could be considered beryliosis, aspergillosis, coccidioidomycosis, Wegener granulomatosis, and several other conditions.

3. The answer is E. Sarcoidosis is more common in African Americans and South Asian Indians. Its onset most commonly occurs when a person is between the ages of 20 and 30 years, and it somewhat more likely in women than in men. Of cases, 90% manifest pulmonary involvement: 50% as bilateral hilar adenopathy, 15% as parenchymal infiltrates, and 25% with both types of involvement of the lungs. Skin lesions occur in 25% and erythema nodosa ranks among the most common, with the other rashes including nonspecific macules, papules, patches, and plaques, and a rash called lupus pernio. The appearance of erythema nodosa portends a more favorable prognosis. Hypercalcemia occurs in about 5% of cases, and the CD4:CD8 ratio is greater than 3:4 in bronchial fluid and other involved organs, as opposed to the normal ratio of 2:1. Despite many theories (including one concerning a possible infectious basis), the etiology remains unknown. The disease may involve virtually any organ with granulomatous lesions.

4. The answer is C. SLE occurs in African American women four times as frequently as in white women and twenty-three times as frequently as in white men. The febrile course that does not follow the normal diurnal variation occurs in inflammatory processes not involving response to infection. Eventually, some two-thirds of patients have arthralgia or arthritis. Nearly three out of four have skin manifestations, of which alopecia is fairly common; of course, the facial butterfly rash, not shown in this patient, is a hallmark of the disease. Renal involvement is found in 16% to 38% of cases. Pulmonary tuberculosis not only would manifest pulmonary symptoms but also a febrile course with normal diurnal variation. Although each of the other choices may be characterized by at least one of the clinical findings in the vignette, none except lupus would manifest all of them.

5. The answer is D. Positive antibody to double-stranded DNA and positive ANA together presumably guarantees the diagnosis of SLE. ANA tests are very sensitive but not very specific. ANA is positive in virtually all cases of SLE but are also positive in several other conditions. Double-stranded DNA is very specific for SLE but only 60% sensitive. In addition, the Sm antibody is also very specific but only 30% sensitive. Each of the other choices is highly prevalent in SLE but not in itself diagnostic. It is recommended that any patient who manifests 2 or more of 11 clinical criteria should be tested for ANA and, if the ANA test is positive, then Sm, SS-A, and SS-B antibodies as well. At some point, for example, if three criteria are met, then it may be wise to test for double-stranded DNA or Sm antibody.

6. The answer is A. Urticaria is not listed by the American College of Rheumatology as a dermatologic criterion for diagnosis of SLE, although, given the protean manifestations of SLE, it may result in urticaria as well as many other dermatologic responses in a given case. The malar rash is the famous butterfly rash. It may be flat or raised, and it usually spares the nasolabial folds. The discoid rash is raised and well demarcated, with keratotic scaling and follicular plugging. Photosensitivity is manifested by exaggerated response to sunlight. It may occur after ingestion of certain drugs (e.g., tetracycline) without being associated with SLE. The oral ulcerations are usually painless.

7. The answer is B. The patient could have a connective tissue disease or drug-induced SLE. The homogeneous

ANA pattern is the most common positive form. It is sensitive but not specific for SLE. The homogeneous pattern may be seen in drug-induced lupus, such as that with hydralazine, isoniazid, and chlorpromazine. The patient has 2 of 11 criteria for clinical diagnosis of lupus. To justify a clinical diagnosis of SLE, there must be 4 of the 11 following criteria: Discoid rash; malar rash; photosensitivity; oral ulcers; arthritis; serositis; renal disorder; neurologic disorder; hematological disorder; immunologic disorder; ANA in the absence of drug-induced positivity.

8. The answer is A. The patient has SLE. The rim pattern of ANA is most specific for SLE. SLE with the rim-type ANA is associated with greater risk of renal and neurologic involvement. Also present may be antibodies to Sm, SS-A, and SS-B, which are present in only 10% to 20% of cases but when positive are virtually pathognomonic for SLE and not seen in rheumatoid arthritis, Sjogren syndrome, polymyositis or dermatomyositis, or Wegener granulomatosis.

9. The answer is D. Positive test for Sm antibodies does not occur in either diffuse scleroderma or limited scleroderma. As may be inferred from the discussion of Question 8, the Sm, SS-A, and SS-B antibodies are specific for SLE. Each of the other listed manifestations is present in scleroderma in fairly high prevalence sooner or later in the course of the disease. Arthralgia is common, as is Raynaud syndrome, neither of which is specific for scleroderma. Pulmonary hypertension occurs as a result of the development of pulmonary fibrosis. Malabsorption occurs secondary to atrophy and fibrosis of the intestinal mucosa.

10. The answer is C. The patient has CREST syndrome, sometimes called limited scleroderma; 80% of scleroderma is of the limited type. CREST stands for calcinosis cutis, Raynaud phenomenon (well described in the vignette in the cold-related fingertip changes), esophageal motility, sclerodactyly, and telangiectasia. Note that the esophageal motility affects the smooth muscle, not the striated muscle that is activated in the initiation of the swallowing mechanism. Of interest and usefulness is that 50% of CREST cases are positive for anticentromere antibodies, whereas only 1% of systemic sclerosis and virtually none of the other connective tissue diseases manifest this laboratory abnormality. CREST syndrome, limited scleroderma, carries a significantly better prognosis than diffuse sclerosis. Tendon friction rubs, usually at the wrist, occur with systemic sclerosis but not in the CREST syndrome.

11. The answer is D. Dermatomyositis, of course, is the disease that causes the "heliotrope" violaceous eyes and the similar discoloration of the periungual areas. On occasion the facial rash involvement mimics the malar rash of SLE. However, SLE does not present a rash that involves the other areas listed in the vignette. The myositic aspects of the disease cause proximal muscle weakness and weakness in the voluntary initiation of swallowing. Although dermatomyositis has muscle symptoms similar to those of polymyositis, biopsy shows recognizable histologic differences. In brief, dermatomyositis manifests perivascular lymphocytic infiltrates whereas polymyositis is characterized by lymphocytic infiltration of the endomysium, the delicate reticular fibrils that surround each muscle fiber.

12. The answer is E. Dermatomyositis is associated with a malignancy in 25% of cases. The most common are lung, breast, ovary, and stomach cancer. Given the clubbing of the nails and the smoking history, lung cancer is far more likely in the presence of dermatomyositis than chronic obstructive pulmonary disease. Each of the other choices presented is or can be associated with nail clubbing but is not likely to appear in the scenario presented in the vignette.

13. The answer is A. Wegener granulomatosis is characterized by multiple organ involvement, like so many of the other connective tissue diseases. However, it is important to be able to differentiate this disease from the others because untreated it is generally fatal within a relatively few years. Of the array of antibody levels usually measured whenever testing for connective tissue diseases, the ANCA level is elevated in virtually only Wegener granulomatosis (except for <1% of SLE). ANCA levels are also elevated in Crohn disease. In Wegener granulomatosis the antibody is present in 93% to 97% and not present in polyarteritis nodosa, some of whose histologic features it resembles. Polyarteritis nodosa, present in only 30 people per million, 10% of whom have hepatitis B, is not a primary care entity for practical purposes.

ANSWERS TO THE MATCHING QUESTIONS

14. Formation of sialoliths (salivary duct stones): **The answer is B,** Sjogren syndrome.

15. Nephrocalcinosis: **The answer is A,** sarcoidosis.

16. Proximal muscle weakness and difficulty in initiation of swallowing: **The answer is C,** polymyositis.

17. Pleural and pericardial effusions: **The answer is D,** SLE.

18. Heliotrope rash about the eye: **The answer is E,** dermatomyositis.

References

Gill JM, Quisel AM, Rocca PV, et al. Diagnosis of systemic lupus erythematosus. *Am Fam Physician.* 2003; 68:2179–2186.

Hellmann DB, Stone JH. Arthritis and musculoskeletal disorders. In: Tierney LM, McPhee DJ, Papadakis MA, eds. *Current Medical Diagnosis and Treatment.* 45th ed. New York: McGraw-Hill/Appleton & Lange; 2006:807–864.

Wu JJ, Schiff KR. Sarcoidosis. *Am Fam Physician.* 2004; 70: 312–322.

SECTION **X**

Sports Medicine

chapter 28

Sports Medicine

Examination questions: Unless instructed otherwise, choose the ONE lettered answer or completion that is BEST in each case. Many items found in Tests 23 and 24 pertain to sports medicine as well.

1 A 35-year-old athletic man complains of pain and tenderness at a point just distal to the right lateral condyle. The man is right-side dominant. He was active in "major" sports in his youth but has only recently taken up tennis. His condition may be caused or aggravated by each of the following activities, except for which one?

(A) Grasping and turning a door knob

(B) Driving a screw with a manual screwdriver

(C) Vigorous hand shaking

(D) Using the overhead tennis serve

(E) Employing wrist extension in the tennis backhand stroke

2 An 18-year-old male senior high school athlete has been training hard early in the spring track season. He complains of pain in the left knee region when he runs over a quarter of a mile (0.4 km), and he wishes to have relief so that he may pursue his goal of repeating his performance as district champion in his long-distance event. The pain had a gradual onset and there has been no identifying moment of injury. There is neither morning stiffness nor "gelling" with afternoon inactivity. Each of the following conditions could be a serious consideration as the cause of the symptoms, except for which one?

(A) Iliotibial band syndrome

(B) Rheumatoid arthritis

(C) Anserine bursitis

(D) Popliteal tendonitis

(E) Patellar tendonitis

3 A 15-year-old boy is going out for football for the first time. His pubescence is accelerating and he has grown 3 in. (7.6 cm) in the past year. You are performing a preparticipation sports physical examination. The aortic second sound is louder than the pulmonic second sound, but the P_2 sound is of normal intensity. You hear a systolic "diamond shaped" murmur along the left sternal border. There is neither precordial heave nor thrill. You ask the patient to perform a Valsalva maneuver and find that the murmur is enhanced. You then ask the patient to squat and then auscultate again, only to find that the murmur disappears. He has no complaint of shortness of breath. He manifests no cyanosis or peripheral edema. Which of the following is the likely diagnosis?

(A) Patent ductus arteriosus

(B) Ventricular septal defect

(C) Hypertrophic cardiomyopathy

(D) Pulmonic stenosis (PS)

(E) Congestive heart failure

4 Assume the sports candidate in Question 3 exhibited a different description of cardiac findings as follows: The systolic cardiac murmur was loudest at the upper left sternal border and is heard in the neck and posterior lung fields. Which of the following would be the most important disposition to determine whether this athlete should proceed to participate in high-exertion competitive sports?

(A) Twelve-lead electrocardiogram

(B) Echocardiogram

(C) Right heart catheterization

(D) Computed tomography scan of the chest

(E) Magnetic resonance image of the chest

5 Regarding athletics, what is the main objective of being a physician to athletes and making a preparticipation (medical) evaluation?

(A) To diagnose hypertrophic subaortic stenosis in high-energy-output athletics

(B) To diagnose exercise-induced asthma and significant cardiac conditions that pose a threat to an exertional athlete or one in a sport of high contact

(C) To identify medical threats to an exertional athlete and to recommend techniques of training that would tend to maximize success in athletics

(D) To identify conditions that will place the athlete at risk of exacerbation of an existing illness or injury or at risk of incurring a new problem

(E) To cover the practitioner against liability lest he or she approve for athletic participation an athlete with a condition that might lead to sudden death

6 Which of the following tests is the one in current use to diagnose (illicit) anabolic steroid use in athletics?

(A) Testosterone-to-epitestosterone ratio

(B) Androstendione level

(C) Testosterone level

(D) Estrogen level

(E) Follicle-stimulating hormone level

7 A 20-year-old star receiver for a Big Ten football team with a reputation for heroic catches leaps into the air and outward nearly 90 degrees to his right in order to effect a reception. His body is rotated so that the right shoulder is positioned straight downward. After catching the pass he falls onto his right shoulder and immediately is seen to writhe in pain, which is located in the shoulder area. He misses the next two games because of the pain. There is no sensory component. Hand strength, including intrinsic muscles, as well as elbow flexion and extension are within normal limits. There is an irregularity to the contour of the right shoulder near the humeral head. An x-ray shows no bone fracture but does reveal an abnormality. The patient is able, upon examination, to abduct, albeit associated with pain, to 150 degrees. Which of the following is the most likely diagnosis?

(A) Rotator cuff partial tear

(B) Rotator cuff complete tear

(C) Fracture of the clavicle

(D) Separation of the acromioclavicular joint

(E) Herniated disc at C4

8 Each of the following may be complications of sports-related activity in female athletes, except for which one?

(A) Osteoporosis

(B) Amenorrhea

(C) Anorexia

(D) Stress fractures

(E) Increased risk of coronary atherosclerosis

For Questions 9 through 11, match the numbered grade of concussion with the defined clinical picture, represented by capital letters.

An 18-year-old senior high school football player fails to arise from the field after being struck helmet to helmet by a tackler. The team physician comes immediately to the boy's side and finds him to be apparently confused. The physician diagnoses a concussion. The boy has never suffered a concussion before.

9 Grade 1 concussion

10 Grade 2 concussion

11 Grade 3 concussion

(A) Dazed without other symptoms

(B) Confusion with amnesia <30 minutes, no loss consciousness (LOC)

(C) Confusion with amnesia and LOC <5 minutes, amnesia <24 hours

(D) Confusion with pupil changes

(E) LOC >5 minutes or amnesia lasting >24 hours

For Questions 12 through 14, match the numbered grade of first concussion with the guideline for when to return the athlete to play, represented by capital letters.

12 Grade 1 concussion

13 Grade 2 concussion

14 Grade 3 concussion

(A) Terminate participation; athlete may return to play if asymptomatic for at least 1 week.

(B) Athlete may return to play only if he remains asymptomatic for the following week.

(C) Terminate contest or practice for the athlete and transport him or her to the hospital; the athlete may return to play 1 month after 2 consecutive asymptomatic weeks; conditioning is allowed after 1 asymptomatic week.

(D) Suspend participation for 1 month; athlete may resume participation if she or he remains asymptomatic for 1 week of play.

(E) Terminate season; strongly discourage the athlete from returning to contact sports.

Examination Answers

1. The answer is D. This patient has, of course, lateral epicondylitis, inflammation of the point of the supinator apparatus at the condyle. It is also called "tennis elbow." The latter term refers to the condition's frequent causation by improper backhand motion, invoking wrist extension and supination instead of the whole arm and shoulder in the tennis backhand. In the correct technique the wrist is splinted in the neutral position and the elbow extension is minimized. The professional-style serving motion puts a stress on the medial epicondyle. This inflammatory syndrome is also referred to as "golfer's elbow," as many players' golf swings employ that medial elbow stress as well. The screwdriver, hand shaking, and doorknob motions all invoke the supinator and wrist extension apparatus.

2. The answer is B. The absence of morning stiffness and afternoon gelling rules out rheumatoid arthritis in this patient who has been training hard and whose onset of pain has been gradual and precipitated by running. The other conditions are each subtly different from one another but may all be lumped into the category of overuse syndromes involving the knee. And despite athletes' desires to the contrary, they all require, first and foremost, a period of rest. Iliotibial band syndrome and popliteal tendonitis both cause pain in the lateral aspect of the knee. Patellar tendonitis causes pain in the area of insertion of the quadriceps into the patella (i.e., the pain is located at the superior aspect of the patella). Anserine bursitis results in pain at the location of the anserine bursa, in the inferior and medial aspect of the knee.

3. The answer is C. Hypertrophic cardiomyopathy results in a choking of the aortic outflow tract, more marked when venous return is diminished as when the subject stands erect, and conversely alleviated when venous return is enhanced as when squatting. The latter displaces blood to the upper body, increasing right-sided return and subsequent left-sided return. Patent ductus arteriosus is seldom discovered and corrected later than infancy, and it causes a continuous "machinery type" murmur. The murmur of ventricular septal defect does not change with position change. The murmur of PS would be expected to remain unchanged or perhaps increase with squatting. PS also causes a left precordial click, and often the murmur obscures the P_2 sound. Congestive heart failure causes dyspnea on exertion, orthopnea, or peripheral edema.

Hypertrophic cardiomyopathy (hypertrophic obstructive cardiomyopathy, once called subaortic infundibular stenosis) is an unusual, but not rare, cause of sudden death (sudden cardiac death) during athletic exertion, accounting for half of nontraumatic athletic deaths. Therefore, diagnosis at the time of a preparticipation physical examination is crucial. The patient should be referred for echocardiogram or cardiac evaluation and athletic activity should be forbidden until the condition is ruled out. Risk factors for this condition include family history of sudden cardiac death and history of syncope.

4. The answer is C. Right heart catheterization is needed to determine whether this candidate has pulmonary stenosis, the most common form being valvular stenosis. The criterion that determines whether this person should participate in competitive sports is the pulmonary artery pressure; it should be <75 mm Hg. Each of the other choices renders the diagnosis or results that are compatible with the diagnosis but will not quantify the pressure that establishes the criterion for acceptability. Similarly aortic valvular stenosis with a gradient >40 mm Hg is a contraindication for physically competitive sports. Other cardiac contraindications are hypertrophic obstructive cardiomyopathy, congenital coronary artery anomalies, and cystic medial sclerosis of the aorta caused by Marfan syndrome.

5. The answer is D, to identify conditions that will place the athlete at risk of exacerbation of an existing illness or injury or at risk of incurring a new problem. This is the mission of the preparticipation examination itself. Further, sports medicine implies that one will become a physician to athletes; thus, the second portion of the answer is important as well. The latter concept carries also the responsibility to be aware of and to teach and counsel in techniques for maximizing success and avoiding injury. All other objectives listed are worthy, including medicolegal mindfulness. However, they are overshadowed by the main theme of protection of the athlete from harm.

6. The answer is A. The testosterone-to-epitestosterone ratio is the current clinical test for anabolic steroid use or abuse. The forms of anabolic steroid that are used include androstendione and testosterone (trade name Dianabol).

The follicle-stimulating hormone level is most directly involved in spermatogenesis rather than testosterone.

7. The answer is D. This injury is typical of the acromioclavicular separation and usually results in a visible and palpable nodule that is the lateral end of the clavicle, no longer tucked into the acromion in its normal position. Extremely painful for as long as it takes to heal soft tissue injuries (3 to 6 weeks, depending on the expected load of the tissues in normal function), this injury does not lend itself to surgical correction; surgery would not be considered. A direct blow such as occurred in the vignette could produce a traumatic rotator cuff tendonitis, though abduction of the shoulder would be more severely affected and that injury would produce no visible contour abnormality. Rotator cuff tears do not occur from the forces portrayed here and a complete tear would produce the phenomenon called "the arm drop," inability to maintain abduction to 90 degrees. The blow described could as easily result in a fractured clavicle, though would be unlikely, given the protection of the football pads, besides which the x-ray has ruled out a fracture. A herniated disc would produce referred pain to the shoulder, unassociated with active or passive movements at the joint and nearly always accompanied by sensory symptoms such as hypesthesia and paresthesia.

8. The answer is E. Exercise for female athletes, as for male athletes, is preventive of atherosclerosis (all other variables being controlled); athletics does not pose an increased risk of coronary atherosclerosis. Osteoporosis, eating disorder (anorexia nervosa), and amenorrhea are known as the female athletic triad. Consequently, it may be not surprising that some studies have shown an increased risk of stress fractures out of proportion to expectations, based on types of activities involved.

MATCHING THE NUMBERED GRADE OF CONCUSSION WITH THE LETTERED CLINICAL PICTURE

9. Grade 1 concussion: **The answer is B,** confusion with amnesia <30 minutes, no LOC.

10. Grade 2 concussion: **The answer is C,** confusion with amnesia and LOC <5 minutes, amnesia <24 hours.

11. Grade 3 concussion: **The answer is E,** LOC >5 minutes or amnesia lasting >24 hours.

MATCHING THE NUMBERED GRADE OF FIRST CONCUSSION WITH THE LETTERED GUIDELINES

12. Grade 1 concussion: **The answer is B,** may return to play if remaining asymptomatic for 1 week, so long as he remains asymptomatic for the following week.

13. Grade 2 concussion: **The answer is A,** terminate participation; may return to play if asymptomatic for at least 1 week.

14. Grade 3 concussion: **The answer is D,** suspend participation for 1 month; may resume if the player remains symptomatic for 1 week of play.

Discussion of Questions 12 Through 14

For second and third concussions, the accepted protocols become increasingly restrictive. For grade 1 concussion, second occurrence, the player is kept out of play for 2 weeks, to return only so long as he or she remains asymptomatic for the first week of return play; third occurrence, out for the season, to return to play only if remaining asymptomatic. For grade 2, second occurrence, the player is out for at least 1 month, returning to play if he or she remains asymptomatic for the first week back; for third occurrence, same as for third occurrence grade 1, that is, the season is terminated. For grade 3 concussion, second occurrence, the season is terminated; athlete is permitted return the following season as long as he or she remains asymptomatic. For ease of memory, the season is terminated for third concussions of any grade and for grade 2 second occurrence.

References

Hellmann DB, Stone JH. Arthritis and musculoskeletal disorders. In: Tierney LM, McPhee SJ, Papadakis MA, eds. *Current Medical Diagnosis and Treatment.* 45th ed. New York: McGraw-Hill/Appleton & Lange; 2006:807–864.

Lombardo JA. Sports medicine. In: Rudy DR, Kurowski K, eds. *Family Medicine: House Officer Series.* Baltimore: Williams & Wilkins; 1997:467–480.

Terrell TR, Leski JL. Sports medicine. In: Rakel RE, ed. *Textbook of Family Practice.* 6th edition. Philadelphia: WB Saunders; 2002:845–890.

SECTION **XI**

Other Infectious Diseases in Primary Care Practice

chapter 29

Adult Acquired Immune Deficiency Syndrome

1 A 25-year-old homosexual man comes to a family physician with a concern as to whether he may have acquired immunodeficiency syndrome (AIDS). After taking a complete history, the physician orders a serologic test for the disease, the enzyme-linked immunosorbent assay (ELISA) screening test. Each of the following may be a criterion for making the diagnosis of AIDS, except for which one?

(A) A positive human immunodeficiency virus (HIV) test consisting of Western blot antigen-antibody test after a positive ELISA

(B) A history of a CD4 T-cell lymphocyte count less than 200/μL in an HIV-positive patient

(C) Dementia and weight loss to the point of wasting in a person with positive HIV serology

(D) Pneumocystis pneumonia, central nervous system lymphoma, and positive HIV serology

(E) CD4 lymphocyte count below 14% and positive HIV serology

2 Which of the following carries the highest risk of contracting AIDS?

(A) Insertive vaginal intercourse with a female partner who is HIV positive

(B) Receptive vaginal intercourse with a male partner who is HIV positive

(C) Accidental needle stick with HIV-infected blood

(D) Sharing of needles for illicit drug use

(E) Insertive anal intercourse with an HIV-positive person participating in receptive anal intercourse

3 A 25-year-old male patient presents with fatigue and weight loss and is found to be positive for HIV, confirmed by the Western blot test. His CD4 count is 500/mm³. Which of the following is the least likely cause of his weight loss?

(A) Persistent diarrhea

(B) Tuberculosis

(C) Malabsorption

(D) Kaposi sarcoma

(E) Pneumocystis pneumonia

4 With CD4 counts at or below 50/μL, each of the following infections is found in greater incidence than expected in the general population, except which one?

(A) Disseminated *Mycobacterium avium* complex

(B) Histoplasmosis

(C) Cytomegalovirus (CMV) retinitis

(D) Primary lymphoma of the brain

(E) Hairy cell leukoplakia

5 A 35-year-old homosexual man has been diagnosed recently with AIDS and manifests spotty bilateral sensory and motor symptoms as well as headaches and altered mental status. Blood pressure levels are within normal limits. A computed tomography (CT) scan of the brain shows scattered bilateral cerebral space-occupying lesions that are enhanced with contrast, which are distributed for the most part peripherally. Which of the following is the most likely diagnosis?

(A) Multiple sclerosis

(B) Non-Hodgkin lymphoma

(C) Multiple infarct dementia

(D) Toxoplasmosis

(E) Metastatic cancer to the brain

6 In evaluating an AIDS patient for visual disturbance, you notice perivascular hemorrhages and white fluffy exudates. Which of the following is the most likely cause?

(A) CMV

(B) Cotton wool exudates

(C) Cataracts

(D) Herpes virus

(E) Toxoplasmosis

7 You are examining a male homosexual patient who has just tested positive for HIV infection in the course of addressing his fears of that possibility. The examination is negative except for white exudates in the oral cavity that leave a raw, slightly bleeding base. Which of the following is a clearly relevant statement regarding this patient's physical findings?

(A) He is presumed to have beta-hemolytic streptococcal pharyngitis and should be treated with penicillin V potassium.

(B) The patient has oral herpes simplex related to his immunodeficient status.

(C) The patient has aphthous stomatitis related to his immunodeficient status.

(D) The patient has oral candidiasis that carries no more significance than is otherwise attendant to HIV infection.

(E) The patient has oral candidiasis and this finding is a relatively significant finding, bearing on the prognosis in an HIV-infected patient.

8 Which of the following is typical of the acute, initial infection with the HIV virus?

(A) Folliculitis

(B) Hairy leukoplakia

(C) Kaposi sarcoma

(D) Lymphadenopathy

(E) Vaginal candidiasis

9 Which of the following poses the least likely medium of contagion for HIV?

(A) Saliva

(B) Shared toothbrush

(C) Blood and blood products

(D) Semen

(E) Cerebrospinal fluid

10 A 28-year-old AIDS patient has begun to complain of intermittent difficulty writing clearly and of bouts of confusion interspersed with periods of lucidity. Neurological examination is otherwise unremarkable, as are a CT scan and magnetic resonance image of the brain. Which of the following is the diagnosis?

(A) Lymphoma of the brain

(B) Toxoplasmosis of the brain

(C) AIDS dementia complex

(D) Multiple infarctions of the brain

(E) Alzheimer disease

11 In the measurement of viral loads as they apply to diagnosis and follow-up of HIV infection, each of the following is correct and relevant, except for which statement?

(A) The test is a measure of active and proliferating HIV virus copies.

(B) The measurements correlate with disease progression.

(C) The measurements correlate inversely with response to antiretroviral drug treatment.

(D) The test may become positive prior to seroconversion of an exposed victim.

(E) A test of viral load before treatment that indicates any number of copies present is the equivalent of a positive HIV serological test confirmed by Western blot.

12 A 26-year-old male intravenous drug abuser has been diagnosed with HIV disease by positive ELISA and Western blot tests and a CD4 count of $440/mm^3$. You have treated him for 6 months with zidovudine and didanosine. In addition, you have treated him for oral candidiasis on two occasions. Otherwise, he has felt well except for increased incidence of seborrhea and has continued to work as a buyer for a large department store. Two months ago, he noted 10 to 15 multilocular buttonlike lesions, 2 to 3 mm in diameter, filled with a thick gelatinous substance on the lower abdominal wall, which were popped off easily with a curette. After being fully rid of the lesions for a 6-week period, the patient has experienced a recurrence of the rash. Which of the following is the diagnosis?

(A) Folliculitis

(B) Smallpox

(C) Varicella

(D) Epidermoid cysts

(E) Molluscum contagiosum

13 Each of the following should signal the institution of prophylactic therapy for pneumocystis in an AIDS patient, except which one?

(A) CD4 counts below 250

(B) Presence of oral candidiasis

(C) Weight loss

(D) Persistent diarrhea

(E) CD4 counts below 14% of total

14 You are considering starting antiretroviral therapy in a 30-year-old male patient who is positive for HIV. Which of the following (and note that the answer has changed since the first edition of this book) would warrant initiating such treatment?

(A) Patient asymptomatic: CD4 count of 740/mm^3, and viral load of 1,000 copies/mL

(B) Patient asymptomatic: CD4 count of 1,000/mm^3 (normal), and viral load of 1,000 copies/mL

(C) Patient asymptomatic: CD4 count of <200/mm^3

(D) Acute symptomatic infection with HIV

(E) Patient has a CD4 count of 1,000/mm^3, but a positive ELISA and Western blot confirmatory test

15 Which of the following meets the requirement for positivity when a physician is reading a tuberculin skin test on an AIDS patient?

(A) ≥2 mm

(B) ≥5 mm

(C) ≥10 mm

(D) ≥15 mm

(E) ≥20 mm

16 Given an HIV-positive patient with a positive tuberculosis skin test conversion, how long should isoniazid therapy be given?

(A) Two months

(B) Six months

(C) One year

(D) Two years

(E) Indefinitely

Examination Answers

1. The answer is A. A positive HIV result consisting of Western blot antigen-antibody test after a positive ELISA is validly confirmed positive serological evidence of infection by the AIDS virus, and the person who exhibits this can pass the disease. However, positive HIV serology does not constitute the disease AIDS. Thus, the relative immune deficiency as evidenced by the low CD4 lymphocyte counts (by absolute number or percentage) and the various syndromes portrayed, each of them quite unusual in immunocompetent individuals, serve as criteria for the clinical diagnosis of AIDS. The latter obtains, of course, when the serology is positive as confirmed by the Western blot. Fortunately, early interventional therapy has made it likely that fewer patients will develop the aforementioned criteria. Such therapy includes the antiretroviral agents, especially those regimens that include protease inhibitors and nonnucleoside reverse transcriptase inhibitors.

2. The answer is D. Sharing of needles for illicit drug use carries an approximately 1:150 risk. This presumably assumes repeated sharing but does not presume specific positivity for HIV in a given incident. The only commonly listed behavior that is riskier than sharing needles and other paraphernalia in illicit drug use is receptive anal intercourse with an infected partner. The risk is between 1:30 and 1:100. Insertive vaginal intercourse carries a 1:10,000 risk (i.e., to the male partner) whereas receptive vaginal intercourse carries a 1:1,000 risk (i.e., to the female partner). Accidental needle stick with HIV-infected blood in a hospital setting carries a 1:300 risk of acquiring the virus.

3. The answer is E. Pneumocystis pneumonia does not enter the picture in HIV disease until the CD4 count falls below 250/mm^3, whereas this patient has a CD4 count of 500. Each of the other conditions mentioned may occur as a result of HIV infection at lesser degrees of severity, wherein CD4 counts are less than the nominal 1,000/mm^3 (but more than 250). Other conditions that may be seen with the CD4 count at or below 200 include the following: toxoplasmosis, cryptococcosis, coccidioidomycosis, and cryptosporidiosis.

4. The answer is E. Hairy cell leukoplakia may be found at fairly moderate levels of suppressions of CD4 T lymphocytes (i.e., in the 500/μL range). The other conditions, all being opportunistic infections, though not unheard of in individuals without immune deficiency, are seen in significant prevalence when the CD4 count drops below 50/μL.

5. The answer is D. Toxoplasmosis is the most common space-occupying lesion of the brain that appears as a complication of AIDS. Toxoplasmosis is a protozoan that may infect immunocompetent people in whom the clinical course usually resembles infectious mononucleosis with a limited and benign course. Often in AIDS patients and other immunocompromised individuals, the infection is not a primary but rather a reactivated disease in the face of the AIDS syndrome. Although multiple sclerosis is multicentric, the demyelinating lesions are not space occupying and visible on CT scan. Non-Hodgkin lymphoma is the second most common space-occupying lesion of the brain associated with AIDS. However, lymphoma is usually unifocal rather than multifocal. Multiple infarct dementia occurs in older people and is associated with long-standing hypertension. Metastatic cancer could be confused with the radiographic picture in some cases but would pose the dilemma of accounting for a clinical picture with more than one major diagnosis. In immunocompromised patients this infection must be treated for 4 to 6 weeks after cessation of symptoms. The first drug of choice is pyrimethamine given 25 to 100 mg daily plus sulfadiazine given 1 to 1.5 g four times daily. Folic acid is added to prevent marrow suppression.

6. The answer is A. CMV retinitis occurs in AIDS patients with CD4 counts under 50/μL. It must be treated to reduce the progression of the retinitis and to prevent retinal detachment. Treatment is by antiviral agents, such as ganciclovir, valganciclovir, and foscarnet. Cotton wool spots, different from the white fluffy exudates of CMV recognized by ophthalmologists, are benign and self-limiting.

7. The answer is E. Oral candidiasis is highly suggestive of immunoincompetence. Of interest is that its presence in an HIV-infected person strongly presages progression to AIDS, even correcting for CD4 count. Candidiasis and all the other choices listed are more strongly likely to occur in HIV infection with CD4 counts of 500 or lower, a count not fitting the definition for AIDS. Exudates associated with beta-hemolytic streptococcal pharyngitis do not particularly leave a raw base after removal. The patient did not have cervical adenopathy, but a rapid strep test would nevertheless constitute good practice. The clinical picture does not include a description of herpetic or aphthous ulcers.

8. The answer is D, lymphadenopathy. Fever, lymphadenopathy, sore throat, rash, and headache are typical symptoms of an acute infection with HIV. During the acute phase, none of the stigmatic conditions associated with HIV infection have yet appeared. The other presented entities are seen in later stages of HIV infection.

9. The answer is A. Saliva, a fluid functionally designed for secretion onto the exterior surface, is not an HIV risk unless there is a break in the mucosa that exudes blood into the saliva; thus, the shared toothbrush is a risk. Blood, semen, vaginal secretions, and synovial, pleural, peritoneal, and cerebrospinal fluids are all felt to contain significant amounts of the virus in an infected individual. Urine, saliva, perspiration, and even vaginal secretions normally (i.e., in the absence of contiguous breaks in skin or mucosa) pose little to no risk as media of transmission. Thus, fluids whose normal function is entirely within the body's envelope of skin and mucosae are not normally media of passage of the HIV virus.

10. The answer is C. AIDS dementia complex is a diagnosis of exclusion (see Question 5 and its discussion). Alzheimer disease may remit regarding cognitive changes, but the motor aspects are not likely to change.

11. The answer is E. A count of any number of copies is not necessarily a confirmation of HIV. If the viral load is reported as a low level, say, <500 copies, it may be a false-positive result. All other statements regarding the use and applications of viral load measurements are true.

12. The answer is E, molluscum contagiosum. This benign infection is caused by a member of the parapoxvirus group of the Poxviridae family. Although it may occur in healthy individuals, its recurrence signifies a connection with the underlying HIV infection.

Smallpox no longer exists in the world, so its presence is highly unlikely in this patient. In any event, smallpox presents as a centrifugally distributed rash of unilocular vesicles, is more generalized, and results in severe systemic febrile illness. Varicella is chickenpox, caused by a member of the Herpesviridae family of viruses. Although varicella is a systemic illness consisting of multilocular vesicles (not fitting the description of the lesions in the present case), it is a centripetally distributed rash of many more lesions. Folliculitis is a pustular rash reminiscent of acne. It could occur in patients such as the one depicted here at a rate greater than expected in healthy people, given all that is known, namely positive HIV status with a CD4 count below 500/mm^3. However, it does not fit the description given. Finally, epidermoid cysts are subcutaneous collections of invaginated keratin from the cornified layer of skin, normally sloughed off in bathing. There is a telltale punctum marking the location of each cyst that represents the point of submergent invagination. The material is contained in semimobile pseudocapsules (merely impacted layered keratin and hence the proper generic category, pseudocyst). Such cysts are common in healthy people and are the subject of many minor office procedures for their removal.

13. The answer is D. Persistent diarrhea occurs in patients with a CD4 count of 500 or below whereas pneumocystis disease is found in association with each of the other conditions listed, in particular a lower CD4 count than is necessary for conditions setting the stage for diarrhea caused by AIDS.

14. The answer is C. When the first edition of this book was published, researchers believed that a patient with confirmed positive serological tests for HIV infection should be treated early while he or she was asymptomatic and the CD4 count was within normal limits. This was in the hope that the disease could be eliminated. However, researchers found that such early treatment would not eradicate the infection and drug side effects were often severe, especially the occurrence of lipodystrophy. Currently, it is recommended that treatment be initiated when the CD4 count falls below 200/mm^3 or the HIV-positive patient manifests symptoms of HIV infection (except for the transient lymphadenopathy that occurs shortly after the primary exposure).

15. The answer is B, ≥5 mm. Note the contrast with adults who are not HIV infected and who have no risk factors (prisoners, intravenous drug users), where ≥15 mm is required to be positive.

16. The answer is C. One year is the length of prophylactic antituberculous treatment in an HIV-positive patient presumed to have had a primary exposure in the past, based on a positive skin test. Note that this also differs from non-HIV-infected individuals, in whom treatment would only be indicated for 6 to 9 months.

References

Katz ML, Zolopa AR, Hollander H. HIV infection. In: Tierney LM, McPhee SJ, Papadakis MA, eds. *Current Medical Diagnosis and Treatment.* 45th ed. New York: McGraw-Hill/Appleton & Lange; 2006:1317–1348.

Weinstock MB, Crane R. Adult acquired immune deficiency syndrome. In: Rudy DR, Kurowski K, eds. Baltimore: Williams & Wilkins; 1997:481–500.

chapter 30

Less Common Infectious Diseases in Primary Care

Examination questions: Unless instructed otherwise, choose the ONE lettered answer or completion that is BEST in each case.

1 A 12-hour-old female newborn has begun to exhibit apathy and poor feeding drive. The mother is 16 years old, gravida 1, para 1; she is single and has had no prenatal care. Her membranes had ruptured about 24 hours prior to her reporting to the emergency department of the hospital. On examination the baby seems to be "floppy." A complete blood cell count reveals a leukopenia and absolute neutropenia of <1,000/mL, thrombocytopenia, and elevated C-reactive protein. Which of the following infections is most likely to be the cause of this clinical situation?

(A) *Escherichia coli* sepsis

(B) Group B streptococcus (GBS)

(C) *Hemophilus influenzae*

(D) *Listeria monocytogenes*

(E) Coagulase negative *Staphylococcus aureus*

2 Regarding the patient in Question 1, each of the following is an established procedure for prevention of GBS, except which one?

(A) Vaginal and rectal cultures of the pregnant female patient at 35 to 36 weeks gestation

(B) Institution of gentamicin 2.5 mg/kg every 12 to 24 hours, beginning with labor

(C) Empiric treatment with penicillin G given to the woman in labor, more than 4 hours prior to delivery for any woman whose predelivery vaginal or rectal culture status is unknown

(D) Intrapartum treatment of the laboring mother with penicillin G more than 4 hours prior to

labor if she was positive for GBS at 35 to 37 weeks gestation

(E) Public education to exhort all pregnant women to seek prenatal care as soon as possible after diagnosis of pregnancy

3 A 24-year-old male injection drug user complains of dry mouth, dysphagia, dysphonia, diplopia, nausea, and vomiting. In the past few hours he has noted shortness of breath. He is alert and oriented. His temperature is normal. Breathing appears to be mildly labored and shallow but the lung fields are "clear" to auscultation and percussion. Of the following that are present in the differential diagnosis of this condition, which one is the most likely?

(A) Tetanus

(B) Botulism

(C) Bowel obstruction

(D) Guillain-Barré syndrome

(E) Myasthenia gravis

4 Regarding the 24-year-old male intravenous drug abusing patient in Question 3, assume different symptomatology as follows: Upon further questioning, the patient mentions that his first symptoms were pain and tingling at the site of one of his "skin pop tracks" on his left forearm. This was followed by stiffness of the jaw and dysphagia, and he felt irritable. The patient is alert and oriented with a temperature of 99.8°F but complains of sudden cramping of various muscle groups in response to minimal stimulation; his deep tendon reflexes are uniformly hyperactive; the sensory examination was normal. Which of the following is the most likely diagnosis?

(A) Tetanus

(B) Botulism

(C) Polymyositis

(D) Hypocalcemia

(E) Myasthenia gravis

5 A 50-year-old diabetic man complains of rapidly developing redness of the right (anatomical) leg over a period of 24 hours. You note a tense edematous area extending 10 to 12 cm along the mid right calf and some bulla formation. The man complains of pain that extends several centimeters beyond the area of visible inflammation while noting hypesthesia at the viable site. The area is warm to touch and the patient manifests systemic symptoms consisting of fever (temperature of 100.8°F), diaphoresis, and tachycardia. Which of the following is the most critical diagnostic test at this time?

(A) Culture and sensitivity of the bullae

(B) Blood culture

(C) Complete blood cell count

(D) Venogram

(E) Surgical exploration and biopsy

6 A 9-year-old boy is brought to you with a 2-day complaint of fever, headache, nausea, vomiting, and a macular rash of pink lesions that appears on the palms, soles, wrists, forearms, and ankles. The lesions blanch with pressure. He had been camping with his family in the western states from 2 weeks ago until about 5 days ago. Today he has also begun to complain of headache, cough, and pleuritic chest pain. The boy has had no gastrointestinal complaints. Examination is unremarkable except for the rash. The neck is supple. A complete blood cell count shows thrombocytopenia, hyponatremia, and hyperbilirubinemia, with mostly the indirect-acting type. Which of the following is the most likely possibility to pursue?

(A) Rubeola

(B) Meningococcemia

(C) Rocky mountain spotted fever (RMSF)

(D) Varicella

(E) Typhoid fever

7 Which of the following is an accepted rational therapy of the disease encountered in Question 6?

(A) Penicillin V potassium

(B) Trimethoprim/sulfamethoxazole

(C) Amoxicillin

(D) Doxycycline

(E) Cefaclor

8 A 4-year-old Chinese American boy has had a fever for 5 days, with temperatures running between 100°F and 101°F. Upon examination he manifests conjunctival injection, sore and fissured lips, palmar and solar erythema with desquamation of the tips of one index and one ring finger, transverse grooves in several fingernails, and enlarged cervical lymph nodes. Aside from the lips, the oral examination is unremarkable. Which of the following must be considered?

(A) Roseola

(B) Rubeola

(C) Scarlatina

(D) Erythema infectiosa

(E) Kawasaki disease

9 A 36-year-old man complains of diffuse macular rash, headache, and reddened eyes developing over 3 days. Today his palms and soles show faintly and finely vesicular changes. He complains also of the recurrence over 4 days of soreness and focal redness on the left side of his nose, manifesting a flame-shaped region of erythema involving the left naris. He denies sore throat, and a rapid flocculation test for beta-hemolytic streptococcus is negative. In the past 24 hours he has developed vomiting and diarrhea. Which of the following is the most likely diagnosis?

(A) Scarlatina

(B) Kawasaki syndrome

(C) Secondary syphilis

(D) Toxic shock syndrome

(E) Cirrhosis of the liver

10 A 25-year-old patient known to you is complaining of fever and malaise for 10 days. He complains also of arthralgia and painful violaceous lesions of the fingers and toes. Upon examination you hear a heart murmur that was never mentioned in your notes, including two "complete physicals" over the past 4 years. His temperature is 101.3°F. He is alert but uncomfortable and manifests no neck stiffness. He says that he visited an urgent care center 2 weeks ago and was given a 7-day prescription for azithramycin and for 1 week felt better and was without fever. However, the fever recurred 5 days ago. You discover, with further investigation, that the young man has been using illicit intravenous recreational drugs. Which of the following is likely the cause of this illness?

(A) Acute hepatitis A

(B) Hepatitis B

(C) Hepatitis C

(D) Meningococcemia

(E) Bacterial endocarditis

11 Regarding the patient in Question 10, which of the following is the most likely cause of the condition?

(A) *Corynebacterium diphtheriae*

(B) *H. influenzae*

(C) *Streptococcus viridans*

(D) *S. aureus*

(E) Enterococcus organisms

12 Regarding the patient in Questions 10 and 11, assume the febrile 25-year-old man had additional complaints of cough and pleuritic chest pain and a chest x-ray shows infectious infiltrates in various places in both lungs. Which of the following sites would be most likely to be the seat of the infection?

(A) Deep veins of the thigh

(B) Aortic valve

(C) Tricuspid valve

(D) Mitral valve

(E) Pulmonic valve

13 Each of the following is a special risk factor for infectious bacterial endocarditis, except which one?

(A) Presence of prosthetic heart valves

(B) Previous bacterial endocarditis

(C) Complex cyanotic congenital heart disease

(D) Status 1 year postrepair of ventricular septal defect

(E) Hypertrophic cardiomyopathy

14 A 35-year-old woman complains of a rash of variable lesions, fever, and headache. She had been camping in the New England states and had been in the wilderness for a week without an opportunity to bathe. This occurred about 3 weeks ago. She does not recall any prior skin lesions since the exposure in the field. Examination reveals a generalized rash of red lesions, some annular, some targetlike, some more intense centrally. Which of the following is the most likely cause of these symptoms?

(A) RMSF

(B) Tinea circinata

(C) Rubeola

(D) Secondary syphilis

(E) Lyme disease

15 Regarding the re-emergence of pertussis, each of the following is true, except which one?

(A) The age grouping of victims is distributed from infancy throughout youth and into young adulthood.

(B) The organism can be cultured from the nasopharynx by using a Dacron swab.

(C) Diagnosis can be made within 48 hours of the culture inoculation.

(D) Timely treatment with macrolide antibiotics reduces the severity and length of the period of symptoms.

(E) Pertussis should be considered in any patient whose cough lasts 2 weeks or more.

16 Each of the following is true regarding genital herpes simplex virus (HSV), except for which statement?

(A) Polymerase chain reaction testing is more sensitive than viral culture.

(B) Viral culture is useful in differentiating HSV-1 from HSV-2 infection.

(C) Early therapy with recently developed antiviral agents can cure the disease.

(D) Suppressant therapy can reduce the recurrence rate by 70% to 80%.

(E) Suppressive therapy reduces significantly the risk of heterosexual transmission in HSV-2 discordant couples.

17 A 57-year-old woman who has smoked 2 packs of cigarettes per day for 40 years has developed fever, headache, cough, and anorexia after spending a lot of time in a new casino that opened in a nearby city. Which of the following would support the most likely diagnosis in this patient?

(A) A Gram stain of the sputum that reveals more bacteria than neutrophils

(B) An incubation period of 2 to 4 weeks

(C) Ear pain

(D) Constipation

(E) Serum creatine kinase test

Examination Answers

1. The answer is B. GBS is the most common infection of neonates. It occurs usually quite early after delivery in the form of pneumonia but may be expressed in more subtle clinical form as in this case, with hypotonia and poor feeding. Risk factors include prematurity, delayed delivery after membrane rupture, and GBS infection in the mother. However, infection may occur as late as at 2 weeks. In the latter case, GBS often presents as meningitis. The other organisms among the choices each may be found in the newborn as well.

2. The answer is B. The institution of 2.5 mg/kg of gentamicin, given to the laboring woman every 12 to 24 hours beginning with labor, is an empiric regimen for prophylaxis against neonatal infection in cases in which the risk is high but specific organisms are not known. It usually is used along with ampicillin, in order to cover not only GBS but gram-negative organisms as well. All other methods mentioned are applicable specifically to the prevention of GBS, except that early and faithful prenatal care is preventative against all types of neonatal infection.

3. The answer is B. Botulism is found in essentially three forms: the foodborne form, as in the ingestion of preformed toxin in canned, smoked, or vacuum-packed foods, which is potentially the most acute and deadly form; infant botulism, which occurs when the ingestion of botulinum spores (usually in honey) causes botulinum toxin to be produced in the gastrointestinal tract of infants; and woundborne botulism. The latter is found most often in injection drug users, probably most likely in those cases in which the addict has run out of functional surface veins and resorted to what is known as skin popping. The symptoms are those of anticholinergic poisoning and there is a curarelike affect on skeletal muscles (i.e., flaccid paralysis in the advanced case). Dyspnea is due to paralysis of the diaphragm and intercostal muscles. Tetanus is not characterized by anticholinergic symptoms and muscle tone is heightened, not reduced. Myasthenia gravis and Guillain-Barré syndrome should be considered but not in the context of intravenous drug abuse.

4. The answer is A. This is a fairly typical clinical picture of tetanus. Here, of course, and unlike in botulism, the muscle tone is hypertonic. Sudden uncontrolled spasms are typical of the symptomatology, and spasms of the muscles of mastication give the problem its name, *lock jaw.* Those at greatest risk are elderly persons, migrant workers, newborns, and injection drug users.

5. The answer is E. Surgical exploration, probable debridement, and biopsy are crucial in the clinical picture shown. Narcotizing soft tissue infection, appreciated increasingly in the past 10 years, usually begins acutely, though on occasion over a more prolonged period. Originally thought to be caused by an evolved virulent strain of beta-hemolytic group A streptococcus, it has been found to be due to infections by several monomicrobial organisms, including *S. aureus* and *Clostridium perfringens* (69%). Often there is polymicrobial infection that is due most frequently to *Staphylococcus epidermidis,* beta-hemolytic strep, Enterococcus organisms, *E. coli, Proteus mirabilis, Klebsiella pneumoniae, Pseudomonas aruginosa,* and species of *Streptococcus, Bacteroides, Prevotella,* and *Clostridium,* as well as anaerobic cocci and fungi. Aerobic and anaerobic organisms may be found in combination. Each of the other studies mentioned are relevant but none is diagnostic. The differential diagnosis includes uncomplicated cellulitis caused by group A beta-hemolytic strep and phlebitis. However, because necrotizing soft tissue infection, also called necrotizing fasciitis, is often so devastating in its course, suspicion must yield to surgical debridement. Biopsy permits the diagnosis of the etiologic organisms and of the pathophysiology. When the diagnosis is made, then the cornerstone of success in prevention of deaths and amputations is early debridement.

6. The answer is C. RMSF is a front-running candidate for the cause of the symptoms and signs portrayed in the vignette, on the basis of the rash, headache, and respiratory symptoms. The blanching macular rash evolves into a petechial eruption. The cause is *Rickettsia rickettsii,* a microorganism that is passed through the bite of a tick with an incubation period of 7 to 14 days. The ticks that carry the rickettsiae are *Dermacentor andersoni* in the western states and *Dermacentor variabilis* in the eastern states. A significant minority of patients do not recall the tick bite. There is a 3% to 5% case mortality, more likely in elderly and infirm individuals. About 10% of cases occur without rash. Diagnosis is made by serial serological studies, a process that may take 2 weeks, or by immunofluorescent antibody. The rash of rubeola is morbilliform (i.e., like measles), not macular or petechial. Meningococcemia, because of its seriousness, must be considered. Meningococcemia runs a rapidly progressive course, with central nervous system symptoms beyond the headaches, and exhibits meningismus. Varicella, chickenpox, presents with a centripetal vesicular rash, as opposed to the mostly centrifugal distribution of the rash of RMSF. Typhoid fever is characterized by a rash but nearly always manifests gastrointestinal symptoms, sometimes early constipation but usually evolving into "soupy diarrhea." Diagnosis of meningococcal meningitis is made by spinal tap for identification of *Neisseria meningitidis*, presumptively by smear and definitively by culture.

7. The answer is D. Doxycycline or tetracycline is the treatment of choice for RMSF, even in children. Chloramphenicol is reserved for pregnant women because of the contraindication to tetracyclines. This plan pertains only if typhoid and meningococcus are ruled out clinically or in the laboratory.

8. The answer is E. Kawasaki disease is the only entity among the choices that fits the clinical picture presented. The disease is an inflammatory response to an unknown agent, perhaps a toxin produced by a staphylococcus organism. Asian individuals are more susceptible than other racial groups. Timely diagnosis is important to prevent vasculitides, especially coronary vasculitis that can lead to myocardial infarction. Roseola affects younger children and is characterized by very high fever for several days that breaks precisely as a morbilliform rash appears. Rubeola features high fever, malaise, and the generalized morbilliform rash that appears along with the first symptoms and persists throughout, as do the Koplik spots that are most often seen opposite the second molars or in the vaginal mucosa. Rubella is also called the "3-day measles" and the adenopathy occurs in the retroauricular and suboccipital regions. Scarlatina is "scarlet fever," a group A beta-hemolytic streptococcal infection that releases the erythrotoxin. With the cervical adenopathy and the desquamation of the fingertips, scarlatina must be considered as well, but this can easily be diagnosed as streptococcal disease with the 10-minute flocculation rapid strep screen from the pharynx. Erythema infectiosa, or fifth disease, occurs in infants younger than 2 years of age and is known for the slapped-cheek appearance, caused by a diffuse flush, as opposed to the other rashes described in this vignette. Therapy for Kawasaki syndrome is based on anti-inflammatory modalities, such as aspirin and, in the opinions of some, glucorticoids. Diagnosis is based on fever lasting at least 5 days and satisfaction of clinical criteria as in other inflammatory conditions.

Four of the following clinical criteria must be met: (a) bilateral nonexudative conjunctivitis; (b) mucous membrane changes of at least one of the following types, that is, injected pharynx, erythema, swelling or fissure of the lips, or strawberry tongue; (c) peripheral extremity changes, palmar or solar erythema, desquamation, induration, or Beau's lines (transverse grooves in the fingernails); (d) polymorphous rash; and (e) cervical lymphadenopathy.

9. The answer is D. Toxic shock syndrome now occurs as frequently in nonfemale menstrual situations as in the originally described association with the retained tampon. The vesicular changes of the palms and soles lead to the well-known desquamation seen in the late stages. Toxic shock, which may carry a case mortality as high as 15% as a result of hypotension and heart failure, is due to the toxin elaborated. Thus, early cultures may be unhelpful. Scarlatina may be considered long enough to rule out quickly because the rash of scarlatina is quite different, described as pampiniform (pinpoint red spots). Kawasaki syndrome occurs nearly always in children 5 years old or younger, albeit characterized by desquamation of the palms and soles. Although secondary syphilis manifests palmar and solar changes, they are nonvesicular and consist of macules papules and pustules. Cirrhosis of the liver is mentioned because of palmar erythema seen in the face of patients with advanced compromise of liver function. Again, however, vesicle formation and desquamation is not characteristic of such a situation.

10. The answer is E. Febrile disease associated with a new heart murmur or a changing heart murmur must be considered to be bacterial endocarditis until proven otherwise, by serial blood culture. The disease is also called infectious endocarditis to distinguish it from autoimmune endocarditis. The major risk factors are previous valvular heart disease and intravenous drug abuse. However, neither of the foregoing need be present for there to be bacterial endocarditis. The painful lesions of the fingers and toes fit the description of Osler nodes. Other stigmata of bacterial endocarditis include Janeway nodes (painless erythematous lesions of the palms or soles), splinter hemorrhages of the nails, and Roth spots (retinal exudates). Although the patient is at risk for hepatitides B and C because of his drug abuse history, and thus they should be ruled out in any febrile illness, they do not present with heart murmurs and are not well known for skin lesions. Meningococcemia is unlikely in the absence of meningismus.

11. The answer is D. *S. aureus* causes 60% of endocarditis cases in intravenous drug users. This has effected a change in the overall concepts of bacterial endocarditis over the past 30 years. This likelihood is reinforced by the relatively acute course of the illness in the case presented, as occurs in staphylococcal disease. Staph disease in endocarditis follows a more acute course than *S. viridans* disease; thus, in the past, the synonym for endocarditis was subacute bacterial endocarditis, or SBE. Not only has the epidemic of drug abuse increased the incidence of endocarditis in patients without previous valve pathology, but such endocarditis, acute and caused by Staphylococcus organisms on previously nondiseased valves, also occurs increasingly in hospitalized patients. In the past the organism well known to cause the great majority of cases was *S. viridans*, the organism that causes the green halo of hemolysis on blood agar. This remains the most likely organism isolated in patients with previous valvular defects, such as those with rheumatic heart disease or congenital heart disease.

12. The answer C. The tricuspid valve is the one most often involved in intravenous drug abuse and, as a right-sided lesion, is apt to loose septic emboli. Deep venous thromboembolic disease may result in pulmonary emboli as well, but the patient is not febrile and the emboli are not; hence, they show up as radiographic densities after a period of delay, rather than seen as infectious infiltrates.

13. The answer is D. The presence of a ventricular septal defect (as well as atrial septal defect) is a risk factor for bacterial endocarditis, but the risk has disappeared 6 months after clinically satisfactory repair. Each of the other conditions is a risk factor (mitral valve prolapse) associated with a murmur (but not mitral valve prolapse with a click if unassociated with a murmur).

14. The answer is E. Lyme disease. Classically, lyme disease consists of three stages. Stage 1 features flulike symptoms (arthralgia, headache, malaise, and weakness) and the typical single skin lesion of erythema migrans at the site of the tick bite. Stage 2, after a latent period, features a rash similar to the one described here and systemic symptoms similar to those of stage 1. Stage 3, after a greatly varying prolonged asymptomatic period, ranging from months to years, features synovitis, arthritis, central nervous system impairment, dermatitis, keratitis, and neurologic and myocardial abnormalities. Stage 3 greatly resembles an autoimmune mechanism. An important point is that a great percentage of cases do not follow this neatly described sequence. Moreover, a significant proportion of afflicted patients give no history of a tick bite. Stage 2 disease may be seen quite early; erythema migrans may not occur or go unrecognized.

15. The answer is C. Diagnosis of pertussis cannot be made within 48 hours of the culture inoculation, though culture is taken from the nasopharynx. Direct fluorescent antibody testing is not available for rapid diagnosis as of this writing. The culture requires at least 7 days for reporting out. All other statements given are true. Although approximately 29% of cases occur in the classic age group, infancy, the remainder are spread throughout all age groups and 20% are found in people over the age of 20 years. Timely treatment with macrolide antibiotics reduces the severity and length of the period of symptoms. In the milieu of 2007, pertussis should be considered in any patient whose cough lasts 2 weeks or more.

16. The answer is C. Early therapy with recently developed antiviral agents cannot cure the disease. HSV remains an incurable disease. Polymerase chain reaction testing is 95% sensitive but not in general use, mostly because of the costs incurred. Viral culture, when positive, is useful in differentiating HSV-1 from HSV-2 infection but is only 70% sensitive. Suppressant therapy, ongoing therapy from any of a number of antiviral agents (e.g., acyclovir, famciclovir, or valacyclovir), can reduce the recurrence rate by 70% to 80% and can also significantly reduce the risk of heterosexual transmission in HSV-2 discordant couples.

17. The answer is E. A recent review of the literature indicates that, of all the common laboratory studies usually performed, only an elevated creatine kinase level separates the other pneumonitides from Legionnaire. This is a typical presentation of Legionnaire disease. A cough may be nonexistent or mild compared to the remaining clinical picture, including chest x-ray. The incubation period for Legionnaire disease is only 2 to 10 days. Diarrhea, not constipation, is an associated finding. Ear pain from an associated otitis media can be seen with mycoplasma pneumonia and even with some streptococcal infections but is not typical of Legionnaire disease. Many more neutrophils than bacteria are usually seen in Gram stains from patients with Legionnaire disease. Anorexia, myalgia, and hyponatremia are also frequently seen. Treatment is accomplished with the macrolides and rifampin.

References

Bauman JG. Genital herpes: A review. *Am Fam Physician.* 2005; 72:1527–1534, 1541–1542.

Bratton RL, Corey GR. Tick-borne disease. *Am Fam Physician.* 2005; 71:2323–2330, 2331–2332.

Campos-Altcalt D. Practice alert—Pertussis: A disease re-emerges. *J Fam Practice.* 2005; 54:699–702.

Chambers HF. Infectious diseases: Bacterial and chlamydial. In: Tierney LM, McPhee SJ, Papadakis MA, eds. *Current Medical Diagnosis and Treatment.* 45th ed. New York: McGraw-Hill/Appleton & Lange; 2006:1400–1442.

Haddy RI. Less common infectious diseases in primary care. In: Rudy DR, Kurowski K, eds. *Family Medicine: House Officer Series.* Baltimore: Williams & Wilkins; 1997:501–512.

Headley AJ. Necrotizing soft tissue infections: A primary care review. *Am Fam Physician.* 2003; 68:323–328.

Moran A, Shandera WX. Infectious diseases: Viral and ricketsial. In: Tierney LM, McPhee SJ, Papadakis MA, eds. *Current Medical Diagnosis and Treatment.* 45th ed. New York: McGraw-Hill/ Appleton & Lange; 2006:1349–1399.

SECTION **XII**

Endocrinology in Primary Care

chapter 31

Diabetes Mellitus

Examination questions: Unless instructed otherwise, choose the ONE lettered answer or completion that is BEST in each case.

1 A 55-year-old obese male patient, known to have diabetes type II, is found to be stuporous after complaining of lethargy for 2 days during a bout of gastroenteritis in which he passed between six and eight loose stools per day. A hemoglobin A1C level taken 2 weeks before was 7.5%. His blood sugar is 600 mg/dL; serum acetoacetate and beta-hydroxybutyrate are normal and serum osmolality is 310. The blood urea nitrogen (BUN) level is 110 mg/dL. Which of the following is the best description of the patient's condition?

(A) Diabetic ketoacidosis (DKA) precipitated by viral infection

(B) Hyperosmolar state precipitated by noncompliance with the antidiabetic medication regimen

(C) Hyperosmolar hyperglycemic state (HHS) precipitated by dehydration

(D) Hyperosmolar state precipitated by acute renal failure

(E) Hyperosmolar state precipitated by inadequate blood sugar control

2 Which of the following statements about the HHS is true?

(A) It carries a mortality rate considerably lower than that of DKA.

(B) It is known for a significant anion gap.

(C) The major precipitants are medication noncompliance, ethanol, and cocaine use.

(D) The presence of gastroparesis effectively rules out hyperosmolar state in favor of ketoacidosis and diabetes type I.

(E) The most rapidly effective therapy is insulin.

3 Which of the following families of oral agents applicable to diabetes type II can facilitate weight loss?

(A) Sulfonylurea agents, such as glyburide

(B) Biguanides, metformin

(C) Nonsulfonylurea secretogogues, such as repaglinide

(D) Thiazolidinediones ("glytizones"), for example, pioglytizone

(E) Alpha-glucosidase inhibitors, such as acarbose

4 A 47-year-old 257-lb (116.4-kg) man whose height is 5 ft, 7 in (1.7 m) has been followed for type II diabetes for the past 2 years. His treatment has consisted of escalating institutions and additions of, first, 10 mg to 20 mg of glyburide; 500 mg to 2 g of metformin daily; and 4 mg of pioglitizone daily. During that time his weight has increased from an initial level of 215 lb (97.4 kg) 2 years ago to the present weight given here. His latest hemoglobin A1C level was 8.5%. He now complains of burning pains in his legs and feet and asks why that would be so and what should be done about it. In order for you to address the base cause, which of the following is the most clearly relevant information?

(A) The pains are caused by noncompliance by the patient.

(B) The pains are caused by ischemic peripheral vascular disease.

(C) The pains are a side effect of the metformin.

(D) The pains are caused by long-standing hyperglycemia.

(E) The pains are caused by lumbar radiculopathy.

5 In performing a routine periodic history and physical examination on a 56-year-old Mexican woman who weighs 175 lb (79.3 kg), you included a glycohemoglobin (HbA1C) study to supplement a complete blood cell count, comprehensive metabolic panel, and fasting lipids. Her fasting glucose level was 115 mg/dL and a 2-hour postprandial blood sugar level was 160 mg/dL. BUN and creatinine levels are normal. The complete blood cell count shows a hemoglobin level of 8 g/L and a hematocrit measure of 31. The HbA1C level was 5.9% (normal is ≤6%). Which of the following factors *does not* explain a lower than expected HbA1C?

(A) Thallassemia

(B) Recent blood loss

(C) Patient's diabetes is not severe enough to create a sustained level of hyperglycemia.

(D) A hemoglobin variant that coelutes with hemoglobin A

(E) Hereditary spherocytosis

6 Which of the following list of factors is included by both the World Health Organization and the Adult Treatment Panel III in defining metabolic syndrome X?

(A) Waist circumference, serum triglyceride level, high-density lipoprotein cholesterol (HDL-C) level, blood pressure, and fasting glucose level

(B) Triglyceride level >150 mg/dL, HDL-C level <40 mg/dL, blood pressure of >130/85

(C) Triglyceride level >150 mg/dL, HDL-C level <35 mg/dL, waist-to-hip ratio >0.9, blood pressure >140/90

(D) Central obesity, Type II diabetes mellitus, and hypertension

(E) Dyslipidemia and diabetes mellitus

7 A 45-year-old type II diabetic patient weighing 240 lb (109 kg) at a height of 5 ft, 10 in. (1.77 m) has not lost weight as mandated by his physician. Recently a co-worker underwent leg amputation as a result of uncontrolled diabetes. Now the patient is newly motivated to lose weight and wishes to review the correct diet for control of his diabetes. Which of the following is the correct diet for control of his diabetes, assuming he has stable weight?

(A) An intake of 3,000 cal as 412 g of carbohydrate (CHO), 113 g of protein, and 113 g of fat

(B) An intake of 2,000 cal as 250 g of CHO, 75 g of protein, and 75 g of fat

(C) An intake of 1,700 cal as 233 g of CHO, 64 g of protein, and 64 g of fat

(D) An intake of 1,200 cal as 164 g of CHO, 45 g of protein, and 45 g of fat

(E) An intake of 800 cal as 100 g of CHO, 40 g of protein, and 30 g of fat

8 Regarding the patient in Question 7, you realize that he should also lose a significant amount of weight in order to facilitate control of his diabetes, perhaps reducing or even reversing the clinical presence of the disease. Thus, you set a course for him to lose 1 lb (0.453 kg) per week. Which of the following would be an appropriate diet to meet the patient's foregoing needs?

(A) Intake of 3,000 cal as 412 g of CHO, 113 g of protein, and 113 g of fat

(B) Intake of 2,000 cal as 250 g of CHO, 75 g of protein, and 75 g of fat

(C) Intake of 1,700 cal as 233 g of CHO, 64 g of protein, and 64 g of fat

(D) Intake of 1,200 cal as 164 g of CHO, 45 g of protein, and 45 g of fat

(E) Intake of 800 cal as 100 g of CHO, 40 g of protein, and 30 g of fat

9 A 25-year-old female type I diabetic comes to you for the first time after moving into the area. She takes NPH human insulin (NPH Humulin, Lilly), 26 units in the morning and 13 units in the evening. You ask her to keep records of home glucose monitoring four times per day for 2 weeks and to return then with the record. You find that blood sugar levels are 110 to 120 mg/dL fasting, 100 to 110 before the noon meal, and 150 to 160 before the evening meal, subsiding to 80 to 90 before bedtime. The HbA1C level taken at the first visit was 7.5%. You consider adding a fast-acting insulin after the noon meal. Which of the following is the fastest acting insulin among those listed?

(A) Regular human insulin

(B) Ultralente human insulin

(C) Lantus insulin

(D) Lispro insulin

(E) Protamine zinc insulin

10 A 16-year-old girl, who weighs normally 140 lb at a height of 5 ft, 8 in., is brought to you with complaints of weight loss, increasing fatigue, thirst, and polyuria accelerating over the past 3 weeks. Her blood sugar is 450 mg/dL and serum bicarbonate level is 19 mmol. You hospitalize her and start fluid therapy (1 L of normal saline for the first 90 minutes), after a 20-unit bolus of regular human insulin and slow infusion of regular insulin at 10 units/hour until the blood sugar has fallen to 250 mg/dL. After slowing the progress of remission, adding 5% dextrose in half-normal saline (0.45% NaCl) intravenously, you find that she emerges from acidosis and is ready for discharge home after 36 hours. Her premorbid weight was 120 lb

(54.4 kg) at a height of 5 ft, 4 in. (1.63 m). Which of the following insulin daily dosages would be the most reasonable for an initial regimen?

(A) 120 units daily

(B) 60 to 120 units daily

(C) 27 to 54 units daily

(D) 25 units daily

(E) 15 units daily

11 Assuming the insulin chosen for use in the patient in Question 10 is a combination of human insulin (e.g., Humulin), both short (R) and intermediate (N) acting, what is the most currently accepted method of dosing the insulin subcutaneously (i.e., short of continuous pumped infusion)?

(A) The day's requirements injected each morning as human N

(B) The day's requirement in the morning as two-thirds human N and one-third human R

(C) The day's requirement as two-thirds of the human N and one-third of the human R requirement in the morning and one-third of the human N and two-thirds of the human R before dinner

(D) The day's requirement as three-fourths of the human N and three-fourths of the human R requirement in the morning and one-fourth of the human N and one-fourth of the human R before dinner

(E) Two-thirds of the daily dosage in the morning as two-thirds human N, one-third human R and a second dose before dinner consisting of the remaining one-third of the day's requirement as two-thirds human N and one-third human R

12 In evaluating a patient regarding his renal status, you now estimate the progress of disease by noting the results of the 24-hour urine collection just received. Which of the following findings in the 24-hour urine specimen should command the most attention in evaluating this patient's renal status?

(A) 10 mg albumin/dL

(B) 295 mg albumin/24 hour

(C) 500 mg protein/dL

(D) Positive urine culture

(E) 3.5 g of protein/24-hour urine output

13 A 35-year-old woman, gravida 3, para 2, is in her 25th week of pregnancy. Although her weight is normal for her period of gestation, her mother has type II dia-betes, as does an older sister who is overweight. She undergoes the 1 hour, 50-g glucose tolerance test and the blood sugar at 1 hour is 155 mg/dL (8.6 mmol/L). You decide to place her on a limited carbohydrate diet in order to prevent the complications in diabetic progeny such as macrosomia and neonatal hypoglycemia. Which of the following ranges is considered the minimum necessary to prevent such complications?

(A) ≤105 mg/dL

(B) ≤190 mg/dL (10.5 mmol/L)

(C) ≤165 mg/dL (9.2 mmol/L)

(D) ≤145 mg/dL (8 mmol/L)

(E) ≤73 mg/dL (4 mmol/L)

14 The patient in Question 13 was treated with diet therapy alone for 3 weeks. You now check her home blood sugar recordings to assess the degree of success on this regimen, and you are prepared to start insulin if control of the diabetes is not satisfactory. At which of the following fasting and 2-hour postprandial limits would you start insulin therapy?

(A) ≤75 mg/dL fasting, 95 mg/dL at 2 hours

(B) ≤105 mg/dL fasting, 120 mg/dL at 2 hours

(C) ≤120 mg/dL fasting, 150 mg/dL at 2 hours

(D) ≤150 mg/dL fasting, 160 mg/dL at 2 hours

(E) ≤100 mg/dL fasting, 105 mg/dL at 2 hours

15 Diabetologists consider three stages of glucose tolerance or intolerance. Which of the following fasting blood sugar levels fits the definition of impaired glucose regulation (vs. normal or diabetes mellitus)?

(A) >90 mg/dL

(B) ≥100 mg/dL

(C) ≥110 mg/dL

(D) ≥140 mg/dL

(E) ≥200 mg/dL

16 A 16-year-old girl who is known to be a type I diabetic has gone through a period of rebellious denial and stopped taking her insulin 7 days ago. Now she is feeling very thirsty and frightened. She wishes to resume her diabetes management. She is alert. Which of the following laboratory findings would indicate that it is safe to manage her case outside the hospital?

(A) Serum bicarbonate level of 10 to 15 mEq/L

(B) Arterial pH of 7.25 to 7.30

(C) High level of beta-hydroxybutyrate; alert patient

(D) Blood sugar of ≤250 mg/dL

(E) Urine ketones positive; alert patient

17 A 36-year-old male insulin-dependent diabetic of 15 years complains of blurred vision in his left eye. You discover that he did not keep his ophthalmologist's appointments over the past 3 years. The eye chart shows his near visual acuity to be 20/50 OS and 20/20 OD; his far visual acuity is 20/40 OS and 20/25 OD. One year ago his visual acuity was 20/25 OU far and 20/20 OU near. Random blood sugar was 130 by finger-stick performed by the office nurse as the patient entered today. A hemoglobin A1C level drawn last week was 8.5%. Which of the following pathophysiologic mechanisms is the cause of this condition?

(A) Retinal surface proliferative changes impede light transmission to the retina.

(B) Microaneurysms interfere with retinal function.

(C) Dot hemorrhages interfere with retinal function.

(D) Cotton-wool exudates interfere with retinal function.

(E) Changes in average blood sugar affect refraction density of the aqueous fluid.

18 For the patient in Question 17, you order a serum creatinine test and 24-hour urine test for creatinine and for total and complete protein. The patient's height is 6 ft, 1 in. (1.85 m) and he weighs 180 lb (81.6 kg). From these data you calculate a creatinine clearance of 50 mL/hour. Each statement is relevant regarding this finding, except for which one?

(A) Closer blood sugar control is indicated.

(B) Among cases of this condition, more are caused by type II diabetes than by type I.

(C) Blood pressure control is important.

(D) Pharmacological means to raise the glomerular filtration rate is indicated.

(E) Dietary protein control is indicated.

Examination Answers

1. The answer is C. HHS precipitated by dehydration is the best description of the pathophysiology of this patient's condition. Required for this development is type II diabetes, a measure of at least temporary poor control, and a clinical stimulus for dehydration. DKA, found virtually only in type I diabetes, is ruled out by the lack of ketosis. The hyperosmolar state is certainly somewhat related to diabetes control, but the latter is not the proximate cause. In the present case, dehydration would have been caused by the gastroenteritis. Even egregiously noncompliant or poorly controlled patients seldom develop the hyperosmolar state. The BUN of 110 mg/dL is common in the hyperosmolar state and does not denote renal failure. The azotemia will respond to aggressive fluid and electrolyte repletion therapy.

2. The answer is C. The major precipitants of HHS, though the final common pathway is dehydration, are medication noncompliance and ethanol and cocaine use. Although it has been written that "causes" include myocardial infarction, stroke, hyperthermia and hypothermia, pulmonary embolus, and many other diseases, no one develops HHS who does not have a type II diabetic diathesis. According to the article by Stoner cited in the references, the case mortality of this syndrome is greater than that of DKA. A significant anion gap is more characteristic of DKA and infarct is not a particular characteristic of HHS. Though gastroparesis is generally thought of as a complication of type II diabetes, it may be found in HHS during the acute phase when dehydration is marked. Because the basic pathophysiology of HHS is dehydration, that is, neither hyperglycemia per se nor acidosis, the quickest response is fluid therapy while using modest means to reduce the blood sugar level, which will fall even without insulin as fluid and sodium repletion proceeds.

3. The answer is B. Only the biguanides, of which the only presently approved example is metformin, facilitate weight loss while reducing blood sugar without stimulating insulin production. It accomplishes the latter by decreasing hepatic glucose production, mainly through reduction of gluconeogenesis. Because of its ability to reduce blood sugar without stimulating insulin production, it functionally reduces insulin resistance. Sulfonylurea agents decrease blood sugar levels by stimulating production of insulin (i.e., they are secretogogues for insulin), hence contributing

to higher insulin levels and ultimate exhaustion of the beta cells of the pancreas. Nonsulfonylurea secretogogues work similarly to sulfonylurea secretogogues but more rapidly. Thiazolidinediones enhance insulin sensitivity by activating a nuclear transcription factor and modulating many genes that regulate carbohydrate metabolism. The net effect is to increase insulin sensitivity. Alpha-glucosidase inhibitors work by delaying intestinal absorption of carbohydrates and thus reducing postprandial glucose levels. Their effectiveness is not impressive and the side effect of flatulence has made the agent acarbose less popular with time.

4. The answer is D. The pains are caused by long-standing hyperglycemia. The patient has diabetic neuropathy (i.e., neuropathy did not cause the pains; the pains were evidence, part and parcel, of diabetic neuropathy). The United Kingdom Prospective Diabetes Study Group results published in four separate journal articles (two in *Lancet* and two in the *British Medical Journal*, all in 1998) showed for type II diabetes the same as the DCCT Group showed for diabetes type I (*Diabetes Care*, 1996); that is virtually all the complications of diabetes, particularly neuropathic complications, are preventable by strict control of blood sugar. Thus, control of diabetes is the route to prevention of complication. Although noncompliance contributes to poor diabetes control, it is neither the direct nor proximate cause.

5. The answer is D. A hemoglobin variant that coelutes with hemoglobin A apparently constitutes an additional substance with an affinity for glucose as the red cell is formed, thus causing a falsely elevated HbA1C level. HbA1C elevation is 91% specific and 85% sensitive. False low levels can be caused by conditions associated with shortened red blood cell life, such as hemolytic anemias (e.g., thallassemia and spherocytosis), or in which red cells are disproportionately recently extruded from the marrow, as in recovery from recent blood loss. Finally, of course, hyperglycemia must be persistent enough to affect a significant proportion of the red cells as they are newly created; that is, the diabetes must be of adequate severity to result in elevation of the HbA1C level. Hemoglobin A1C is but one of three A1 hemoglobins. The other two, hemoglobins A1a and A1b, involve phosphorylated glucose and fructose, respectively. They are not measured in clinical medicine.

6. The answer is A. The point of the question is to show that, although there may be differing opinions and details in varying definitions as to what constitutes the metabolic syndrome, qualitatively, there is wide agreement; waist circumference (related to hip circumference), serum triglyceride level, HDL-C level (HDLC), blood pressure, and fasting glucose are listed in the definitions of metabolic syndrome X by both the World Health Organization and Adult Treatment Panel III. These items constitute risk factors that tend to occur together in the same individuals and families, such as dyslipidemia, hypertension, and diabetes. Obviously, the definition is thus arbitrary. However, all agree that insulin resistance exists and that it is characterized by increased central obesity, elevated triglyceride levels, decreased HDL-C levels, tendency to or existing hypertension, and some degree of compromised glucose tolerance. Of greatest clinical significance is that the syndrome in full expression presents an array of vascular risk factors. Diagnosis neither requires all the elements to be present nor needs to be official in order for the syndrome to be treated by diet and medications as appropriate to management of the separate disease manifestations. Each of the other choices as answers to the question is relevant to the syndrome, but few choices are present in all cases.

7. The answer is C. The correct maintenance diet for diabetes (or for anyone) is based on the following information. At 70 in. (1.77 m) of height, the patient's ideal weight is 106 lb (48 kg) + 6 lb (2.7 kg) for each inch over 5 ft (1.52 m), or 100 lb (45.3 kg) + 5 lb (2.3 kg) for each inch over 5 ft (1.52 m) for women; for the patient in this vignette, this is 166 lb (75.2 kg). Total maintenance caloric requirement is ideal weight in pounds × 10 = (rounded), or 1,700 calories for this patient. Of these calories, 55% should be in carbohydrates, that is, 935 cal. Grams of CHO = 935/4 cal/g, or 233 g. Of the calories taken in, 15% should be in protein (1,700 × 0.15), that is, 255 cal; grams of protein = 255 cal/4 cal/g, or 64 g. This leaves 30% of calories, or 510 cal, to be consumed as fat: 510 cal/8 cal/g = 64 g.

8. The answer is D. To lose 1 lb (0.453 kg) per week, a fairly ambitious plan, requires a deficit of 3,500 cal per week, or 500 cal per day. For this patient we begin with his maintenance needs and subtract 500 cal per day, from the 1,700-cal maintenance diet, to result in a 1,200-cal diet, allocated in the same proportions of CHO, protein, and fat as in the maintenance diet. Thus, a 500 cal/day dietary deficit of which 55% are CHO = 275 cal/4 cal/g = 69 g of CHO subtracted from the 233 g, which is 164 g of CHO in the reduction diet. Subtracting the calories as protein leads us to 500 cal, of which 15% = 75 cal/4 cal/g = 19 g to be subtracted from 64 g of protein in the maintenance diet, or 45 g of protein. Finally, 30% of the calories to be subtracted

out are in fat or 500 cal × 0.3 = 150 cal/8/cal/g = 19 g of fat to be subtracted from 64 g of fat, or 45 g of fat content in the reduction diet. The final product is 1,200 cal as 164 g of CHO; 45 g of protein; and 45 g of fat.

Another method, assuming 1,200 cal is the target reduction diet for this patient, is to work directly on that starting figure: 1,200 cal as 55% CHO (660 cal/4 cal/g = 165 g); 15% protein (180 cal/4 cal/g = 45 g); 30% fat (360 cal/8 cal/g = 45 g of fat).

9. The answer is D. Lispro insulin is the most rapidly acting, commencing to function in the blood within less than 30 minutes. Package insert instructions state that this injectable insulin should be given either with or immediately after a meal. In the case presented in the vignette, lispro is chosen to cover immediately the blood sugar "spike" after the noon meal. Because the HbA1C was not in the optimal zone (normal is <6%) the lispro insulin could be added as opposed to supplanting an equal number of units of NPH human insulin. That said, it should be started at a low number of additional units out of prudence, say, 2 to 3 units for a brief trial period. Regular insulin is the insulin with next most rapid action, followed by NPH ultralente, Lantus, and, the longest of all, protamine zinc insulin.

10. The answer is C; giving 27 to 54 units daily fits the guideline of 0.5 to 1 unit of insulin/kg. Thus, 120 lb/2.2 = 54 kg.

11. The answer is E. The most conventional method of insulin delivery for the patient in Question 10 is two-thirds of the daily dosage in the morning as two-thirds human N, one-third human R and a second dose before dinner consisting of the remaining one-third of the day's requirement as two-thirds human N and one-third human R. For the 140-lb pound (63.6 kg) person in Question 10, we might have chosen a starting dosage of 45 units/day (in the range given, 0.5 to 1 units/kg/day). Thus, 30 units would be given in the morning as 20 units of human N, 10 units of human R, and the 15 units in the evening would be given as 10 units of human N, 5 units of human R. The evening dose is given generally before dinner, but may be further divided on certain occasions by some practitioners, depending on the patient's individual needs, by administering the second human R insulin before dinner and the second human N insulin at bedtime.

12. The answer is B; 150 to 300 mg albumin/24 hours is the earliest diabetic clinical sign of diabetic nephropathy coming after the initial formation of Kimmelstiel–Wilson basement membrane lesions in the glomeruli. Note the distinction between protein and albumin in this definition: Microproteinuria is defined in milligrams per 24 hours of albumin, a component of urinary protein. This amount on a single voided specimen is as little as 20 mg/dL on urinalysis. A similar but only slightly more liberal figure is 200 to 500 mg/24 hours, employed in hypertensive renal disease. The definition of nephrotic syndrome is 3.5 g/24 hours. Renal parenchymal tissue can be preserved by dietary protein restriction to 0.75 to 1 g/kg of body weight, closer glycemic control, and close blood pressure control if hypertension coexists.

13. The answer is A; $\leq$105 mg/dL (5.8 mmol/L) is the accepted level above which the blood sugar in a 50-g 1-hour glucose tolerance test, done at 24 to 28 weeks of pregnancy, should call for aggressive diet therapy for diabetes. Generally, although some feel that sulfonylurea agents are safe for the fetus, most believe that if dietary therapy alone does not control diabetes in pregnancy, the next level of therapy is insulin.

14. The answer is B. Blood sugar reaching above 105 mg/dL fasting or 120 mg/dL at 2 hours are two criteria for starting insulin therapy for gestational diabetes if dietary therapy does not yield the results stipulated in the discussion for Question 13.

15. The answer is C; $\geq$110 mg/dL ($<$125 mg/dL) is the level above which a patient is considered to have impaired glucose regulation. This may appear to be an academic exercise because any patient with prediabetes, diabetes, or simply harboring risk factors for diabetes deserves qualitatively similar therapeutic approach. However, research has been devoted to the prevention or delay of the onset of diabetes type II and has shown that the stage of impaired regulation yields success through lifestyle change that rivals that of metformin.

16. The answer is B. An arterial pH level of 7.25 to 7.30 is only mildly depressed and is compatible with an alert person in early DKA. At this level of acidosis the patient may be managed as an outpatient. A moderately acidotic pH level is defined as 7 to 7.224 and severe is defined as $<$7. Urine ketones would be positive in all three degrees of severity. Similarly, hydroxybutyrate might be elevated to high levels in all three categories of severity, and blood sugar levels above 120 mg/dL are to be found in all three categories. Bicarbonate levels of 10 to 15 mEq/L are in the moderately acidotic category and $<$10 is considered severe. Mild DKA is reflected by a bicarbonate level of 15 to 28 mEq/L.

17. The answer is A. Retinal surface proliferative changes are directly related to visual loss (and distinctly so compared with the other factors mentioned). The fact that the visual loss is unilateral (OS = left eye) and that random blood sugar determination is nearly normal rules out a change in refraction brought about temporarily by hyperglycemia. The elevated glycolated hemoglobin allows the inference that long-term control, however, has been less than optimal. Thus, the patient likely suffers from retinopathy. Such retinopathy occurs in approximately one-half of all diabetics after 10 years of living with type I disease and after a variable duration in type II. This retinal lesion is the reason that diabetes is the leading cause of blindness in the United States. For this reason the standard of care is for routine ophthalmologic examination scheduled annually after 5 years of disease or after a proliferative lesion has been seen. The other changes, that is, microaneurysms, dot hemorrhages, and cotton-wool exudates, as well as hard exudates, are commonly seen in diabetes; microaneurysms are virtually pathognomonic of the disease, but no authors have stated that they are causes of blindness. Finally, if the doctor does not know for 3 years that the patient has not seen the ophthalmologist, then the doctor is remiss unless the patient has failed to return for primary care follow-up as well.

18. The answer is D. This man's creatinine clearance is significantly less than would be expected for a man of his age and size. If this problem is not acted upon, he is likely to be headed ultimately for endstage renal disease. One-third is the approximate proportion of cases of endstage renal disease that are caused by diabetes. The following table puts diabetes, hypertension, and renal disease into a perspective of their clinical interaction.

Diseases	Percentage
Diabetes mellitus	31
Hypertension	27
Glomerulonephritis	14
Obstructive uropathy	5.7
Polycystic renal disease	3.6
Others	5.7
Unknown	13

Used with permission from Rudy and Kurowski (1997). The diseases listed in the left column are responsible for the corresponding percentages of endstage renal disease.

References

Kimmel B, Inzucchi SE. Oral agents for type 2 diabetes. *Clin Diabetes*. 2005; 23:65–75.

Masharani U. Diabetes mellitus and hypoglycemia. In: Tierney LM, McPhee SJ, Papadakis MA, eds. *Current Medical Diagnosis and Treatment*. 45th ed. New York: McGraw-Hill/Appleton & Lange; 2006;1194–1239.

Rudy DR. Hypertension. In: Rudy DR, Kurowski K, eds. *Family Medicine: House Officer Series*. Baltimore: Williams & Wilkins; 1997:513–544.

Stoner GD. Hyperosmolar hyperglycemic state. *Am Fam Physician*. 2005; 71:1723–1730.

Turok DK, Ratcliffe SD, Baxley EG. Management of gestational diabetes. *Am Fam Physician*. 2003; 68:1967–1972, 1075–1076.

Tzagournis M, Rudy DR. Diabetes mellitus. In: Rudy DR, Kurowski K, eds. *Family Medicine: House Officer Series*. Baltimore: Williams & Wilkins; 1997:513–542.

chapter 32

Thyroid Problems in Primary Care

Examination questions: *Unless otherwise instructed, choose the ONE lettered answer or completion that is BEST in each case.*

1 In screening for primary thyroid disease (hypothyroidism or hyperthyroidism), which of the following serum tests is the most sensitive?

(A) Free tetraiodothyronine (FT_4)

(B) Tri-iodothyronine (T_3) resin uptake

(C) Total tetraiodothyronine (T_4)

(D) Thyroid-stimulating hormone (thyrotropin, or TSH)

(E) Antithyroglobulin antibodies

2 A 25-year-old woman complains of fatigue and cold intolerance increasing over the past 3 months. On examination she manifests a somewhat dry skin, which she says is a change from her usual. She admits to being puzzled and saddened over the situation. Her apical heart rate is 68 in a regular rhythm. Blood pressure is 110/68. The TSH level is 0.3 μIU/mL (0.4 to 4.8). She gives a further history of being on bromocriptine for a microprolactinoma. Which of the following is the likely cause of her condition?

(A) Hashimoto thyroiditis

(B) Panhypopituitarism

(C) Secondary hypothyroidism

(D) Primary hypothyroidism

(E) Primary hyperthyroidism

3 A 45-year-old white woman is undergoing a routine annual preventive health examination. After reviewing the routine mammogram and before performing the routine breast and pelvic examination, you proceed to a head-to-toe brief physical examination. You discover a palpable thyroid nodule that seems to be about 2.5 cm in diameter. Which of the following blood tests would be the most logical, in addition to certain routine medical profiles?

(A) Serum lipids

(B) Free T_4 and TSH

(C) Protein-bound iodine

(D) T_3 resin uptake and total T_4

(E) Timed Achilles heel reflex

4 The results of routine testing of the patient in question 3 are FT_4, 3 ng/dL (0.2 to 2.1) and TSH, 0.2 μIU/mL (0.4 to 4.8). Which of the following would be the next most logical action?

(A) Order serum antithyroperoxidase antibodies

(B) Order exploratory surgery of the thyroid

(C) Order a bone scan for metastatic lesions

(D) Order sodium iodide I^{123} thyroid uptake

(E) Perform a fine-needle aspiration (FNA) biopsy

5 Regarding the patient in Question 3, if the thyroid function studies had indicated a euthyroid state, what would be the best next action?

(A) Order serum antithyroperoxidase antibody test

(B) Order exploratory surgery of the thyroid

(C) Order a bone scan for metastatic lesions

(D) Order I^{123} thyroid uptake

(E) Perform FNA biopsy

6 A 25-year-old woman manifests a single palpable nodule and it has tested out to be euthyroid by FT_4 and TSH. An FNA biopsy is planned. Her mother inquires as to which of the results would be most favorable if the finding were to be cancer. Which of the following is the least aggressive thyroid cancer?

(A) Papillary thyroid carcinoma

(B) Follicular thyroid carcinoma

(C) Medullary thyroid carcinoma

(D) Anaplastic carcinoma

(E) Metastatic melanoma

7 Regarding the patient in Question 6, the diagnosis is found to be follicular carcinoma. A decision is made that I^{131} will be employed in the treatment of the cancer. Which of the following must be accomplished in order to maximize the effect of therapy in obliterating primary, residual, and metastatic disease?

(A) Treat with beta-blocking agents to prevent thyroid storm

(B) Treat with levothyroxine for enough time to increase metabolism to a point where the I^{131} may have the greatest effect

(C) Complete a course of glucocorticoids

(D) Render the patient hypothyroid

(E) Perform an excisional biopsy to verify the findings of the FNA biopsy

8 Each of the following clinical or laboratory findings may be found as statistically more likely in hypothyroidism, except which one?

(A) Hyponatremia

(B) Amenorrhea

(C) Menorrhagia

(D) Delayed recovery of deep tendon reflexes

(E) Onset of obesity

9 A 25-year-old woman, gravida 1, para 0, is in her eighth week of pregnancy when she reports to you for referral for an obstetrician. She is known to be hypothyroid and is taking 100 μg of levothyroxine daily. Each of the following statements is relevant and true regarding pregnancy and hypothyroidism, except for which one?

(A) Maternal hypothyroidism is a risk for fetal central nervous system development in the second trimester.

(B) Dosages of thyroid hormone adequate to control TSH at normal levels in the pregravid state are satisfactory for continuation during pregnancy.

(C) TSH should be monitored regularly during pregnancy associated with primary hypothyroidism.

(D) The fetal thyroid is not completely developed until term in pregnancy.

(E) The increased level of estrogen in pregnancy causes an increase in thyroid-binding globulin.

10 You have been following a 45-year-old man for hypothyroidism for the past 2 years without significant complaints. He was prescribed 100 μg of levothyroxine 1 year ago, when the diagnosis was made, and his TSH fell to normal levels at the 3-month and 6-month visits. He returns for a routine annual recheck and manifests a normal blood pressure and apical heart rate of 80, regular. As he has a family history of adenomatous colon polyps, you arrange for colorectal cancer screening annually this decade. Then you draw routine fasting lipids because he has gained 5 lb (2.26 kg) during the past year and also draw in the same specimen serum TSH. The test results return normal except for TSH, whose level is 6.2 μIU/mL (normal is 0.4 to 4.8). Each of the following may constitute explanations for this finding, except which factor?

(A) Failure of patient to comply with the prescribed dosage of levothyroxine

(B) Inadequate dosage of levothyroxine prescribed

(C) The prescribed levothyroxine is malabsorbed.

(D) The patient has secondary hypothyroidism.

(E) There may be a comorbid autoimmune condition.

11 A 45-year-old white woman complains of an 8-lb (3.6-kg) weight loss, despite eating normally, if not more than her usual amount, over the past 3 months. She admits to being more irritable than is her custom. Upon examination she exhibits a stare and lid lag. The thyroid gland is diffusely palpable. Her skin is moist and velvety and her peripheral and apical pulses are identical: 104 and regular. Blood pressure is 140/60. Her deep tendon reflexes are uniformly hyperactive, including the presence of the Hoffman reflex bilaterally. Which of the following combinations of test results distinguishes this as thyroiditis as opposed to primary hyperthyroidism?

(A) Suppressed TSH, elevated FT_4, abnormally low I^{123} uptake

(B) Suppressed TSH, elevated FT_4, elevated I^{123} uptake

(C) Elevated TSH, elevated FT_4

(D) Suppressed TSH, normal FT_4, normal T_3

(E) Suppressed TSH, elevated FT_4

12 Which of the following is the most likely precipitating cause of hyperthyroidism in an iodine-deficient patient (or iodine-deficient geographic area)?

(A) Toxic nodule

(B) Hashimoto thyroiditis

(C) Iodine ingestion or injection

(D) Prior treatment with beta-blocking agents

(E) Treatment with lithium

13 A 55-year-old white woman has noted for the past month an increasing tightness in her neck when wearing certain high-buttoned clothing. The thyroid gland is diffusely palpable, somewhat enlarged, and finely nodular. She denies changes in heat or cold tolerance; her vital signs are unremarkable and there are no other physical findings. TSH and FT_4 levels are within normal limits. Which of the following is the most logical next step among those mentioned?

(A) FNA biopsy

(B) Temperature graph recorded at home, to be returned in a week

(C) Serum T_3 determination

(D) Open biopsy

(E) Serum antithyroglobulin test

14 A previously healthy 35-year-old man complains of painful neck for the past 2 weeks, along with malaise and night sweats. In addition he notes increased nervousness and irritability. He manifests a sinus tachycardia at 108 beats per minute. He denies treatment for cancer and human immunodeficiency virus (HIV) disease and risk factors for HIV. The thyroid is diffusely palpable and mildly tender. The eyes exhibit a mild stare but exophthalmos is not present. The TSH level is 0.2 μIU/mL (0.4 to 4.8) and the FT_4 level is 3 ng/dL (0.9 to 2.1). A radioactive iodine (RAI) uptake and scan shows a very low uptake. Which of the following is the diagnosis?

(A) Graves disease

(B) Riedel struma

(C) Hashimoto thyroiditis

(D) Ludwig angina

(E) Subacute thyroiditis

15 Which of the following is the most reasonable therapeutic approach for the patient in Question 14, at the present time?

(A) Institute methimazole treatment as 30 mg daily by mouth

(B) Start propylthiouracil 300 mg daily

(C) Start propranolol 20 mg daily

(D) Treat with I ^{131}

(E) Consult and arrange for subtotal thyroidectomy

16 The patient in Question 14 has responded symptomatically to the treatment prescribed and returns for a third follow-up visit in 3 months. Now, however, he complains of decreasing energy and increased sleep requirements. His skin is dry and the eyes mildly "puffy" compared with his former appearance, even before the acute phase of the recent illness. Each of the following statements regarding this development is true except for which one?

(A) The patient's case has evolved into hypothyroidism.

(B) Treatment of this condition will remain in place for life.

(C) This complication occurs in nearly one-half of patients.

(D) The patient may, at a later date, develop hyperthyroidism.

(E) A significant proportion of patients with this condition will have persistent elevations of antithyroperoxidase antibodies.

17 A 35-year-old woman enters your office complaining of a 20-lb (9-kg) involuntary weight loss over a period of 4 months. At 5 ft, 4 in. (1.63 m), she weighs 110 lb (50 kg), down from her usually stable weight of 130 lb (59 kg). Her skin is moist and velvety in texture. Her sclerae are visible above her corneae and she shows an asymmetrical ocular proptosis. Her thyroid gland is diffusely palpable and nonnodular. She is at risk for each of the following diseases, except which one?

(A) Alopecia areata

(B) Diabetes mellitus type I

(C) Vitiligo

(D) Coronary atherosclerosis

(E) Adrenal insufficiency

18 Regarding the patient in Question 17, which of the following tests is most specific for the disease represented in the vignette among those mentioned?

(A) Antithyroperoxidase antibody

(B) Antithyroglobulin antibody

(C) Antinuclear antibody

(D) TSHR-Ab [stim] test

(E) Serum FT_4

19 The patient in Question 17 appears to be agitated. Her heart rate is 125 and regular and her blood pressure is 150/60. She has had three children, the youngest of whom is 10 years old. Which of the following is the *least* favored choice of treatment for this woman, assuming she wants no more children and is not pregnant?

(A) Methimazole

(B) Propythiouracil

(C) I^{131}therapy

(D) Thyroidectomy

(E) Short-term propranolol

20 A 45-year-old white man complains of weight loss for several weeks and his wife complains that he often sets the heating system down, a change from his prior comfort zone in which the two had always had agreement. He has lost weight from his usual 185 lb (84 kg) at 5 ft, 10 in. (1.78 m) to 165 lb (74.7 kg) over the past 3 months. His wife reminds him that while they were living in another city several years ago, he was diagnosed as having a goiter, which was treated with thyroid hormone but his prescription lapsed after they had moved and he had not sought further treatment. His thyroid gland is enlarged and palpably nodular in both lobes. Examination of his eyes externally is normal. This entity is preceded by which of the following conditions?

(A) Single "cold" thyroid nodule

(B) Single "hot" thyroid nodule

(C) Autoimmune thyroiditis

(D) Nontoxic multinodular goiter

(E) Factitious hyperthyroidism

21 Regarding the patient in Question 20, which of the following is the most likely treatment of choice?

(A) Respective surgery

(B) I^{131} therapy

(C) Propylthiouracil

(D) Methimazole

(E) Propranolol

Examination Answers

1. The answer is D. TSH, sensitive assay, is the most sensitive screening test for overactive and underactive thyroid disease. Although not a direct measurement of metabolism, as total and free T_4 (tetraiodothyronine) and T_3 (tri-iodothyronine), the TSH responds in suppression before T_3 and T_4 begin to rise in hyperthyroidism and by elevation before T_3 and T_4 begin to fall. Obviously, in both the foregoing instances the patient would be asymptomatic.

2. The answer is C, secondary hypothyroidism. Abnormally low or suppressed TSH occurs most often in Graves disease or other forms of primary hyperthyroidism, as a result of suppression by the feedback on excessive circulating thyroid hormones. However, this patient manifests symptoms and signs of hypothyroidism rather than thyrotoxicosis. Abnormally low TSH occurs, of course, in hypopituitarism as well, causing secondary hypothyroidism. In this case, rather than panhypopituitarism, the patient most likely has secondary hypothyroidism that is due to suppressed TSH as a side effect of bromocriptine. Hashimoto thyroiditis presents in several phases but generally results in the long term in primary hypothyroidism, with TSH elevation.

3. The answer is B. Free T_4 and TSH are generally thought of as constituting the best combination of initial tests of thyroid physiology. TSH is the most sensitive screen for both hyperthyroidism and hypothyroidism. Free T_4 is the metabolically active form of tetraiodothyronine, which in turn accounts ultimately for the overwhelming proportion of hormone output by the gland, with tri-iodothyronine accounting for the remainder. I^{123} thyroid uptake is unnecessarily involved for an initial investigation of the activity status of the thyroid gland, if the TSH is suppressed and the FT_4 is elevated. Protein-bound iodine is an outmoded test for thyroid hormone activity, being directly related to the T_4 content. It is no longer in use because not only is it not a direct measurement of hormone, but it also is subject to too many inaccuracies. Similarly, the Achilles tendon reflex exhibits time of recovery inversely related to the state of metabolism regulated by the thyroid. It too has inadequate sensitivity and specificity. T_3 resin uptake is an indirect measurement that has also fallen out of use, in favor of the free T_4 and TSH.

4. The answer is D. I^{123} thyroid uptake is indicated in a solitary palpable thyroid nodule with hyperthyroid functional status. The rachorodine radioidine (RAI) uptake can distinguish a hot nodule from an incidental or cold nodule in a hyperthyroid gland.

5. The answer is E. FNA biopsy is indicated for most solitary nodules, the exception being a hot nodule, as judged by the I^{123} thyroid uptake and scan. This is the only way to rule out carcinoma, short of open exploration.

6. The answer is A. Papillary thyroid carcinoma is the least aggressive and happily the most common, comprising 76% of all thyroid cancers. Follicular thyroid carcinoma is the most well differentiated of the thyroid cancers; the second most well differentiated is papillary carcinoma. Medullary carcinoma of the thyroid occurs equally frequently in male and female individuals, whereas anaplastic carcinoma occurs 56% of the time in female individuals. Follicular carcinoma constitutes 16% of all thyroid carcinomas. Because of good differentiation, follicular carcinoma is also amenable to I^{131} therapy after total thyroidectomy. To a lesser degree, this applies to papillary carcinoma as well. Patients with medullary carcinoma have a 6% chance of dying of the disease; those with follicular carcinoma have a 24% chance of dying of the disease. Although papillary carcinoma is the least aggressive, it tends to be multifocal and presents frequently with lymph node metastases. These, however, tend to respond to I^{131} therapy.

7. The answer is D. Rendering the patient hypothyroid before instituting I^{131} produces an elevation in TSH. TSH then acts on the thyroid cells, including the well-differentiated malignant cells, to stimulate them to take up the iodine, including I^{131}. Often and especially in the case of follicular carcinoma, this is effected by a surgical thyroidectomy that precedes I^{131} therapy. The distracters are clinically nonsensical as far as this author knows.

8. The answer is E. Contrary to popular lore, hypothyroidism, although rendering it more difficult to lose weight because of reduced basal requirements, does not cause true obesity. Along with reduced basal energy requirements, the appetite appears to be reduced proportionately. Each of the other choices is well known to be powerfully associated with hypothyroidism except for amenorrhea. Conventional wisdom as taught to medical students is that thyrotoxicosis is associated with oligomenorrhea or amenorrhea whereas hypothyroidism is associated with menorrhagia. Actually, either amenorrhea or menorrhagia may be found in hypothyroidism. Thus, any form of menstrual irregularities warrants routine thyroid function studies.

9. The answer is B; this is the incorrect statement. Dosages of thyroid hormone adequate to control TSH at normal levels in the pregravid state are *not* satisfactory for continuation during pregnancy. Thyroid replacement dosages (T_4) are increased in pregnancy by an average of 36 μg in absolute terms or by 47%. This is due to many causes, but the most significant appears to be the increase in thyroid-binding globulin effected by the higher levels of estrogen evoked during pregnancy, serving to reduce free T_4 levels. This physiological phenomenon also explains why thyroid-replacement dosages are reduced after delivery, after cessation of estrogen therapy, and after menopause. The fetal thyroid begins development at about 18 weeks of pregnancy but requires full-term incubation to be fully formed. Fetal hypothyroidism has a potentially devastating effect on infant central nervous system development. Likewise, inadequately treated maternal hypothyroidism can retard fetal central nervous system development. Consequent to the foregoing, the TSH should be monitored every 4 to 6 weeks during pregnancy.

10. The answer is D: "The patient has secondary hypothyroidism" is an incorrect statement. Secondary hypothyroidism occurs as a result of failure of the pituitary gland, specifically, inadequate TSH production, and hence it manifests lower than normal TSH levels, not elevated levels. Each of the other choices results in elevated TSH in primary hypothyroidism. Malabsorption of thyroid medication can occur because of concurrent administration of binding substance, sprue or diarrhea of any kind, or bile acid-binding agents like cholestyramine. However, in Choice E, the elevation is spurious and could occur also in relative secondary hypothyroidism (i.e., where TSH, though inadequate, could be responsive enough to be elevated) or in euthyroid states. Thus, in some autoimmune conditions, false elevations of TSH may occur through interference with the laboratory assay.

11. The answer is A. Suppressed TSH, elevated FT_4, and an abnormally low I^{123} uptake are typical of acute thyroiditis. However, for confirmation, thyroglobulin should be checked and found to be elevated. Otherwise, the diagnosis may be hypermetabolism caused by exogenous thyroid

hormone. Acute thyroiditis causes a release of thyroid hormone resulting in a suppression of TSH, all of which occurs in the absence of active production of hormone by the parenchyma; thus, there is no increase and may be a decrease in I^{123} uptake. Choice B, suppressed TSH, elevated FT_4, and increased I^{123} uptake, is typical of primary hyperthyroidism. If the increased uptake is diffuse, the picture is that of classical Graves disease. A nodular I^{123} uptake scan result may be multiple in toxic multinodular goiter or single in the case of a toxic adenoma. Choice C, elevated FT_4 and elevated TSH, assuming no spurious cause of TSH elevation, can occur only in secondary hyperthyroidism (i.e., increased production of pituitary TSH). Choice D, suppressed TSH, normal FT_4, and normal T_3, is evidence of subclinical hyperthyroidism, treated hyperthyroidism (perhaps dosed slightly above therapeutic), pregnancy, or rarely nonthyroid illness. Choice E, suppressed TSH, elevated FT_4, indicates exogenous thyroid hormone, as may occur in Choice D.

12. The answer is C. Iodine ingestion or injection may cause thyrotoxicosis, especially in an iodine-deficient patient. This may occur after radiographic iodine-containing contrast media or after treatment with the iodine-rich drug amiodarone or with treatment by interferon or interleukin-2. Iodine apparently precipitates thyrotoxicosis in a gland that is primed by a long period of iodine deficiency and consequent chronically elevated TSH. This is doubly so if the gland has developed multiple hyperplastic nodules. After withdrawal of the iodine or amiodarone, the thyrotoxicosis may last for several months in the absence of treatment with an antithyroid drug, usually methimazole. The disease is otherwise self-limited and will not recur after the antithyroid treatment results in subsidence of the toxicosis. Lithium treatment, used in bipolar disorder, causes hypothyroidism. All other choices are meaningless distracters.

13. The answer is E. Serum antithyroglobulin, taken on a blood sample, if elevated, makes the diagnosis of Hashimoto thyroiditis, the most common thyroid disorder in the United States. RAI uptake with I^{123}, in the subacute phase, as with all thyroiditides, will be very low as opposed to Graves disease or normal. However, as the disease becomes chronic, in euthyroid or hypothyroid patients, the RAI uptake tends to be normal or elevated with an uneven distribution. FNA biopsy would be indicated if there were a single prominent nodule. In the absence of thyrotoxicosis, T_3 determination is not indicated and then only if TSH is suppressed and FT_4 is normal. Hashimoto thyroiditis (also called lymphocytic thyroiditis or, archaically, struma lymphomatosa) uncommonly causes a thyrotoxic phase but often leads to hypothroidism, remitting then in 5% of cases.

14. The answer is E. Subacute thyroiditis, accounting for about 5% of clinical thyroid disease, is usually painful but may be silent, the latter understandably causing confusion with Hashimoto thyroiditis. It is often associated with systemic symptoms of virallike illness during the early phase. It has been called also de Quervain thyroiditis. Graves disease causes exophthalmos in addition to other signs of hyperthyroidism and manifests an increased RAI uptake. Riedel struma does not cause thyrotoxicosis. Hashimoto thyroiditis does not present with a tender gland and only rarely manifests hyperthyroidism. Ludwig angina is a streptococcal infection of the floor of the mouth and descending inferiority. Though anterior neck pain would be characteristic, hyperthyroidism would not.

15. The answer is C. Start propranolol at 20 mg daily. In subacute thyroiditis, the thyrotoxic phase usually is mild and lasts about 2 months. Therefore, thiourea drugs (e.g., methimazole and propylthiouracil) are not necessary and would not be effective because their action depends on active hormone production by the gland. The same statements are true for I[131]. From the foregoing it is clear that thyroidectomy is not warranted.

16. The answer is B. Typical of subacute or de Quervain thyroiditis is not only a brief thyrotoxic phase but also 6 to 9 months of hypothyroidism that follows virtually on the heels of the toxic phase. Thus, treatment of this condition will rarely remain in place for life. The complication occurs in nearly one-half of patients, although the vast majority revert to a euthyroid state without elevated antithyroid antibodies. Approximately 5% of patients will not remit from the hypothyroid phase; a few will have recurrent subacute phases, and uncommonly some will undergo change to Graves disease. About one-third of subacute thyroiditis patients will have persistent elevations of antithyroperoxidase antibodies and a persistent goiter.

17. The answer is D. Coronary atherosclerosis is not a particularly strong risk in Graves disease, the most common cause of hyperthyroid disease, illustrated in the vignette presented. As an autoimmune disease, Graves is associated statistically with all the other diseases mentioned among the choices and as well with coeliac disease, myasthenia gravis, cardiomyopathy, and hypokalemic periodic paralysis. The female-to-male ratio among those afflicted with Graves disease is approximately 8:1. Lifetime incidence (sometime prevalence of this disease) is thus 2.2% for female individuals and about 0.3% for male individuals. Indeed, the vast majority of all thyroid problems occur more in female than in male individuals.

18. The answer is D. TSHR-Ab [stim] stands for TSH-receptor antibody, stimulating (to set it apart from the blocking antibody). Although it is the most specific test, it is hardly the most sensitive one, as it occurs in only 66% of cases of Graves disease. Antithyroperoxidase antibody, antithyroglobulin antibody, and antinuclear antibody each or all may be present in Graves disease but are not specific. Serum FT$_4$ is, of course, virtually always elevated in Graves disease as it is in all forms of thyroitoxicosis.

19. The answer is D. Thyroidectomy is the least likely choice, with the patient having the final vote, assuming she is well informed of all side effects and contraindications. In the short term, when the patient is uncomfortable or seriously in jeopardy because of the severity of the thyrotoxicosis, nonselective beta-adrenergic blocking drugs such as propranolol are used while the definitive therapy takes effect. I[131] therapy is well tolerated but is usually followed ultimately by hypothyroidism and the need for replacement therapy. The thiourea drugs have the advantage of often succeeding after finite periods of 1 to 2 years. Between the two most often utilized, propylthiouracil is safe even in pregnancy, if kept below 200 mg/day to avoid fetal hypothyroidism. Thyroidectomy is less and less frequently elected because of its obvious invasiveness and the fact that it too must generally be followed by permanent hypothyroidism and the need for replacement therapy.

20. The answer is D. This patient has toxic nodular goiter. This disorder is not characterized by exophthalmos, unlike Graves disease, though the eyes may manifest the stare and the lid lag of thyrotoxicosis. It occurs most frequently in older individuals (i.e., $\geq$55 years) and begins as a grouping of autonomous nodules, apparently under the influence of an elevated TSH caused by incipient hypothyroidism. In a certain proportion of cases the nodules become autonomous and hyperfunctional. This form of thyrotoxicosis is a less severe form of hyperthyroidism, whether measured in terms of clinical symptoms and signs or laboratory measurement of FT$_4$, T$_3$, or I[123] uptake.

21. The answer is B. Therapy with I[131] is ideal in this disease because it occurs most frequently in older people (but would be the best choice in any adult with toxic multinodular goiter, as will be clear from subsequent commentary). Surgery is eschewed for the same reasons as discussed elsewhere, unless there is reason to expect a cancerous nodule or nodules. Thiourea agents are not effective over the long term, as they are followed by a 95% chance of recurrent multinodular disease. Beta-blocking agents are not needed during the early treatment phase in most cases because in the vast majority the degree of thyrotoxicosis is mild.

References

Fitzpatrick PA. Endocrinology. In: Tierney LM, McPhee SJ, Papadakis MA, eds. *Current Medical Diagnosis and Treatment.* 45th ed. New York: McGraw-Hill/Appleton & Lange; 2006: 1098–1193.

Larsen PR, Davies TF, Hay ID. The thyroid gland. In: Wilson JD, Foster DW, Kronenberg HM, et al., eds. *William's Textbook of Endocrinology.* 9th ed. Philadelphia: WB Saunders; 1998: 00–00.

Reid JR, Wheeler SF. Hyperthyroidism: Diagnosis and treatment. *Am Fam Physician.* 2005; 72:623–630, 635–636.

Rudy DR, Tzagournis M. Thyroid problems in primary care. In: Rudy DR, Kurowski K, eds. *Family Medicine: House Officer Series.* Baltimore: Williams & Wilkins; 1997:543–566.

chapter 33

Problems of the Adrenal and Parathyroid Glands

Examination questions: Unless instructed otherwise, choose the ONE lettered answer or completion that is BEST in each case.

1 A 34-year-old type I diabetic man had been controlled on 36 units daily of human insulin, both short (R) and intermediate (N) acting, in the form of 16 units of human N and 8 units of human R in the mornings and 8 units of human N and 4 units of human R after the evening meal. Three days ago the man was involved in an auto accident in which he incurred abdominal blunt trauma and was hypotensive several hours before undergoing transfusion and splenectomy for rupture. There had been no apparent head injury. Yesterday, in the hospital, he began running a fever, with a temperature of 39°C (102.2°F). There are no apparent sites of infection. Blood cultures were drawn and are incubating. This morning, 3 hours after his morning insulin, he experienced a severe episode of hypoglycemia with a blood sugar measurement of 45 mg/dL. The fasting blood sugar before the morning insulin doses was 85 mg/dL. The patient complains of nausea, vomiting, and diarrhea. Initial laboratory results show a mild eosinophilia and hyperkalemia at 5.3 mEq/L. Which of the following is the most likely explanation of these developments?

(A) Sepsis secondary to surgical wound infection

(B) Sepsis secondary to primary wound infection at the sites of abdominal trauma.

(C) Viral gastroenteritis

(D) Acute adrenal insufficiency

(E) Neurologic complication of the trauma involving temperature control

2 Adrenal insufficiency may be primary or secondary (i.e., secondary to pituitary failure). In addition to abnormally low levels of corticotropin (adrenocorticotropic hormone, or ACTH), which of the following findings would favor secondary adrenal insufficiency?

(A) Abnormally low level of serum cortisol

(B) Hypovolemia, hyponatremia, and hyperkalemia

(C) Physical findings of hyperpigmentation in the skin creases, skin over extensor surfaces (e.g., knuckles, elbows), and posterior neck

(D) Abnormally low level of serum cortisol, moderate neutropenia, lymphocytosis, and neutrophilia

(E) Hypovolemia, normal sodium concentration, normal serum potassium, and normal skin color

3 Your 33-year-old female patient has been diagnosed with primary adrenal insufficiency. She had manifested, among other things, hyperkalemia. Which of the following would be the most likely acceptable regimen for replacement therapy?

(A) Dexamethasone 0.75 mg daily, given in divided doses as 0.5 mg in the morning and 0.25 mg in the afternoon

(B) Prednisone 5 mg daily

(C) Hydrocortisone 24 mg daily, given as 16 mg in the morning and 8 mg in the afternoon, plus fludrocortisone 0.3 mg daily in the morning

(D) Prednisone 10 mg daily and fludrocortisone

(E) Prednisone 15 mg daily, given as 10 mg in the morning and 5 mg in the afternoon

4 A 12-year-old boy is brought to the family doctor by his parents, who are concerned that he is exhibiting early pubescence. This was manifested by pubic hair growth at the age of 11 and genital enlargement during the past year along with deepening of his voice. Laboratory studies are performed and results include findings of elevated dihydroepiandrosterone. Which of the following laboratory studies will diagnose the most common form of adrenal hyperplasia, which is deficiency of cytochrome $P450_{c21}$ (21-hydroxylase deficiency)?

(A) Elevated follicle-stimulating hormone levels

(B) Elevated 17-hydroxypregnenolone

(C) Elevated 11-deoxycortisol

(D) Increase in 17-hydroxyprogesterone after ACTH

(E) Low levels of 17-alpha-hydroxysteroid

5 Regarding the patient in Question 4, which of the following is the basis of standard treatment for that condition?

(A) Conjugated estrogens

(B) Orchidectomy

(C) Hydrocortisone in replacement dosages

(D) Fludrocortisone

(E) Syntropin

6 A 35-year-old woman complains of weakness, fatigability, polyuria, and polydipsia. She had become hypertensive during the past few months and has been treated with a combination of hydrochlorothiazide/triamterene with fair results. Her most recent blood pressure readings have averaged 120/88. A spot blood sugar test 3 hours after her latest meal showed a level of 95 mg/dL. She complains also of muscular weakness, on occasion exhibiting paralysis for brief periods. Which of the following routine chemistries is likely to be the most critical in making a diagnosis that encompasses the hypertension and the weakness?

(A) Blood urea nitrogen

(B) Serum potassium

(C) Serum creatinine

(D) Serum sodium

(E) Serum bicarbonate

7 The results of testing for the patient in Question 6 show hypokalemia. In order to precisely confirm the diagnosis, what is the next action that is most appropriate?

(A) Hold all antihypertensive medications

(B) Measure blood pressure in all four extremities

(C) Repeat the electrolyte measurements

(D) Order a magnetic resonance image of the adrenal glands

(E) Add a beta-adrenergic blocking agent for better control of the blood pressure

8 A 45-year-old woman has been followed for four visits for hypertension (blood pressure of 150 to 160/90 to 100) discovered during a routine examination, at which time she was also found to have type II diabetes. Initially an angiotensin-converting enzyme inhibitor failed to effect a fall in blood pressure from her baseline measurements. On the third visit the blood pressure had responded to hydrochlorothiazide/triamterene and her blood sugar had fallen to 120 to 130 at 2 hours postprandially as prescribed glipizide took effect. You notice that she is not only obese but also that her obesity is centripetal with proximal muscle wasting, associated with a plethoric face and purple striae about the trunk, and that she complains of menstrual irregularity. She manifests also supraclavicular fat pads. Which of the following is the most likely comprehensive clinical diagnosis?

(A) Metabolic syndrome

(B) Essential hypertension

(C) Type II diabetes

(D) Cushing syndrome

(E) Morbid obesity

9 Regarding the patient in Question 8, which of the following tests will differentiate Cushing disease (Cushing syndrome caused by pituitary overproduction of ACTH) from Cushing syndrome caused by an ectopic source, primary adrenal disease, or extrinsic origin?

(A) Serum cortisol test

(B) 24-hour urine catecholamine test

(C) Dexamethasone suppression test

(D) Serum prolactin test

(E) Melanocyte-stimulating hormone test

10 A 56-year-old ambulatory white woman undergoes routine periodic physical examination and evaluation that includes mammogram, Pap smear, review of systems and medications, and routine laboratory hemogram and chemistries. All results are normal except that the serum calcium level is confirmed to be elevated. Which of the following is the most likely cause of the hypercalcemia, assuming no other information is available?

(A) Carcinoma of the breast

(B) Hypervitaminosis D

(C) Hypervitaminosis A

(D) Sarcoidosis

(E) Primary hyperparathyroidism

11 Regarding the patient in Question 10, a parathyroid hormone (PTH) level and urinary calcium-to-creatinine clearance ratio (Ca/CC) were ordered. At that time you found the patient had been taking vitamin D supplements. Which of the following results would you expect if the cause of hypercalcemia were vitamin D intoxication?

(A) Elevated PTH and Ca/CC >0.02

(B) Normal PTH and Ca/CC >0.02

(C) Low PTH and Ca/CC >0.02

(D) Low PTH and Ca/CC <0.01

(E) Normal PTH and Ca/CC <0.01

12 Regarding the patient depicted in Question 10, you find that the condition has occurred in other family members. You wish to seek further the possibility of coexistence of each of the following diseases, except for which one?

(A) Colonic adenomatous polyps

(B) Pheochromocytoma

(C) Parathyroid adenoma

(D) Facial angiofibromas

(E) Medullary carcinomas

13 Primary adrenal insufficiency, as distinct from secondary disease, is characterized clinically by hyperpigmentation, among other stigmata. Which of the following other endocrinopathies is also associated with hyperpigmentation and also with hyperkalemia?

(A) Thyrotoxicosis

(B) Parathyroid adenoma

(C) Adrenocortical adenoma

(D) Nonpituitary adenoma

(E) Pancreatic adenoma

14 For which of the listed clinical effects might the following medications, namely, ketoconazole, mitotane, metyrapone, and aminoglutethamide, be applicable?

(A) Each may be utilized in serious mycotic injections (ketoconazole).

(B) Each may be indicated for medical control of primary aldosteronism (spironolactone).

(C) Each blocks the production of cortisol from 11-beta-deoxycortisol (metyrapone).

(D) Each may be used to treat hypercortisolism in the short term (i.e., a glucocorticoid inhibitor).

(E) Each inhibits the production of ACTH.

15 A 35-year-old man has been having bouts of palpitations, pounding heart, and headaches, lasting several minutes. Last evening he had such an attack during intercourse. He denies flushing during the attacks. During one attack his wife, a medical assistant, measured his peripheral pulse at 130 beats per minute, but the pulse was easily counted and regular. Looking back, the man feels he has had at least one attack daily for the past 2 weeks. Vital signs are normal, with blood pressure being 115/75 and pulse 78 and regular. Temperature was 97.8°F at 9 AM. The doctor considers first that the patient has had panic attacks as a part of panic disorder. However, feeling that panic disorder should be considered only after ruling out organic causes of the attacks, which of the following would be the most reasonable diagnosis for the doctor to investigate and pursue?

(A) Thyrotoxicosis

(B) Carcinoid syndrome

(C) Pheochromocytoma

(D) Supraventricular tachycardia

(E) Sepsis

Examination Answers

Handwritten annotation (top):
↑ACTH → ↑17-OH-progesterone
↓ → Androgenic cmpds.
↓ ← 21-OH-lase deficiency → (P450$_{c21}$)
Cortisol   Aldosterone   ↓ Hy

1. The answer is D. Acute adrenal insufficiency may be precipitated by hypotension, trauma, or hemorrhage. The fact that this is an acutely ill patient, who is a type I diabetic yet manifests hypoglycemia, as opposed to markedly increased insulin requirements, rules against, if not eliminates, sepsis or other infectious causes. Neurologic sequelae from trauma would be unexpected in a person who suffered neither loss of consciousness nor symptoms of concussion.

2. The answer is E. Hypovolemia, normal sodium concentration, normal serum potassium, and normal skin color, in association with abnormally low levels of cortisol, are all signs of adrenal insufficiency that is due to pituitary failure as opposed to primary adrenal insufficiency. In primary disease, ACTH is elevated and increased skin pigmentation is an indirect result of this. Also, in primary adrenal insufficiency, most often as a result of destructive processes in the physical site of the adrenal glands, the zona glomerulosa is destroyed as well so that hyperkalemia, resulting from absence of aldosterone, occurs; this is not so in secondary adrenal insufficiency. Peripheral blood cell changes, neutropenia, relative eosinophilia, and lymphocytosis occur in primary or secondary adrenal insufficiency.

3. The answer is C, hyrocortisone 24 mg daily, given as 16 mg in the morning and 8 mg in the afternoon, plus fludrocortisone 0.3 mg daily. Important points to remember are (a) that the glucocorticoid should be given as two-thirds of the replacement dosage in the morning with the remainder in the afternoon, and (b) that many patients with primary adrenal insufficiency require replacement of the mineralocorticoid as well. In this example, fludrocortisone replaces aldosterone. The dexamethasone replacement dosage is 0.75 mg daily in divided doses, with two-thirds in the morning and one-third in the afternoon. However, as the most pure synthetic product among those presented, it has the least mineralocorticoid activity. Thus, nearly always there must be mineralocorticoid replacement, if dexamethasone is used to treat primary adrenal insufficiency. If prednisone is used for glucocorticoid replacement then the dosage is 5 mg, but also in divided doses (two-thirds and one-third). From the foregoing it is easily inferred that prednisone is five times as potent, milligram for milligram, as hydrocortisone and that dexamethasone has thirty-three times the potency of hydrocortisone.

4. The answer is D. Increase in 17-hydroxyprogesterone after ACTH stimulation allows the diagnosis of 21-hydroxylase deficiency, also called P450$_{c21}$ deficiency, the cause of 90% of adrenal hyperplasia. The prerequisite for this test is an elevated baseline 17-hydroxyprogesterone level. This compound rises as a result of metabolic arrest in the pathway toward production of cortisol. Thus, androgenic compounds are overproduced and the feedback process, through elevation of ACTH, results in androgenization. The effects depend on how severe is the metabolic arrest and upon the sex of the patient. Severe cases result in salt wasting and hyperkalemia during the newborn or infancy period. The latter occurs because the normal pathway to production of aldosterone is interrupted to varying degrees as well. Thus, salt wasting in the most severe cases results in hyponatremia and hyperkalemia. The three other types, all rare, manifest elevated 17-hydroxypregnenolone (3-beta-hydroxy) and decreased 17-alpha-hydroxysteroid (17-hydroxylase deficiency).

5. The answer is C. Hydrocortisone in replacement dosages not only repletes the serum cortisol that tends to be insufficient but also, through negative feedback, suppresses ACTH, removing the stimulus for driving the aberrant pathway. Little known is that polyuria and polydipsia may accompany this disease.

6. The answer is B. Serum potassium may explain the combination of hypertension and weakness as being caused by primary aldosteronism.

7. The answer is A. Holding all antihypertensive medications for up to 2 weeks is necessary in order to validate the hypokalemia. Assume the serum potassium result returns as 3.0 mEq/L (3.5 to 4.5), supporting the diagnosis of primary aldosteronism. Usually, but not in all cases, serum potassium is depressed in primary aldosteronism. In fact hypokalemia in the face of hypertension, in the absence of extrinsic cause or pathologic loss as in diarrhea or vomiting, should be considered to be primary aldosteronism until proven otherwise. Although hypokalemia is typical in primary aldosteronism, spurious low results can result when potassium-losing diuretics have been in use, though in this case the hydrochlorothiazide is titrated fairly well by the triamterene. Besides diuretics, calcium channel blocking

Handwritten annotation (bottom):
Dexamethasone → Prednisone → Hydrocortisone
33X   5X   X potency
                         ÷4 mg

agents tend to normalize otherwise elevated levels of aldosterone and beta-blockers suppress renin levels, also depressed in primary aldosteronism. Once hypokalemia is confirmed, then the diagnosis of primary aldosteronism is confirmed by first placing the patient on a diet consisting of a minimum of 120 mEq sodium per day (about three times the amount contained in a no-salt-added diet). Then a 24-hour urine sample is assayed for aldosterone, free cortisol, and creatinine. More than 20 mEq in 24 hours gives the diagnosis of primary aldosteronism. Although adenoma is the cause of primary aldosteronism in 60% of cases, the remainder are secondary to bilateral adrenal hyperplasia. Renin levels are almost always low in physiologic response to sodium retention and hypervolemia, and low renin is characteristic of primary aldosteronism.

8. The answer is D, Cushing syndrome. Cushing syndrome is associated with and precipitates, if not causes, both hypertension and diabetes type II. The purple striae are not specific for Cushing syndrome, as they are associated with recent and rapid development of obesity. However, Cushing syndrome brings with it not only recent and rapid obesity but also the protein catabolic aspects of the syndrome, and attendant weakening of protein structures allows a significantly lower threshold for development of the striae. The same may be said for the facial plethora but to a lesser degree. The metabolic syndrome is also associated with hypertension and diabetes type II, but the purple striae and rubor are a virtual stigma of Cushing syndrome when seen with hypertension and diabetes. On occasion, in a primary care setting, a physician may encounter seemingly mysterious supraclavicular fat pads in a patient seen for unrelated reasons. In such cases one needs to be mindful of the possibility of Cushing syndrome. Morbid obesity, weight equal to or exceeding 100 lb (45.3 kg) in excess of the ideal, would not explain proximonal muscle wasting.

9. The answer is C. There are several levels of precision and sensitivity in the dexamethasone suppression tests. In Cushing disease, cortisol precursors and their metabolic by-products are responding to excessive production of ACTH by the anterior pituitary. In the overnight dexamethasone suppression test, the baseline plasma cortisol level is measured before administration of 1 mg of dexamethasone and should be suppressed to less than 50% of that value on the next morning. In addition, baseline ACTH is measured and expected to be similarly suppressed, and the same with 24-hour urine 17-hydroxycorticosteroids. Another version of the overnight dexamethasone suppression test employs administration of 1 mg of dexamethasone orally at 11 AM and the collection of serum cortisol on the following morning at 8 AM. A morning cortisol level of <5 μg/dL by fluorometric assay or of <2 μg/dL by

high-performance liquid chromatography is 98% specific to rule out Cushing syndrome. Thus, cortisol was suppressible. This would not apply to Cushing disease caused by exogenous hydrocortisone (medication). Thus, Choice A, serum cortisol, is part (but only part) of the test. None of the other choices is relevant to this case.

10. The answer is E. Primary hyperparathyroidism is the most common cause of hypercalcemia in ambulatory patients. However, there are numerous causes of elevated serum calcium, and they include not only the other choices given here but also several more. Sarcoidosis would be more likely in a person of black African descent. Carcinoma of the breast is associated with extreme hypercalcemia in late, virtually always metastatic, disease, and can be life threatening. Malignancy is the most frequent cause of hypercalcemia in hospitalized patients. Both hypervitaminoses D and A are causes of hypercalcemia. In addition to the foregoing, other causes and concurrent conditions include prolonged immobility (especially in a patient with Paget disease of the bone), thiazide diuretics, severe thyrotoxicosis, aluminum toxicity (usually with renal dialysis), and, for reasons not understood, Addison disease.

11. The answer is D, low PTH and Ca/CC <0.01. Elevated PTH and Ca/CC >0.02 are what one would find in primary hyperparathyroidism. Even with a normal PTH level, a Ca/CC of >0.02 constitutes strong evidence for primary hyperparathyroidism. Low PTH levels are generally secondary, through the feedback mechanism, to other causes of hypercalcemia. Normal PTH and Ca/CC <0.01 is the normal state.

12. The answer is A. Colonic adenomatous polyps are not associated with hyperparathyroidism. Each of the others is among the conditions associated with hyperparathyroidism in the multiple endocrine neoplasia (MEN) syndromes, types I and II (MEN I and MEN II, respectively). Besides hyperparathyroidism, MEN I has the strongest associations with facial angiofibromas and collagenomas, pancreatic and pituitary adenomas, and, to a lesser extent, adrenocortical adenomas and subcutaneous lipomas. In MEN II, medullary carcinoma is associated with hyperparathyroidism and pheochromocytoma in 20% to 50% of the cases and 20% to 35% of the cases, respectively. Hyperparathyroidism is not a part of MEN III, which is a cluster, more or less, of mucosal and gastrointestinal ganglioneuromas, medullary carcinomas, and pheochromocytomas.

13. The answer is D. Nonpituitary ACTH-producing adenomas, the most prominent example of which is from a small-cell lung carcinoma, may produce ACTH at quantities that dwarf the average pituitary adenoma. In those situations, melanocyte-stimulating hormone may be activated and hyperpigmentation ensues.

14. The answer is D. Each is an adrenal glucocorticoid inhibitor. Their common clinical usefulness is that they may be used therapeutically for temporary suppression of hypercortisolism in preparation for surgical approach to pituitary adenoma to remove the source of excess ACTH. Ketoconazole is also an antifungal agent. Mitotane is an inhibitor of ACTH production; thus, it indirectly shuts down production of cortisol in true Cushing disease. Metyrapone blocks the production of cortisol from 11-beta-deoxycortisol. This action is utilized in the metyrapone test to probe the pituitary response to hypocortisolism.

15. The answer is C. Pheochromocytoma, though uncommon, best fits the clinical picture presented. Although all other diagnoses listed may be considered to some degree and would in reality be ruled out, their likelihoods would be small. Carcinoid syndrome is the second in consideration because it causes cataclysmic bouts, not unlike pheochromocytoma, and is generally tested for at the same time as pheochromocytoma. However, carcinoid is famous for causing flushing during attacks. Thyrotoxicosis rarely occurs without sinus tachycardia or atrial fibrillation, as the former is steady, not paroxysmal; the latter perhaps occurs in bouts. For that matter, any type of supraventricular tachycardia is unlikely, given the regular rhythm found at home by the spouse. Sepsis would be unlikely, given the basically well state in which the patient presented to the office the morning after an attack.

References

Fitzpatrick PA. Endocrinology. In: Tierney LM, McPhee SJ, Papadakis MA, eds. *Current Medical Diagnosis and Treatment.* 45th ed. New York: McGraw-Hill/Appleton & Lange; 2006: 1098–1193.

Sandarum V, Falko JM. Triage of problems of the adrenal gland. In: Rudy DR, Kurowski K, eds. *Family Medicine: House Officer Series.* Baltimore: Williams & Wilkins; 1997:567–576.

chapter 34

Problems of Growth and Development

Examination questions: Unless instructed otherwise, choose the ONE lettered answer or completion that is BEST in each case.

1 You are approached by the parents of a 15-year-old boy who is concerned that he is not as sexually developed as his class peers. Upon inspection you see that pubic hair is only lightly pigmented and elongating but not curly. The penis is only slightly enlarged as compared with that expected in the preadolescent state. Which of the following should be your next disposition?

(A) Order serum follicle-stimulating hormone (FSH) level test

(B) Order serum luteinizing hormone (LH) level test

(C) Order x-rays for bone age

(D) Reassure the parents that the boy's level of sexual maturation is within normal limits

(E) Start the boy on testosterone at a dosage of 50 mg daily

2 A 5-year-old girl presents as being behind in her growth, as she is more than 3 SD below the mean height for age and sex. Her parents' achieved heights do not make it clear that she has constitutional short stature; trisomy 21 and Turner syndrome karyotype have been ruled out, being chromatin negative; she displays no stigmata of achondroplasia; diabetes, rickets, and hypothyroidism have been ruled out; bone age is normal for height; she manifests no arthritic processes; urinalysis is within normal limits; and interviews of the family fail to yield evidence of psychosocial short stature. Which of the following tests would be the most appropriate at this time?

(A) Thyrotropin (thyroid-stimulating hormone, or TSH), tri-iodothyronine (T_3), and free tetraiodothyronine (FT_4)

(B) Chest x-ray

(C) Electrocardiogram

(D) Computed tomography scan of the hypophysis

(E) Overnight growth hormone test

3 You are treating the 5-year-old girl introduced in Question 2 for growth hormone deficiency. You have been treating her with growth hormone injections six times a week. She has no other complaints and feels well. Her physical examination remains normal except for her small size. When reassessing her 1 year later, you find that her growth remains poor. Besides checking for compliance and rechecking her bone age, which of the following would you recommend?

(A) Stop growth hormone treatment, as this must be constitutional growth delay

(B) Check the serum cortisol level

(C) Perform the dexamethasone suppression test

(D) Repeat the karyotype testing

(E) Check TSH, T_3, and FT_4

4 Given that the pubertal maturation scale before puberty is defined as stage I, on the Tanner scale, in which stage is a female who manifests breast bud development, as opposed to enlargement of the breasts?

(A) Tanner I

(B) Tanner II

(C) Tanner III

(D) Tanner IV

(E) Tanner V

5 At which Tanner stage is a male who has penile enlargement and pubic hair limited to the area immediately surrounding the base of the penis?

(A) Tanner I

(B) Tanner II

(C) Tanner III

(D) Tanner IV

(E) Tanner V

6 You are examining an obese 16-year-old girl who has never had a period and is at Tanner I on examination. She has no complaints. She is 2 SD below mean height for her age. A TSH test is normal. A urine pregnancy test is negative. Her bone age is appropriate for her short stature. Her dehydroepiandrosterone sulfate level is appropriate for her age. Her FSH and LH levels are elevated. Among the options presented, which of the following accounts for her condition?

(A) Prader–Willi syndrome

(B) Prolactinoma

(C) Gonadal failure

(D) Constitutional delay

(E) Dramatic recent weight loss (≥20% of body weight)

7 Regarding the patient featured in Question 6, there are other possible causes not mentioned among the choices given. Each of the following is an additional possible etiology for the disorder of the patient described in Question 6, except for which one?

(A) Polycystic ovary syndrome

(B) Over 3,000 rads of radiation to the ovaries

(C) Autoimmune gonadal failure

(D) Alkylating agent chemotherapy

(E) Turner syndrome

8 During your examination of a 19-month-old female infant, you note unilateral breast bud development in the right breast. The child has otherwise been well and is on no medications. The vaginal mucosa appears as expected at 19 months. She remains at about the 50th percentile for both height and weight. Which of the following do you recommend?

(A) Reassure the parents that this can sometimes be seen at this age and have them contact you if any other secondary sex characteristics develop

(B) Order a right breast ultrasound

(C) Order a bilateral mammogram

(D) Suggest a breast surgeon consultation for surgical excision of lesion

(E) Check estradiol, FSH, and LH levels

9 You are evaluating a 14-year-old girl who is manifesting virilization. She otherwise has no complaints and has not been ill. She used to take an albuterol inhaler but has not needed this in the past 2 years. She has clitoral enlargement and facial hair, but motor and sensory examination, including deep tendon reflexes, are normal. Visual fields are intact to gross confrontation. You appreciate no masses on abdominal examination. Which of the following would be part of your *initial* work-up?

(A) Serum testosterone level

(B) Serum progesterone level

(C) Karyotype testing

(D) Serum estrogens (total) level

(E) A magnetic resonance image of the pituitary gland

10 A 25-year-old man and his 23-year-old wife express their concern regarding failure to achieve pregnancy after 2 years of marriage and monthly attempts at conception. An initial screening sperm count shows significant azospermia. The husband possesses an elongated lower body segment but otherwise is of normal weight for height. His education level was high school. His testicles measure 3 cm and 3.5 cm, respectively. Otherwise, secondary sex characteristics are normal except for a suggestion of gynecomastia. His past development was normal in regard to secondary sex characteristics and the timing of their onset. LH and FSH levels are within normal limits. Which of the following is the most likely diagnosis?

(A) Kallmann syndrome

(B) Prader–Willi

(C) Klinefelter syndrome

(D) Laurence–Moon syndrome

(E) Bardet-Biedl syndrome

11 A phenotypical male newborn shows no testicles in the scrotum. Which of the following should be the most timely action to be taken in the newborn period in regard to this finding?

(A) Consult a surgeon for possible orchiopexy

(B) Consult a surgeon for orchiectomy

(C) Observation for likely descent of the testicles within the first 3 months

(D) Ascertain the presence of testes in the abdomen

(E) Early institution of hormonal therapy to bring about descent of testes

12 The parents of the newborn referred to in Question 11 inquire regarding the prognosis of undescended testicles if they have had to be brought down into the scrotum medically or surgically. Your best thoughtful response is which of the following?

(A) Fertility can be expected to revert to normal when the child comes of age if correction is made by time the child reaches the age of 1 year.

(B) Potential for malignancy in an undescended testicle reverts to normal after medical or surgical correction if accomplished by the time the child reaches the age of 1 year.

(C) Neither fertility nor potential for malignancy can be expected to be comparable with those in males without the affliction, even if the condition is corrected by the time the child reaches the age of 1 year.

(D) Both fertility and potential for malignancy will revert to normal after correction if it is made by the time the child reaches the age of 1 year.

(E) Surgical or medical correction of cryptorchidism serves only a cosmetic function, as it has no effect on the long-term course of the individual who suffered from the condition.

13 The parents of a 7-year-old boy bring him to you for evaluation. They have noted bilateral breast development. There is no history of exogenous estrogen use. His vital signs are normal, including a regular heart rhythm at a rate of 88. He has otherwise been well and is on no mediations. There is no history of ambiguous genitalia at birth. On examination the testes are approximately 1 cm each bilaterally. The penis is small. Breast tissue is palpable bilaterally with discernible areola development. There are no abdominal masses. The boy is 40th percentile for height and weight. Which of the following do you recommend?

(A) Reassure parents that his is just benign gynecomastia and is probably transient

(B) Begin treatment with testosterone enanthate 50 mg IU each month

(C) Begin search for estrogen-secreting tumor

(D) Obtain surgical consultation for excisional biopsy of breast masses

(E) Review the family history for similar occurrences

14 An 8½-year-old boy is brought to you by his parents who are concerned about his deepening voice and early growth of facial hair. His testicles measure 2.8 cm bilaterally. Bone age is advanced for his height and chronological age. FSH and LH levels are in the pubertal range; that is, they are above the low prepubertal levels. Which of the following conditions does this boy have?

(A) True precocious puberty

(B) Prader–Willi syndrome

(C) Kallmann syndrome

(D) Pseudoprecocious puberty

(E) Normal variant of puberty onset

15 Regarding the patient featured in Question 14, which of the following medications would be appropriate for treatment of the condition depicted?

(A) Gonadotropin-releasing hormone (GnRH) agonist

(B) Human chorionic gonadotropin

(C) Cyproterone acetate

(D) Medroxyprogesterone acetate

(E) Spironolactone

Examination Answers

1. The answer is D. Reassure the parents and the boy that the boy's level of sexual maturation is within normal limits. Delayed puberty is defined as the onset of puberty at an age later than the age onset of puberty for the sex type. For boys that is 13.5 ± 4 years. For girls the mean age ± SD is 13 years ± 7. Thus, although the 15-year-old boy is in an age above average for the time of clear progress in development of puberty, he does not warrant expensive and anxious measures of diagnosis at this time.

2. The answer is E, overnight growth hormone test. The main point to convey is that virtually all the many other causes of growth retardation should be ruled out, as much more statistically likely than failure of growth hormone. Although hypothyroidism is a cause of growth retardation, it has already been ruled out according to the vignette. Failure of growth hormone, unlike pituitary gigantism and acromegaly, does not manifest masses in the hypophysis. Chest x-ray and electrocardiogram hold no special meanings in the evaluation of growth retardation.

3. The answer is E, thyroid function studies. That hyothyroidism was ruled out before embarkation on growth hormone therapy notwithstanding, growth hormone sometimes induces hypothyroidism and this is a significant possible etiology of poor growth of patients *on therapy.* Even patients who are growing normally should have thyroid function testing every year. Stopping growth hormone treatment would be self-defeating because the girl's growth rate remains an issue. Cortisol levels would be relevant only if she exhibited signs or symptoms of adrenal insufficiency or excess, as would the dexamethasone suppression test. The karyotype (XO karyotype) was already tested and found to be normal.

4. The answer is B, Tanner II. Sparse pubic hair can also be noticed just on the labia during this stage. Tanner III is best defined as breast enlargement without separation of the contours of the areola and the papilla, in formation of a single mound. Stage IV features contour development, with the nipple being the only projection of the breast but without the full adult pattern (i.e., triangular form). Stage V thus is defined by full pubic hair development.

5. The answer is B, Tanner II. In keeping with the theme that Tanner I is prepubertal, Tanner II is the first identifiable stage of pubertal development. Stages III and IV in the case of males are definable only by degree of testicular, penile, and pubic hair growth (i.e., without clear-cut boundaries). Tanner V in males, as in females, is defined by the full adult pattern of public hair (i.e., for males, spread of the hair onto the thighs). Arbitrary as the Tanner stage definitions may be, they provide the language necessary for communication among physicians when questions of growth and development arise.

6. The answer is C. The increased LH and FSH levels indicate primary ovarian failure; in other words, the fact that gonadotropins were in the stimulatory range, yet the gonads failed to respond, shows that gonadal failure was the basis for the abnormality. Turner syndrome is one likely cause of primary ovarian failure. Weight loss, prolactinoma, and Prader–Willi syndrome can all cause a delay in puberty, but through insufficient hypothalamic release of LH and FSH (and thus low levels are detected). Constitutional growth delay also results in *low* FSH and LH levels (i.e., the cause of delays being a hypothalamic–pituitary cause as opposed to ovarian failure).

7. The answer is A. Polycystic ovary syndrome (PCOS) is a potential etiology of infertility, but not of ovarian failure. FSH and LH have not failed. Other aspects of PCOS include amenorrhea, androgenization, and insulin resistance, leading to type II diabetes. Weight loss is the single best therapy for PCOS. Radiation to the ovaries, autoimmune gonadal failure, alkylating chemotherapy, and Turner syndrome can each account for ovarian failure. Viral infections (such as mumps or coxsackie B virus) also can produce acute gonadal failure.

8. The answer is A. Reassure the parents that this can sometimes be seen at this age and have them contact you if any other secondary sex characteristics develop. This case demonstrates premature thelarchy, which is most commonly seen at ages younger than 2 years or older than 6 years. Reassurance alone is required unless there is evidence of pubertal development in other tissues or if growth or bone age is affected. Breast ultrasound mammogram, surgical consultation, and serum estradiol, FSH, or LH level testing are not called for, given the foregoing facts.

9. The answer is A, serum testosterone. Virilization is likely to be secondary to an androgen-secreting tumor, congenital adrenal hyperplasia, hyperprolactinemia, hypothyroidism, or drugs. It is not produced by an estrogen or progesterone deficiency, so checking these levels is not appropriate. Checking testosterone, testosterone-binding globulin, and prolactin levels is appropriate. A magnetic resonance image would be indicated only if laboratory studies showed hyperprolactinemia or a suspected gonadotropin-dependent disorder. A general rule in endocrinology is to first define the hormonal abnormality before ordering imaging studies.

10. The answer is C. Klinefelter syndrome is the most common cause of male infertility. As a matter of economics, the evaluation of couple infertility should begin with a sperm count on the male partner. Normal secondary sex characteristics and pubertal timing are typical of Klinefelter syndrome. Unlike Turner syndrome, testosterone levels and growth are normal in Klinefelter syndrome patients until about age 14. Klinefelter syndrome is a congenital disorder, classically with an XXY karyotype. Each of the other choices is a form of hypogonadotropic hypogonadism. Kallmann syndrome features delayed puberty, anosmia, and small genitalia. Prader–Willi syndrome is characterized by childhood obesity. Laurence–Moon syndrome manifests hypogonadotropic hypogonadism and spastic paraplegia with developmental delay in virtually all cases. Bardet–Biedl syndrome shows hypogonadotropic hypogonadism, polydactyly, and obesity.

11. The answer is D. Ascertaining the presence of testes in the abdomen is crucial to ruling out the possibility of the newborn being a fully virilized female with potentially fatal salt-losing congenital adrenal hypoplasia as opposed to a case of undescended testicles. This can be effected by measurement of plasma testosterone level after human chorionic gonadotropin stimulation. After that has been accomplished, watchful waiting is justified for as long as 1 year before the commitment to surgery must be made. Fifty percent of cryptorchid testes will descend by the time the child reaches the age of 3 months; 80% will descend by the time the child reaches the age of 1 year.

12. The answer is C. Neither fertility nor potential for malignancy can be expected to be comparable with those in males without the affliction, even if the

affliction is corrected by the time the child reaches the age of 1 year. Thus, the abnormalities attendant to cryptorchidism are part of the cause of the condition; the nondescent is not the cause in itself. In fact, when one side descends within the medically satisfactory time interval of 1 year, even the opposite testicle, normally descended, will exhibit malignant potential, greater than normal, accounting for 25% of malignancies of the testicles in cases of cryptorchidism. Nevertheless, the recommendation is for medical or surgical correction to occur in time for at least partial amelioration of infertility and malignant potential, improved opportunity for close observation over time, and for cosmetic effect.

13. The answer is C. Begin search for an estrogen-secreting tumor. In contrast to boys in puberty, in which over 50% have at least a transient gynecomastia, breast development in males before puberty causes concern about estrogen exposure, either from an estrogen-secreting tumor (adrenal, testicular, or bronchogenic) or exogenous estrogen exposure. Interesting is that fact that hyperthyroidism is sometimes associated with excess estrogen, but not hypothyroidism. Besides the obvious difference in setting between benign transient gynecomastia and an endocrinologically significant condition (pubertal vs. prepubertal), there may be the question of gynecomastia versus enlarged breast in an obese male. In case of obesity, there is neither palpable breast bud nor particular areola development. Thus, reassurance is inappropriate; treatment with testosterone is premature, as is surgical consultation for excisional biopsy. This condition is associated with no identifiable familiality. Thyroid function is not feasibly an issue in this case.

14. The answer is A. True precocious puberty, sometimes called central precocity, makes its onset before the age of 9, is characterized by pubertal levels of FSH and LH (or low levels that rise with GnRH to pubertal levels, i.e., >10 IU/L). Pseudoprecocity, sometimes called peripheral precocity, occurs as a result of sex hormone production independent of the hypothalamic–pituitary axis, as in adrenal hyperplasia or Leydig cell hyperplasia (testotoxicosis), and as a result FSH and LH are suppressed and do not respond to GnRH. Prader–Willi and Kallmann syndromes are types of hypogonadotropic hypogonadism. A normal variant of puberty onset would have to occur within 2 SD of the mean age of onset of normal puberty.

15. The answer is A. Leuprolide, a GnRH agonist, when administered in a steady (as opposed to pulsing) dosage, suppresses the GnRH pulsating release, which is necessary for the physiologic stimulation of FSH and LH. Use of human chorionic gonadotropin has no application in precocious puberty. Cyproterone is a testosterone antagonist, which is appropriate for peripheral precocity (pseudoprecocity). Medroxyprogesterone acetate is the most widely prescribed progestogen, which is not relevant in this case. Spironolactone is, of course, the sole clinically applied aldosterone; it is used in primary and some secondary forms of aldosteronism.

References

Schuster DP, Falko JM. Problems of growth and development. In: Rudy DR, Kurowski K, eds. *Family Medicine: House Officer Series.* Baltimore: Williams & Wilkins; 1997:577–590.

Zeitler PS, Travers SH, Barker J, et al. Endocrine disorders. In: Hay WW Jr, Levin MJ, Sondheimer JM, et al., eds. *Current Pediatric Diagnosis and Treatment.* 17th ed. New York: McGraw-Hill; 2003:961–1005.

SECTION **XIII**

Allergies

chapter 35

Atopic, Food, and Contact Allergies

Examination questions: Unless instructed otherwise, choose the ONE lettered answer or completion that is BEST in each case.

1 A 30-year-old woman develops wheezing, throat tightness, and urticaria 2 minutes after being stung by a yellow jacket. Her pulse is 104. Her respiratory rate is 30 and her blood pressure is 110/70. She appears in significant distress. There is diffuse expiratory wheezing. Which of the following best describes the pathophysiology of her situation?

(A) Circulating antigens reacting with tissue-based antigen, producing inflammatory injury

(B) Deposition of circulating immune complexes into the tissues, where they produce inflammatory injury

(C) Immunoglobulin G (IgG) response to injected antigen

(D) Mast cell granule release in response to membrane-bound IgE that is cross-linking with a specific allergen

(E) A so-called late-phase reaction produced through inflammation

2 Regarding the patient in Question 1, which of the following therapeutic measures is the best clinical response?

(A) Epinephrine 1:100 injected subcutaneously

(B) Epinephrine 1:100 injected intravenously

(C) Diphenhydramine 50 mg injected intramuscularly

(D) Epinephrine 1:1,000 injected intramuscularly

(E) Cromolyn/nedocromil by nasal inhalation

3 Regarding the patient featured in Questions 1 and 2, which of the following might be a cause for increasing the dosage of epinephrine?

(A) Increased body mass index of the patient

(B) Blood pressure rising to 170/110

(C) Current medications being taken by the patient include propranolol

(D) Patient has a past history of frequent attacks of allergic symptoms.

(E) The patient has Celtic ethnicity.

4 The patient featured in Questions 1 and 2 responded to therapy for the acute anaphylactic syndrome. Twelve hours later she manifests angioneurotic edema and urticaria. Which of the following is the most reasonable approach to treatment of this development?

(A) Diphenhydramine 25 to 50 mg given orally every 6 hours

(B) Repeated injections of epinephrine

(C) Increase the volume of fluid therapy per unit time by 50%

(D) Theophylline 0.5 mg/kg/hour after a loading dose

(E) Beta-adrenergic medication given orally

5 A 35-year-old female patient has begun experiencing hives at various times, usually within 30 minutes after a meal. If you were to actuate a trial of food eliminations, adding back one eliminated food every 5 days until occurrence of allergic symptoms, which of the following groups of four foods would you choose first, to obtain the earliest conclusion as to cause?

(A) Beef, rice, apples, bananas

(B) Tomatoes, peaches, wheat, potatoes

(C) Peanuts, tree nuts, vertebrate fish, shellfish

(D) Chicken, green beans, peas, corn

(E) Kidney beans, lima beans, lettuce, radishes

6 A white 18-year-old young woman who lives in the Midwest (Ohio valley; northwest of the Appalachian mountains, east of the Mississippi River) complains of rhinorrhea and sneezing that begins during the months of May and June, peaks at about July 4, and then tapers off in September and October. Which of the following is true regarding this condition?

(A) The condition is precipitated by exposure to *Cladosporium* (previously known as *Hormodendrum*) and *Alternaria* mold spores.

(B) The symptoms are caused by exposure to ragweed pollen.

(C) The peak age for symptoms is between 10 and 15 years of age.

(D) Females are twice as likely to be affected as males.

(E) Symptoms will respond to antibiotics.

7 A 35-year-old man has been your patient since moving into the area from his lifelong home in California. He comes to you in the first week of September complaining of coryza and occasional wheezing that seems not to evolve through the various stages of a cold. It occurred about this time last year but it is now more severe; it has lasted more 2 weeks since its onset in the last half of August. The nasal discharge is thin and watery, without yellowish mucus or mucosanguinous characteristics. He has tried taking the antihistamine loratidine (Claritin), which did not give him significant relief; you prescribed cetirazine (Zyrtec), which also failed to relieve his symptoms. You then suggested over-the-counter diphenhydramine (Benadryl) and chlorpheniramine. The latter two antihistamines relieved his symptoms but caused intolerable drowsiness. Which of the following is the most practical approach for his acute symptoms, assuming he has no other significant medical problems?

(A) Skin testing to confirm the offending allergen, followed by allergen immunotherapy (desensitization)

(B) Prescription of clarithromycin 500 mg XL tablets, two daily times for 7 days

(C) Prescription of prednisone, given orally at a starting dosage of 40 mg daily, reduced every 2 days to taper off over a 2-week period

(D) An increase in the dosage of Benadryl

(E) Counseling the patient to remain indoors in an air-conditioned environment for the duration of the allergy season

8 The patient in Question 7 was found to be reactive to ragweed and you plan on initiating desensitization in the coming year. Meanwhile, which of the following foods, if any, would you advise he avoid while attempting other means to give relief of symptoms?

(A) Peanuts

(B) Shellfish

(C) Vertebrate fish

(D) Chocolate

(E) Bananas

9 From the physiological point of view, which of the following is the goal of immunotherapy in the treatment of atopic allergies, for example, rhinitis and conjunctivitis, in regard to allergen-specific antibodies?

(A) Increase IgE antibodies specific to the allergen

(B) Decrease IgG antibodies specific to the allergen

(C) Increase in IgE, decrease in IgG

(D) Increase in IgG, decrease in IgE

(E) Decrease in both IgG and IgE

10 Regarding the patient in Questions 7, 8, and 9, in what period of time might you expect his symptoms to remit on immunotherapy if he were to respond?

(A) 1 month

(B) 6 weeks

(C) 6 months

(D) 1 year

(E) 5 years

11 A 34-year-old man has noticed increasing incidents of being stung by bees and increasingly severe reactions from the stings. Instead of normal erythema and swelling, when he was stung 2 weeks ago on the ankle, the whole leg became swollen with an angry redness. At that time he went to another doctor, who diagnosed cellulitis and treated with antibiotics. Then today he was stung on the arm with rapid development of the same type of response as last week, and this time he is experiencing hives and having some shortness of breath. The sting occurred an hour ago. He appears to be in mild distress with the dyspnea and discomfort at the sting site. Auscultation of the lungs reveals bilateral wheezes with adequate respiratory excursion. You opt for an intramuscular injection of 1:1,000 epinephrine and the patient's dyspnea responds rapidly. Which of the following is the best long-term management plan for this patient?

(A) Prescribe 5 years of specific venom immunotherapy

(B) Prescribe epinephrine unit-dose syringes (EpiPen Auto-Injector) for use immediately after he is stung

(C) Prescribe prednisone in 2-week tapering dosages for initiation whenever he is stung

(D) Prescribe 8 mg of chlorpheniramine given orally whenever he is stung

(E) Prescribe cromolyn for inhalation at the time of a bee sting

(D) Prescribe diphenhydramine 50 mg for oral use immediately upon being stung

12 A 12-year-old boy has been followed for asthma for the past 2 years. Until recently he has been satisfied with self-treatment with albuterol inhalations once or twice per week and they are needed once or twice per month at night. However, in the past 2 weeks he has required albuterol three or four times per week. His forced expiratory volume in 1 second (FEV_1) is measured at 85% of normal. Which of the following would be an accepted therapeutic adjustment to this development?

(A) Increase albuterol inhalations to every 6 hours as needed

(B) Start oral albuterol at a dosage of 8 mg every 12 hours

(C) Start inhaled glucocorticoids

(D) Start both inhaled cromolyn and inhaled glucocorticoids

(E) Start long-acting beta-2 agonist, inhaled glucosteroids, and oral glucosteroids

13 The patient in Question 12 has responded well to the escalation of therapeutic measures until his season of (mold-spore) allergies began. Since then he has developed symptoms requiring his albuterol daily and once or twice weekly in the night. His FEV_1 and peak expiratory flow (PEF) have fallen to 65% of predicted levels. In addition, the variability of his PEF ranges from 20% to 30% of predictability. What should be the next therapeutic regimen?

(A) Perform skin testing and prepare for immunotherapy

(B) Start oral albuterol at a dosage of 8 mg every 12 hours

(C) Start inhaled glucocorticoids

(D) Start both inhaled glucocorticoids and a long-acting beta-2 agonist

(E) Start a long-acting beta-2 agonist, inhaled glucosteroids, and oral glucosteroids

14 Considering infectious precipitants, which of the following organisms is thought to be most often implicated in the initiation of an asthmatic diathesis?

(A) Adenoviruses

(B) Herpes viruses

(C) Arboviruses

(D) Respiratory syncytial virus

(E) *Streptococcus pneumoniae*

15 A 17-year-old with a long-standing history of asthma (since age 5) has been on short-acting beta-agonist inhalers or cromolyn inhalers (step 2) with fair daytime symptom control, but he is now awakening almost every night with attacks of wheezing and dyspnea. The PEF is 75% of the predicted level. In keeping with recategorizing the stage of asthma, hence the care step, which of the following inhalers has the longest duration of action and thus specifically would be the best choice to control his nocturnal symptoms?

(A) Albuterol

(B) Terbutaline

(C) Pirbuberol

(D) Ipratropium

(E) Salmeterol

16 A 35-year-old factory worker who works around detergents and organic solvents has developed an erythematous, pruritic rash on the forearms that first appeared 3 days ago and today has formed vesicles that have begun to weep with clear serous fluid. Which of the following is the most likely offending agent?

(A) Machine oil

(B) Industrial strength degreasing soap

(C) Organic solvents

(D) Poison ivy

(E) Cosmetics

Examination Answers

1. The answer is D, mast cell granule release in response to membrane-bound IgE that is cross-linking with specific allergen. This is a classic immediate hypersensitivity response. This individual must have had prior exposure to the antigens (but may not recall the first uneventful sting), which previously led to the production of these IgE antibodies on the mast cell surface. The early-phase response is characterized by capillary permeability and fluid leakage. It is invoked in allergy skin testing as another example of its applicability. Late-phase responses include local invasion by basophiles, eosinophiles, monocytes, and lymphocytes. Analogous clinical situations include the rapid onset and recovery (15 to 30 minutes) of bronchospasm in asthmatic exposure to inhaled allergenic antigens. The late response in asthma occurs 3 to 8 hours later and can last up to 24 hours. There are mucosal and conjunctival counterparts to these reactions. The late phase resembles the actual clinical picture in asthma, resulting in air trapping, for example. Circulating immune complex deposition such as occurs in lupus erythematosus or glomerulonephritis results in chronic inflammation but not anaphylaxis. Serum sickness is an example of IgG response to injected antigen. Rash, endocarditis, synovitis, and glomerulonephritis may result, but anaphylaxis is not a late-phase sequela.

2. The answer is D. Epinephrine 1:1,000 injected intramuscularly, or on occasion intravenously, is the treatment for anaphylaxis. The greatest single error made in the management of acute anaphylaxis is timidity; there is a failure to act in a timely and aggressive manner. Epinephrine 1:100 injected subcutaneously would be a dangerous overdose of this powerful sympathomimetic drug (and has occurred by accident with fatal consequences). Epinephrine 1:100 injected intravenously would be an even greater overdose. Diphenhydramine 50 mg injected intravenously would be too mild a response, given the rapidly developing systemic involvement of the anaphylaxis. Cromolyn/nedocromil by nasal inhalation is a preventive treatment for allergic rhinitis and has no application in anaphylaxis. To combat hypotension, besides the epinephrine, fluid therapy and other vasopressors (e.g., dopamine, norepinephrine, and phenylephrine) may be employed. Specific therapy for persistent bronchospasm should be treated with beta-agonists, such as albuterol, by inhalation.

3. The answer is C. If the patient with anaphylaxis has been taking the nonselective beta-adrenergic blocking agent, propranolol, the effective dosage of epinephrine for reversing the pathophysiology may well be increased. This occurs, of course, because of the blocking effect on the beta-adrenergic portion of the action of epinephrine. None of the other choices has any bearing on treatment of anaphylaxis.

4. The answer is A. Late occurrence of anaphylactoid symptoms and signs are frequent after anaphylaxis, as a result of the late-phase reaction discussed in Question 1, manifestations of which are possible for up to 24 hours and are the basis for continued monitoring of anaphylaxis patients for that period of time. If these include angioneurotic edema and urticaria, then oral diphenhydramine (Benadryl) is appropriate. If late manifestations involve bronchospasm, a frequent part of the acute syndrome, then albuterol or theophylline (Aminophylline) are appropriate, although the latter is less frequently used because of the narrow therapeutic versus toxic range rations. Fluid therapy applies only in the case of hypotension, a development not to be expected during the late-phase reaction.

5. The answer is C. Peanuts, tree nuts, vertebrate fish, and shellfish account for 90% of all food allergies. An elimination diet is a practical technique available in primary care. Additional foods that are often involved in food allergic situations include beer, chocolate, tomatoes, and egg (albumen). In practice it may be helpful to include all eight of the foregoing groups in an elimination diet. Foods are added back individually with 2 days between each addition. When the urticaria or angioneurotic edema reappears, the most recently added food item is assumed to be at least one of the causes of the symptoms. That food can then be avoided. Food allergies in many cases appear for a certain epoch of a patient's life, followed by remission. The period of the most intense symptoms, in some cases, may seem to coincide with life stressors, such as crises in a marriage or child rearing.

6. The answer is A. The condition is precipitated by exposure to mold spores, that is, *Cladosporium* and

Alternaria organisms, in a person specifically to the antigens. These are the second and third most intense and prevalent pollen allergens in the United States, generally confined to the eastern half of the country. Ragweed, the most prevalent and severe offending allergen, has a season that begins on approximately August 15 at the 40th parallel, occurring earlier as one moves north (the allergic season is timed with the drying ripened flower). The peak age group for allergic rhinitis is between 15 and 25 years. There is no particular difference in the prevalence of allergic rhinitis between the sexes.

7. The answer is C. Prednisone, given orally at 40 mg daily, with the dosage reduced every 2 days to taper off over a 2-week period, is a regimen justified in cases such as the one presented, which is typical for allergic rhinitis that is due to ragweed allergy in the eastern half of the United States. Skin testing and desensitization will not be able to address and relieve symptoms in the year in which the program is initiated. However, the need to employ glucocorticoids in a given season for relief of severe, otherwise nonresponsive symptoms should be the trigger to initiate skin testing, as systemic glucocorticoids should not be prescribed lightly. The patient had no symptoms of sinusitis or of any other bacterial infection; thus, clarithromycin is not indicated and any other antibiotic would not be justified. Benadryl was already shown to cause drowsiness at a therapeutic dosage, and increasing the dosage would only be expected to worsen the drowsiness. Avoidance may be effective in cases of animal dander allergy but is not practical for the management of pollen allergy.

8. The answer is E. Bananas and also melons cross-react with ragweed and therefore should be avoided during the season of allergic symptoms (mid-August until the temperature drops below 40°F). Other cross-reacting foods include apples and carrots with birch pollen. These foods may increase the symptoms of rhinitis. The other foods presented as choices are prominent classic food allergens. Symptoms of classic food allergies are more likely to be angioneurotic edema or urticaria, rather than coryza.

9. The answer is D, an increase in IgG and decrease in IgE antibodies specific to ragweed, in this case. The immediately reacting IgE is the offending antibody. Successful immunotherapy (desensitization) leads to a transient slight rise in IgE followed by a fall to much lower levels than beforehand and a rise in the blocking antibody IgG. (Remember: The "G" in IgG is "good," applying to

immunity to both allergens and infections in virtually all disease states to which it is relevant.)

10. The answer is D, 1 year. If patients do not respond at least partially to 1 year of treatment, then they are unlikely to respond to further immunotherapy. In patients who do respond, treatment is often continued for up to 4 or 5 years. The efficacy of immunotherapy depends on the protocol, typically consisting of a series of three successive vials containing graduated concentrations of the antigen(s) in the "vaccine." The skin testing should be done well in advance of the season of allergic symptoms, say, in June or July in the case of ragweed allergy, whose symptoms begin in August in the eastern half of the country. The first vial may contain the involved antigen or antigens in a dilution of 1:10,000. Typically the patient receives 0.1 mL on a twice weekly schedule, with the volume increasing by 0.1 mL weekly until 1 mL is being given, and the volume is held at that level until the end of the vial is reached. The second vial contains the antigens in a 1:1,000 dilution and the same schedule of injections is followed. In the first season all three vials are completed. After the first season and series of vials ends, typically in January of the year (about 6 months), the patient may be "furloughed" until June or July of the following year. Some allergists recommend carrying the patient through the off season on biweekly injections of the full-strength injections. If a patient has an exacerbation of symptoms or local swelling at the injection site during the acceleration phase of injections, the dose should be held flat (without being increased) until no symptoms occur after the shot. Obviously the patient is kept in the office for at least 15 minutes after each injection. Severe systemic reactions to immunotherapy shots against pollen allergy are rare. However, animal dander desensitization is another story and, on the part of this author, is not recommended (simple avoidance is favored here, as it is always possible in the case of animal dander allergy).

11. The answer is A, 5 years of specific venom immunotherapy. This program is 98% effective in preventing systemic reactions to specific stinging insects, such as honey bees, wasps, hornets, yellow jackets, and immigrant fire ants. Epinephrine unit-dose syringe injections are necessary for the acute reaction after the sting but should not comprise the long-term management. Prednisone (or other oral glucocorticoids) is not suited to acute-phase (IGE) reactions and is not suited to long-term prevention. Both antihistamines chlorpheniramine and diphenhydramine are inadequate for acute treatment and have no place in prevention. Cromolyn by inhalation is a preventative, specific for reactive airway disease, that must be taken three times daily for effect but, unlike immunotherapy, does not have preventive effects for longer than the term of administration.

12. The answer is C. Start inhaled glucorticoids (or inhaled cromolyn). The patient has progressed from the mild, intermittent stage (symptoms requiring use of a beta-2 agonist inhaler no more than twice weekly and no more than twice in the night monthly), which could be called stage 1. When he began having symptoms more than twice weekly (but not as frequently as daily), he entered the stage called mild persistent, or stage 2. In the first two stages described, the FEV_1 and the PEF should be greater than 80% of those predicted for age. The foregoing and the complete spectrum of the staging of asthma are based on guidelines published by the National Asthma Education and Prevention Program (NAEPP).

13. The answer is D. Start both inhaled glucocorticoids and a long-acting beta-2 agonist (e.g., salmeterol or formoterol). The inhaled glucocorticoids, dosed mildly in the second step of therapy, are prescribed as a medium-dosed product at step 3 and a high-dosed product at step 4. The patient has entered the third stage of asthma, which is moderate persistent asthma. It is defined as symptoms that occur daily and more than once per week at night. Either the FEV_1 or the PEF is between 60% and 80% of the predicted values. Stage 4 is defined as continuous symptoms and limited physical activity caused by asthma. Because long-acting beta-2 agonists and inhaled steroids are not rapidly acting, they must still be supplemented with the rapid-acting medications such as albuterol. As stated previously, albuterol alone is not adequate in persistent asthma. Immunotherapy would have no application for treating symptoms in the present or near future. Albuterol alone is not appropriate as a stable plan, as was pointed out in the definition of stage 2 asthma. Long-acting beta-2 agonists, inhaled high dose glucosteroids, and oral glucosteroids, all three, would be appropriate in stage 4 disease (i.e., as step 4 therapy). Below is a table outlining the stages of asthma.

14. The answer is D, respiratory syncytial virus. Up to 50% of children with bronchiolitis caused by respiratory syncytial virus will have recurrent wheezing until they reach the age of 3 years, though most children with this combination of circumstances have atopic constitutions and family histories of similar problems. Bacteria are less likely than viruses to provoke asthma. In the case of *S. pneumoniae*, the organism is the most likely bacterium to complicate symptomatic lower respiratory tract infections, especially those that are community acquired, and sometimes asthma, but it is not an initiator of reactive airway disease. However, the 50% rate of such sequelae to respiratory syncytial virus is far above the expected rate in the population.

15. The answer is E, salmeterol, a long-acting beta-2 agonist. The patient has moved to the moderate persistent stage or, one could say, stage 3. The effects of salmeterol may last up to 30 hours and salmeterol is many times stronger than albuterol as a beta-2 agonist. Terbutaline and pirbuterol are beta-2 agonists that are intermediate in their duration of activity. Anticholinergic medications (e.g., ipratropium) are rather short in length of activity (4 to 6 hours). The following is a table outlining step care that corresponds to the four stages of asthma.

Stage	Symptoms	Night Symptoms	Lung Function
1. Mild	≤2×/wk	≤2×/mo	FEV_1 or PEF intermittent none; normal PEF ≥80%; PEF between bouts var <20%
2. Mild	>2×/wk <1 daily	>2×/mo	FEV_1 or PEF persistent ≥80 PEF var 20%–30%
3. Moderate persistent	Daily short beta-2 Ag Activity affected Attacks ≥2×/wk May last for days	>1×/wk	FEV_1 or PEF >60%, <80% PEF var >30%
4. Severe persistent	Contin symptoms Limited physical activity	Frequent	FEV_1 or PEF <60% PEF var >30%

Table is modified slightly from the scheme shown by the National Asthma Education and Prevention Program (1997).
Notes: var, variability; beta-2 Ag, beta-2 agonist.

Therapeutic Modalities for Steps Analogous to the Stages of Asthma

Step	Long-Term Control	Quick Relief
Step 1	None	Short beta-2 Ag
Step 2	Daily inh Ster LD	≤2×/wk ≥beta-2 Ag/ day signifies or cromolyn or nedocromil move to step 3
Step 3	Daily MD inh Ster, Long beta-2 Ag Or both	See step 2
Step 4	Same as step 3 + PO Ster	See step 2

Notes: beta-2 Ag, beta-2 agonist; inh, inhaled; Ster, (gluco)steroid; LD and MD, low and medium dose (steroids); PO, oral.

16. The answer is D, poison ivy. Poison ivy contact dermatitis is an allergic contact dermatitis, as opposed to an irritant contact dermatitis. Only allergic dermatitides lead to vesiculation. The differentiating point here is that machine oil, degreasing soap, and organic solvents are irritant contactants. Although cosmetics do sometimes cause allergic contact reactions, these seldom appear on the forearms for obvious reasons.

References

Boguniewicz M. Allergic disorders. In: Hay WW Jr, Levin MJ, Sondheimer JM, et al., eds. *Current Pediatric Diagnosis and Treatment.* 17th ed. New York: McGraw-Hill; 2003: 1080–1111.

Kishyama JL, Adelman DC. Allergic and immunologic disorders. In: Tierney LM, McPhee SJ, Papadakis MA, eds. *Current Medical Diagnosis and Treatment.* 45th ed. New York: McGraw-Hill/ Appleton & Lange; 2006:788–806.

National Asthma Education and Prevention Program. Expert Panel Number 2. Washington, DC: National Institutes of Health/National Heart, Lung, and Blood Institute; 1997. NIH publication 97–4951.

Schwer WA. Atopic, food, and contact allergies. In: Rudy DR, Kurowski K, eds. *Family Medicine: House Officer Series.* Baltimore: Williams & Wilkins; 1997:591–604.

SECTION **XIV**

Preventative Care and Health

chapter 36

Preoperative Clearance and Evaluation and Management

Examination questions: Unless instructed otherwise, choose the ONE lettered answer or completion that is BEST in each case.

1 A 45-year-old male patient is scheduled for elective cholecystectomy and common duct exploration. He has neither history nor finding of hypertension, diabetes, heart disease, or bleeding diathesis, nor any other significant system review. Specifically, he denies and manifests on examination no excessive bruising. He underwent general anesthesia for emergency appendectomy in the past. He is athletic and runs routinely without symptoms of chest pain or undue dyspnea. Which of the following would be the minimally acceptable set of ancillary studies to order for preoperative clearance?

(A) Complete blood cell (CBC) count, Prothrombin time (PT), partial thromboplastin time (PTT), electrocardiogram (ECG), routine liver and kidney function blood studies, and chest x-ray

(B) CBC count, PT, PTT, and routine liver and kidney function blood studies (no chest x-ray)

(C) CBC count, PT, PTT, and kidney function studies (neither liver function studies nor chest x-ray)

(D) CBC count, PT, and PTT

(E) No ancillary testing

2 A 55-year-old white man is scheduled for abdominal surgery to resect a segment of colon from which was snared an adenomatous polyp that revealed at least stage B carcinoma (tumor in muscularis or serosa). All but which one of the following situations significantly increases the risk of a myocardial infarction or other coronary event during or after surgery?

(A) Angina symptoms with strenuous physical activity, such as shoveling dirt at a rapid pace

(B) Angina when walking one or two blocks on level ground

(C) History of congestive heart failure (CHF)

(D) Anginal pains with any significant physical activity

(E) Insulin treatment for diabetes

3 A 58-year-old man with a history of angina treated successfully with percutaneous transluminal angioplasty 3 months ago is now asymptomatic. He must undergo a femoropopliteal graft for peripheral vascular disease. For a low-risk patient with known coronary artery disease, the perioperative cardiac mortality risk is 4%. Each of the following preoperative measures can reduce that risk, except for which one?

(A) Atenolol

(B) Metoprolol

(C) Clonidine

(D) Albuterol

(E) Atorvastatin

4 A 60-year-old woman has been diagnosed with cholelithiasis without evidence of common duct involvement. Although she has had several moderately severe attacks of abdominal pain after meals, currently she is asymptomatic. Elective surgery is indicated but she has a history of an uncomplicated myocardial infarction 2 months ago. Which of the following is the best preoperative strategy for maximizing her cardiovascular safety through the period of surgery and the 2-week postoperative period?

(A) Institute preoperative beta-adrenergic blocking agents for 2 weeks before and 30 days after surgery

(B) Start calcium channel blocking agents in the preoperative and 4-week postoperative period

(C) Postpone surgery for 2 to 4 months

(D) Start atorvastatin and maintain it throughout the postoperative period

(E) Institute an alpha-adrenergic agonist before surgery and throughout the postoperative period

5 A 56-year-old male patient with cholelithiasis has had two attacks of abdominal pain caused by gallbladder disease. Currently he has been abdominal symptom free for 2 weeks, but upon system review he is shown to have a history of anginal pains precipitated by climbing a single flight of stairs and by walking one block. His course had been stable and he has apparently been in denial of his chest pains until the history was extracted as a part of preoperative clearance for his gallbladder problem. In fact, the anginal pains appear to be precipitated with increasingly less activity. Which of the following is the best strategy for minimizing his perioperative cardiovascular risk?

(A) Institute preoperative beta-adrenergic blocking agents for 2 weeks before and 30 days after

(B) Proceed with evaluation for coronary revascularization

(C) Postpone surgery for 2 months

(D) Start atorvastatin and maintain it throughout the postoperative period

(E) Prescribe nitroglycerin sublingually and a long-acting nitrate for 2 weeks before proceeding with surgery

6 A 67-year-old black female patient has been treated for 3 months for CHF caused by uncontrolled hypertension; her blood pressure readings have been running 180 to 220/100 to 140. She had been in pulmonary edema that responded to after-load reducing agents and loop diuretics. Her blood pressure readings are now under control, through the use of a combination of angiotensin-converting enzyme inhibitors and a potassium-sparing combination of a thiazide diuretic and triamterene. Now she is to undergo a semiurgent uterine suspension for stress incontinence. For the past 8 weeks she has not been dyspneic and she exhibits no peripheral edema, hepatomagaly, or neck vein distention. Which of the following is true or correct regarding the upcoming surgery?

(A) The patient should undergo her surgery after an aggressive program of loop diuresis.

(B) The patient will be at increased risk for myocardial infarction.

(C) The patient will be at increased risk of the onset of angina.

(D) The patient will be at increased risk of pulmonary edema.

(E) Because the patient is well compensated, she will be subject to no excess risk.

7 A 55-year-old man must undergo laparotomy to resect a descending colon segment at the site of a malignant polyp discovered at routine colonoscopy. He had a myocardial infarction 6 months ago, which was diagnosed too late for successful thrombolytic therapy. However, his course has not been complicated by symptoms of CHF and he has had no chest pains since then during an orderly cardiac rehabilitation program. Because of this history, the patient's preoperative clearance included measurement of the cardiac ejection fraction, whose result was 45%. Which of the following is true or correct regarding the patient's upcoming surgery and postoperative period?

(A) He should be anticoagulated prior to surgery.

(B) The patient will be at increased risk for myocardial infarction.

(C) The patient will be at increased risk for the onset of angina.

(D) The patient will be at increased risk of CHF.

(E) Because the patient is well compensated, he will be subject to no excess risk.

8 A 45-year-old man with hypertension must undergo abdominal exploration for an asymptomatic mass that was suggestive of lymphoma. His blood pressure readings, on hydrochlorothiazide/triamterene and lisinopril, have averaged 145 to 150/95 to 98 over the past 7 days. CBC count and serum electrolyte levels are within normal limits. Which of the following decisions regarding his preoperative and intraoperative management is correct in light of current thinking?

(A) Continue the current medications, including the dose(s) that is due on the day of surgery, and proceed with the surgery

(B) Delay surgery and add a calcium channel blocking drug; proceed with surgery when the blood pressure is consistently below 140/90

(C) Add a ganglionic blocking drug for 2 days and proceed with surgery

(D) Order an ECG and proceed with surgery if there is no evidence of left ventricular hypertrophy

(E) Consult a cardiologist for preoperative clearance and advice on management of the blood pressure

9 If the patient in Question 8 had had a blood pressure of 190/115 without symptoms, which of the following would have been the most acceptable therapeutic approach?

(A) Continue the current medications, including the dose(s) that is due on the day of surgery, and proceed with the surgery

(B) Delay surgery and step up the care of the hypertension, such as adding a calcium channel blocking drug; proceed with surgery when the blood pressure is consistently below 140/90

(C) Order a thallium stress test

(D) Consult cardiology and anticipate coronary angiography before proceeding with the elective surgery

(E) Consult a cardiologist for preoperative clearance and advice on management of the blood pressure

10 A 45-year-old white man with a 50 pack-year history of smoking has been diagnosed with Barrett esophagus and is being considered for an aggressive esophageal surgical procedure. He has symptoms of chronic obstructive lung disease. You order pulmonary function studies to determine whether it is safe to proceed without subjecting the patient to chronic maintenance on a ventilator. Which of the following criteria or combinations comprises a safe cutpoint for pulmonary function testing to clear the patient for pulmonary or upper abdominal surgery without further testing?

(A) Forced expiratory volume in 1 second (FEV_1) >1 L/minute; forced vital capacity (FVC) >50% of predicted value; and maximal voluntary ventilation (MVV) >50% of predicted value

(B) MVV >50% of predicted value and diffusion capacity of the lungs for carbon dioxide (DLCO) >40% of predicted value

(C) FEV_1 >500 mL

(D) DLCO >40% of predicted value

(E) FVC >60% of predicted value

11 Regarding the patient in Question 10, he survived the esophageal surgery. One year later he presents with a left upper lobe mass on a chest x-ray, ordered because of bloody mucus production from his previously long-standing cough. The patient has resumed smoking after a period of cessation lasting 3 weeks. Spirometry is repeated because of the passage of a year since this ongoing smoker was cleared for surgery and operated upon. It now shows a FEV_1 of 2.2 L; a MVV of 45% of predicted value; and a DLCO of 45% of predicted value. Because of these findings, a ventilation–perfusion (V/Q) scan is ordered. Which of the following is a criterion that must be met in order for this patient to qualify for a pulmonary resection without leading to the probability of ventilator dependency?

(A) The contribution of the lobe being considered for resection must not exceed 1,400 mL.

(B) A V/Q mismatch must not be found.

(C) A diagnosis of pneumonia constitutes a permanent contraindication for lobectomy.

(D) The V/Q criterion for resectability depends on the tissue diagnosis of the mass.

(E) V/Q results may be interpreted only in the context of the spirometric findings.

12 A 52-year-old white man has suffered from crushing chest pain that lasted 4 hours before he came to the hospital emergency department. There were elevated ST segments and Q waves that were 10 mm deep in leads V_5 and V_6. Myocardial enzymes were elevated. His course remained uncomplicated and he was discharged for convalescence at home today, 10 days after his pain. He and his surgeon canceled an elective inguinal herniorrhaphy at the time of his hospitalization. What is the minimum time after the event that this patient should wait for rescheduling that elective surgery?

(A) 6 weeks

(B) 3 months

(C) 9 months

(D) 12 months

(E) 18 months

13 A 43-year-old male alcoholic is scheduled for biliary surgery after discovery of an impacted common bile duct stone. Which of the following preoperative parameters is the most significant prognostic indication of his postoperative hepatic status in regard to ascites, encephalopathy, and gastrointestinal bleeding?

(A) Direct-acting bilirubin

(B) Presence or absence of ascites

(C) Level of serum albumin

(D) Preoperative Child–Turcotte–Pugh classification of cirrhosis score

(E) Presence or absence of encephalopathy

14 A 34-year-old woman is being prepared for hysterectomy, indicated by menometrorrhagia in a woman who is gravida 4, para 4 and desires no more pregnancies. In preparing for surgery you are aware that her hemoglobin may be decreased as a result of an iron deficiency, which at various periods over the past 3 years has required iron therapy. She has been inconsistent in her compliance with the prescriptions. Which of the following is felt to be the point below which the risk of perioperative complications in otherwise healthy individuals is significantly increased?

(A) 12 g/dL

(B) 10 g/dL

(C) 8 g/dL

(D) 6 g/dL

(E) 4 g/dL

15 Besides risk of cardiac complications in those with risk factors, in patients with preoperative hemoglobin <10 g/dL or hematocrit <30%, which of the following complications occurs with a greater than expected rate?

(A) Urinary tract infection

(B) Postoperative atelectasis

(C) Pneumonitis

(D) Pancreatitis

(E) Postoperative delirium

16 A 65-year-old man has been diagnosed with a symptomatic ventricular septal defect (VSD) but surgical correction is indicated because of the emergence of concentric cardiomegaly (diastolic dysfunction). The blood pressure is 140/65. The patient is also diagnosed, in the course of his overall evaluation and the discovery of a bruit over the right carotid artery, as having a 75% right carotid artery stenosis caused by atherosclerosis. While awaiting repair of the septal defect, the patient experiences a 2-minute bout of a visual scotoma involving the right lower quadrant of the field, with no visual disturbance on the left. Which of the following is the most logical sequence of actions?

(A) Perform repair of the VSD followed by carotid endarterectomy

(B) Perform a coronary bypass grafting procedure followed by repair of the VSD

(C) Perform carotid endarterectomy followed by repair of the VSD

(D) Perform carotid artery bypass graft followed by the indicated cardiac procedure

(E) Treat the cardiac hypertrophy aggressively medically, followed by carotid endarterectomy when the cardiac status is stable and satisfactory

17 Which of the following ranks as the most specific and earnest preoperative preparation for an elective abdominal operation on a 55-year-old man who is in chronic renal failure on dialysis?

(A) Preoperative ECG within 24 hours of the operation

(B) Blood urea nitrogen and creatinine levels within 24 hours of the surgery

(C) CBC within 1 week of surgery

(D) Dialysis within 24 hours and electrolytes studies just before surgery

(E) Renal biopsy within 30 days of surgery

18 A 35-year-old female patient with chronic diarrhea has been diagnosed as having Crohn disease and is being considered for exploratory laparotomy. Considering the recent severe diarrhea, the patient's state of nutrition is a factor in preparing for surgery and planning postoperative care. Below what level of serum albumin may she be considered to be severely malnourished?

(A) ≤4 g/dL

(B) ≤3.5 g/dL

(C) <2 g/dL

(D) <1.5 g/dL

(E) <3.0 g/dL

19 A 63-year-old woman is being scheduled for an operation to relieve partial bowel obstruction that is due to a descending colon carcinoma. Her symptoms consist of alternating constipation (cessation of movements, normally daily) for periods of 2 to 3 days, followed by diarrhea for 1 to 2 days. She says her appetite has waned during the period of these symptoms, approximately 6 weeks. Her weight is 120 lb (54.4 kg) at a height of 5 ft, 6 in. (1.68 m). In evaluating her for the possible need of supplemental feeding, at least orally, prior to surgery to take place in 1 week, you find what dietary intake that she should be able to ingest (caloric and percentage of protein oral intake) that would be adequate to obviate the need for an oral supplement (e.g., Ensure)?

(A) 35 kcal/kg, of which 20% should be protein

(B) 30 kcal/kg, with 30% protein

(C) 40 kcal/kg, with 80 g of protein

(D) Adequate oral intake as confirmed subjectively by the patient will suffice to ensure that the patient is taking in an adequate amount to carry her through major surgery.

(E) This calculation is not needed as long as the patient's serum albumin and transferrin levels are within normal limits.

20 The foregoing patient canceled her semielective surgery for personal reasons and presented 3 weeks later with total large bowel obstruction. She has been anorectic and in colicky pain for the past 7 days. Now the surgeon states the patient will require a temporary colostomy. Her weight is 110 lb (50 kg). Her skin turgor is normal but her mucosae are "sticky," though not dry. Laboratory studies include the following: serum albumin, 2.9 g/dL

(3.5 to 5.5 g/dL); serum transferrin, 150 mg/dL (250 to 430 mg/dL); total lymphocyte count, 1,200/mm^3 (1,500 to 3,000/mm^3). She is scheduled for surgery tomorrow morning. What is the most appropriate nutritional program for this patient prior to surgery?

(A) Oral supplement 200 mL qid now and for 10 days postoperatively

(B) Nasogastric tube feedings to ensure 2,100 calories per day for the first 7 days postoperatively

(C) Low-residue diet commencing 2 days after surgery

(D) Total parenteral nutrition now and for 7 days postoperatively

(E) Dietary consultation

21 Prophylactic antibiotics after surgery have become a much more accepted practice over the past 20 years. However, there are guidelines and a theme for this practice. Which of the following *does not* merit prophylactic antibiotic therapy after surgery?

(A) Lymph node biopsy in the neck area

(B) Thoracotomy

(C) Hysterectomy

(D) Biliary surgery

(E) Urinary cystotomy

22 For which of the following pre-existing conditions is preoperative antibiotic prophylaxis against bacterial endocarditis recommended?

(A) Patients who have undergone coronary bypass surgery

(B) Patients with cardiac pacemakers

(C) Patients with hypertrophic cardiomyopathy

(D) Patients with previous Kawasaki disease

(E) Patients with implanted defibrillators

Examination Answers

1. The answer is E. No ancillary testing is recommended for healthy patients under the age of 50, given the complete historical and physical findings given in the vignette. There has been a steady reduction in the routine tests recommended for preoperative testing on young and healthy individuals. In the first edition of this work, the age cutoff was given as 40 years. To be sure, this presupposes a careful history for cardiovascular health and exercise tolerance and care in exposing liability for hemorrhagic diathesis. Regarding the latter group, a checklist of historical and physical information should include whether there have been unprovoked bruising on the trunk >5 cm in diameter; frequent epistaxis or gingival bleeding; menorrhagia with iron deficiency; hemarthrosis with mild trauma; history of excessive surgical bleeding; family history of abnormal bleeding; or presence of severe kidney or liver disease.

2. The answer is A. Angina symptoms with strenuous physical activity, such as shoveling dirt at a normal pace, is not considered to be severe and is classified in the Canadian Cardiovascular Society system as level II. Level I is angina that appears with rapid strenuous but not with ordinary walking or climbing stairs. Levels I and II pose low risk of intraoperative and postoperative cardiac complications. Levels III and IV pose significant risks and call for noninvasive preoperative testing. Angina when a person is walking one or two blocks on level ground is classified as level III; level IV is characterized as angina with any significant physical activity. CHF uncompensated within 1 year of elective surgery increases the risk of cardiovascular complication significantly, as does the presence of insulin-dependent diabetes.

3. The answer is D. Albuterol, of course, is a beta-2 agonist. Coronary disease risk in surgery would more likely be increased by the use of this class of drugs. In contrast, beta-adrenergic blocking drugs, such as atenolol, metoprolol, and clonidine, an alpha-2 agonist, have been shown to reduce such perioperative risk significantly. In addition, 45 days of a statin, such as atorvastatin, beginning 2 weeks before surgery has also effected a markedly reduced perioperative coronary disease risk status.

4. The answer is C, postpone surgery for 2 months. A myocardial infarction within 3 to 6 months poses a significant risk of perioperative cardiovascular mortality and morbidity. If the planned surgery is elective, delaying the operation is the correct strategy, rather than instituting risk-reducing agents, effective though they may be.

5. The answer is B. One should proceed with evaluation for coronary revascularization. This is another example of a high-cardiovascular-risk situation in that the patient has class III angina, according to the Canadian Cardiovascular Society system (see the discussion of Question 2), that is now accelerating. Although there have been some recently published data that might shed doubt on correcting stable coronary artery disease before elective noncardiac surgery, all agree that patients with clear-cut indications for a revascularization procedure without regard for contemplated surgery must have such a procedure before proceeding with elective surgery. A patient with evidence of operable coronary artery disease should be investigated for that and revascularization should be accomplished before the patient proceeds with elective noncardiac surgery. Nitroglycerin and long-acting nitrates have their place in maintaining the patient's stability before definitive evaluation, but operability should be determined, even if noncardiac elective surgery were not contemplated.

6. The answer is D. The patient will be at increased risk for pulmonary edema but not for other cardiac events. This applies specifically to patients who have a history of CHF but are well compensated.

7. The answer is D. The patient will be at increased risk of CHF on the basis of the preoperative ejection fraction of <50%. Such patients have four times the chance of CHF (12% vs. 3%) compared with those patients with ejection fractions >50%.

8. The answer is A. Continue the current medications, including the dose(s) that is due on the day of surgery, and proceed with the surgery. Current thinking and inferences from certain studies suggest that mild to moderate hypertension does not pose a significant cardiac risk in the perioperative period. By the same token, however, it is felt that antihypertensive medications should be continued into the day of surgery and postoperatively as required for control of the blood pressure.

299

9. The answer is B. Delay surgery and take more aggressive steps to control the blood pressure, such as adding a calcium channel blocking drug; proceed with surgery when the blood pressure is consistently below 140/90. One should put this or another effective method of lowering the blood pressure into play before allowing the operation to proceed. This is the thinking of experts for repeated blood pressure readings >180/110.

10. The answer is C; FEV_1 <500 mL appears to be the sole criterion among those presented that is valid in predicting a high risk of prolonged dependence on a ventilator after surgery involving the thorax or upper abdomen. This recommendation differs from what was given in the first edition in that, in the past, the MVV and DLCO were given significant weight at that time.

11. The answer is A. The contribution of the lobe being considered for resection must not exceed 1,400 mL. This is based on the fact that the postoperative FEV_1 must be at least 800 mL. Thus, as the preoperative FEV_1 was 2.2 L, the contribution of the tissues to be resected being greater than 1,400 mL would leave less than 800 mL after the surgery. (One may encounter a more liberal opinion, i.e., that the FEV_1 may be as low as 500 mL after surgery.)

12. The answer is B. This patient had a lateral wall myocardial infarction. Three months is the minimum time after myocardial infarction that one should wait for elective surgery. Preferably, this time period should be as long as 6 months. This is based on the statistic that, during the first 3 months after a myocardial infarction, the risk of perioperative recurrent myocardial infarction or death is 8% to 30%; after 6 months, such risk falls to 3.5% to 5%.

13. The answer is D, preoperative Child–Turcotte–Pugh classification score. This score is a combination of graduated scores regarding several manifestations of cirrhosis. Five conditions are listed, each with a score from 1 point to 3 points (1 is normal, 2 is moderately abnormal, and 3 is severe). The normal score is thus 5; the worst score is 15. The risk of postoperative hepatic complications is reasonably directly related to the Child–Turcotte–Pugh score. The following table is a representation of the Child–Turcotte–Pugh scoring.

Parameter	Numerical Score		
	1	2	3
Ascites	none	Slight	Moderate to severe
Encephalopathy	none	Slight to moderate	Moderate to severe
Bilirubin (mg/dL)	<2	2–3	>3
Albumin (g/dL)	>3.5	2.8–3.5	<2.8
PT(seconds increased)	1–3	4–6	>6

The table is modified from Friedman (2006); used with permission.

14. The answer is C; 8 g/dL is the accepted level below which the hemoglobin should be corrected before elective surgery in those patients with no major risk factors for coronary artery disease or factors of age, nutrition, or alcohol. However, for those with baseline risk factors, risk of coronary disease perioperatively is significantly increased if the hemoglobin falls below 10 g/dL.

15. The answer is E. Postoperative delirium is a greater possibility in patients whose hematocrits are <30%, which is the equivalent, in a normochromic state, of 10 g/dL. Other risk factors for postoperative delirium are age >70 years, alcohol abuse, poor premorbid cognitive status, poor physical condition, markedly abnormal sodium, potassium, or glucose, and noncardiac thoracic or aortic surgery.

16. The answer is C; perform carotid endarterectomy followed by VSD repair. The main point to be made is that the carotid stenosis is not only severe enough to indicate a repair but also that the repair was made more urgent when the carotid stenosis became symptomatic (ipsilateral quadrantanopsia, a variant of amaurosis fugax). Although there is less than a 1% chance of stroke fatality after noncardiac surgery, it occurs in up to 6% of cases after cardiac surgery. Such perioperative stroke carries up to a 22% mortality rate. If both cardiac surgery and carotid endarterectomy are indicated, the first to be performed is a matter of judgment. In the vignette, the carotid procedure became more urgent with the advent of the symptom. The cardiac condition, with concentric hypertrophy, must be repaired as well, but it does not represent decompensation such as systolic dysfunction would manifest and thus is not in an unstable stage. In contrast, symptomatic carotid stenosis poses an urgent situation because of the possibility of an early major stroke.

17. The answer is D, dialysis within 24 hours and electrolytes studies just before surgery. Patients on renal dialysis exhibit a 20% to 30% risk of postoperative hyperkalemia requiring emergency dialysis. Another complication particularly likely in such patients is fluid overload, a condition amenable to timely dialysis. Other problems seen at a rate greater than in patients not on dialysis include pneumonia and bleeding.

Def n Malnutrition

18. The answer is C; <2g/dL is one of the definitions of severe malnutrition. Others are a recent weight loss of >20 lb (9 kg); transferrin <100 mg/dL; prealbumin <7 mg/dL; and absolute lymphocyte count <1,000 cells/mm^3. A serum albumin level <3.5 (>3) g/dL is considered mildly malnourished and a level of ≤3 but >2 is considered moderately malnourished, assuming no special circumstances to account for the measurement as an isolated finding.

19. The answer is A; 35 kcal/kg, of which 20% should be protein, is the minimum caloric (and percentage protein) oral intake criterion that the physician should expect from the patient before ruling out at least oral supplementation given preoperatively.

20. The answer is D, total parenteral nutrition now and for 7 days postoperatively (or for as long as it takes for the patient to take in adequate calories, protein, and fluid). This patient is moderately malnourished (10% to 20% weight loss; albumin <3; transferrin <170; lymphocyte <1,500) and, based on the contemplated surgery, will not be able to take in orally for at least 7 days after surgery. An oral supplement, low-residue diet, and tube feedings are ruled out because of the projected enteral malfunction for the early postoperative period. Dietary consultation without thinking through the foregoing issues is inappropriate.

21. The answer is A. Lymph node biopsy in the neck area is considered a "clean" procedure as long as it does not involve entering the foregut or other part of the gastrointestinal tract. Any procedure that enters the gastrointestinal tract, the urinary tract, the respiratory tract, or biliary tract, or any procedure that involves operating on an inflamed area, requires prophylactic antibiotics.

22. The answer is C. Surprisingly, patients with hypertrophic cardiomyopathy warrant preoperative antibiotic prophylaxis against bacterial endocarditis. *In none of the other conditions is prophylactic antibiotic indicated.* Other indications (not presented as choices here) are not surprising and include the presence of prosthetic cardiac valves, previous bacterial endocarditis, rheumatic and other valvular dysfunction, and the presence of significant congenital cardiac malformations, even if they have been repaired.

References

Adler JS, Goldman L. Preoperative evaluation and perioperative management. In: Tierney LM, McPhee SJ, Papadakis MA, eds. *Current Medical Diagnosis and Treatment.* 45th ed. New York: McGraw-Hill/Appleton & Lange; 2006:35–49.

Friedman, LS. Liver, biliary tract and pancreas. In: Tierney LM, McPhee SJ, Papadakis MA, eds. *Current Medical Diagnosis and Treatment.* 45th ed. New York: McGraw-Hill/Appleton & Lange; 2006:649–701.

Vanderhoff BT. Preoperative clearance and preparation. In: Rudy DR, Kurowski K, eds. *Family Medicine: House Officer Series.* Baltimore: Williams & Wilkins; 1997:617–636.

chapter 37

Obesity and Dyslipidemia

Examination questions: Unless instructed otherwise, choose the ONE lettered answer or completion that is BEST in each case.

1 A 45-year-old man sees you for a "checkup," having not seen a physician since the age of 35. His older brother died recently after a myocardial infarction at the age of 49 and his father died at the age of 55 of heart disease. The patient has smoked for 25 years but quit after the death of his brother. His weight is 165 lb (74.8 kg) at a height of 5 ft, 9 in. (1.75 m). His blood pressure is 135/88. You measure his lipids and find the following: total cholesterol (TC), 240 mg/dL; high-density lipoprotein cholesterol (HDL-C), 37 mg/dL; low-density lipoprotein cholesterol (LDL-C), 155 mg/dL; triglycerides, 300 mg/dL. Which of the following is the best therapeutic plan for this patient?

(A) Advise weight loss to the ideal, 160 lb (72.5 kg), and repeat lipid screen after 2 months

(B) Start a lipid-lowering agent and repeat the lipid screen after 1 month

(C) Start the patient on a low-carbohydrate diet to prevent diabetes

(D) Start the patient on a low-fat diet and repeat the lipid screen in 2 months

(E) Reassure the patient that because he has stopped smoking he need not be further concerned about his cardiovascular status

2 For the patient in Question 1, which of the following would be the best pharmacological approach to his health problems?

(A) Nicotinic acid

(B) Fibric acid derivative

(C) Metformin

(D) An HMG-coenzyme A (HMG-CoA) inhibitor

(E) Cholestyramine

3 A 23-year-old man weighs 180 lb (81.5 kg) at a height of 5 ft, 10 in. (1.78 m). The patient has no family history of cardiovascular disease and there is no dyslipidemia in his or his family's history. He has never smoked. He is concerned about his weight because his mother is significantly overweight and his father is modestly overweight. His TC is 240 mg/dL; his HDL-C is 53 mg/dL; his LDL-C is 110 mg/dL; and his triglyceride level is 130 mg/dL. His blood pressure is 128/78 ± 5/2 mm Hg. What is your best advice regarding this patient's weight?

(A) Reassure the patient that he has no weight-related health problem

(B) Place the patient on a diet consisting of 1,300 calories, with 175 g of carbohydrate, 50 g of fat, and 50 g of protein

(C) Place the patient on a very-low-calorie diet (VLCD)

(D) Start sibutramine for appetite control

(E) You cannot formulate a plan based on the information given.

4 A young mother brings to you her 18-month-old boy who weighs 30 lb (13.6 kg). This is at the 95th percentile for his height and sex. She is concerned because her family has many members who are overweight and she worries that the child's future health is at risk. Your best advice is which of the following?

(A) She should commit the child to a weight-reduction program forthwith.

(B) The child's weight-related health is not an issue until he reaches adolescence.

(C) The child should be committed to a weight-loss program but not before he reaches the age of 2 years.

(D) A child's obesity-related health issues involve vascular disease, diabetes, and joint health only, and these problems do not begin until adulthood.

(E) Obesity in early childhood is not a health issue.

5 A 50-year-old woman consults you for weight loss. She weighs 200 lb (91 kg) at a height of 66 in. (1.68 m). Her body mass index or BMI is 31; she is well into the obese range and 48% above the ideal weight. She says she has tried on her own for several years to lose weight but has never consulted a physician, and recently she was told of the health risks attendant to her status. Which of the following is a workable program *for her*?

(A) Reassure the patient that she is not in a health risk status as a result of her weight

(B) Refer her to Over Eaters Anonymous

(C) Place the patient on a VLCD

(D) Start fluoxetine

(E) Enroll the patient in a commercial weight-loss program

6 A 40-year-old mother of a teenaged daughter complains to you that her daughter is significantly obese and that her own parents and two sisters are obese and have diabetes mellitus type II. She asked you to brief her as to what caveats she might point out to her daughter so as to persuade her to take seriously her obesity as a health risk and to stimulate her to commit herself to a weight-loss program. You answer that each of the following occurs at increased incidence in obese individuals, except which one?

(A) Breast cancer

(B) Uterine cancer

(C) Chronic obstructive pulmonary disease

(D) Osteoarthritis of the knees

(E) Gallstones

7 A 50-year-old white man weighs 240 lb (109 kg) at a height of 5 ft, 10 in. (1.78 m). Which of the following is this man's ideal weight?

(A) 133 lb (60.2 kg)

(B) 144 lb (65.2 kg)

(C) 166 lb (75.2 kg)

(D) 180 lb (81.5 kg)

(E) 200 lb (91 kg)

8 Regarding the patient in Question 7, what is his calculated BMI?

(A) 22

(B) 24

(C) 34

(D) 44

(E) 55

9 Regarding the patient in Question 7, which of the following is true regarding his status compared with that of nonobese people?

(A) He probably consumes more calories than nonobese individuals.

(B) He has a 30% chance of having a binge-eating disorder.

(C) His rate of energy expenditure is probably the same as that of nonobese individuals.

(D) His rate of physical activity is likely the same as that of nonobese individuals.

(E) He is expected have a greater likelihood of psychological problems even when not dieting.

10 A 45-year-old man has a family history of diabetes mellitus, is 25% overweight, has a pretreatment blood pressure of 145/92 averaged over three determinations, an LDL-C level of 160 mg/dL, and an HDL-C level of 35 mg/dL. You placed him on aspirin 81 mg daily and atorvastatin (Lipitor) eventually at a dosage of 80 mg once daily. His LDL-C has fallen to 130 mg/dL and his HDL-C has risen only to 38 mg/dL. He has not been able to lose weight. Which of the following changes in the treatment regimen is the most logical?

(A) Increase the atorvastatin to 120 mg/dL

(B) Add niacin at an initial dosage of 100 mg daily

(C) Add gemfibrozil (Lopid) at an initial dosage of 600 mg daily

(D) Change to lovastatin (Mevacor) starting at a dosage of 40 mg daily

(E) Change to colestipol (Colestid) starting at 5 mg daily

11 A 35-year-old female mail carrier is a nonsmoker with blood pressure levels on repeat in the 145 to 150/90 to 95 range. Her weight is 130 lb (58.9 kg) at a height of 5 ft 5 in. (1.65 m). She has a TC level of 250 mg/dL, and HDL-C of 30 despite being on a diet with less than 200 mg of cholesterol and 30% fat (<7% saturated fat). She has family history of myocardial infarction on her father's side and stroke on her mother's side of the family. Which of the following is the most appropriate step to rectify her dyslipidemia?

(A) Start therapy with niacin or an HMG-CoA reductase inhibitor

(B) Repeat lipid panel in 6 to 12 months. Defer interventions

(C) Reduce dietary cholesterol to <100 mg/day and fat to ≤10% of all calories

(D) Encourage her to drink a small amount of alcohol each day to raise her HDL-C

(E) Start bile acid sequestrant therapy

12 A 45-year-old man weighs 180 lb (81.5 kg) at a height of 5 ft, 11 in. (1.8 m). His TC is 180 mg/dL; his HDL-C is 35 mg/dL and his LDL-C is 105 mg/dL; his serum triglyceride level is 220 mg/dL. The patient's father died of coronary artery disease at the age of 55 years. Neither the patient nor his father ever smoked cigarettes. He has followed your diet of limited saturated fats, limited cholesterol content, and net calories balance for the past year, and the foregoing lipid profile represents a 10% improvement in the HDL-C and triglycerides. Which of the following pharmacological approaches to his dyslipidemia would be the most effective?

(A) Nicotinic acid

(B) Simvastatin

(C) Gemfibrozil

(D) A bile sequestrant

(E) Atorvastatin

13 You are treating a 55-year-old man with a history of angina and a previous coronary angiogram that shows an 80% stenosis of his left anterior descending artery. He has been on a step II low-cholesterol diet for 3 months. You recheck his lipid profile and his LDL-C is 195 mg/dL with an HDL-C of 30 mg/dL and a triglyceride level of 220. He states he has been fully compliant with his diet and his wife confirms this. You have previously evaluated him for secondary causes of dyslipidemia and found none. (Assume he is on nitroglycerin as needed and aspirin 80 mg by mouth each day.) Which of the following is most appropriate for him?

(A) Continue the low-cholesterol diet and recheck panel in 3 months

(B) Start colestipol

(C) Start niacin

(D) Start gemfibrozil

(E) Start an HMG-CoA reductive inhibitor (a "statin")

14 Assume a patient is already following a low-fat, low-cholesterol diet. Also assume this test was done with the patient fasting. Which of the following lipid profiles would be most appropriate for treatment with gemfibrozil?

(A) TC of 200 mg/dL, HDL-C of 40 mg/dL, triglyceride level of 200 mg/dL

(B) TC of 230 mg/dL, HDL-C of 30 mg/dL, triglyceride level of 1,000 mg/dL

(C) TC of 290 mg/dL, HDL-C of 40 mg/dL, triglyceride level of 150 mg/dL

(D) TC of 290 mg/dL, HDL-C of 40 mg/dL, triglyceride level of 280 mg/dL

(E) TC of 320 mg/dL, HDL-C of 50 mg/dL, triglyceride level of 300 mg/dL

15 A 22-year-old woman is 5 ft, 6 in. (1.68 m) in height and weighs 148 lb (67 kg) and is asking you about pharmacologic approaches to weight loss. You calculate her ideal weight to be 130 lb, or 61 kg (100 lb at 60 in. or 5 ft, plus 5 lb/in. for every inch over 5 ft). Which of the following plans best fits her weight status?

(A) Reassure the patient that she is not in a health risk status as a result of her weight

(B) Place the patient on a diet consisting of 1,300 calories, with 175 g of carbohydrate, 50 g of fat, and 50 g of protein

(C) Place the patient on a VLCD

(D) Start fluoxetine

(E) You cannot formulate a plan based on the information given.

16 A 33-year-old man weighs 350 lb (159 kg) at a height of 5 ft, 10 in. (1.78 m). He has lost up to 100 lb (45 kg) on various diets but has always regained his lost weight after 1 to 2 years. He has been morbidly obese since he was 25 years old. He wishes to discuss bariatric surgery (e.g., gastric by-pass surgery). You reply that each of the following is true, except for which one?

(A) This patient is more than 110% above ideal weight.

(B) Indications for bariatric surgery include being 100 lb (45 kg) overweight.

(C) Indications for bariatric surgery include a BMI of ≥40.

(D) Indications for bariatric surgery include a BMI of 35 to 40 when associated with sleep apnea.

(E) Indications for bariatric surgery include osteoporosis.

Examination Answers

1. The answer is B. The patient is within 5 lb (2.27 kg) of his ideal weight (at 69 in. or 1.75 m, ideal weight is 106 + 6 lb for each inch over 5 feet in height = 160 lb, or 72.5 kg). Therefore, even if the patient were very sensitive to the relationship between weight and hypertension, dyslipidemia, and prediabetes (metabolic syndrome), this man cannot be expected to change his vascular risk profile to a significant degree by losing less than 5% of his present weight. Thus, specific methods of weight loss, such as low carbohydrate or low fat, are equally inapplicable at this time, though low-fat maintenance is always advisable. Most authorities have moved to the position of advising pharmacologic therapy for virtually anyone with pre-existing heart disease or with strong family history of atherosclerotic vascular disease and present significant risk factors, including a significant recent history of smoking.

2. The answer is D. The patient deserves a pharmacologic approach. Of all the agents presented as choices in Question 2, an HMG-CoA inhibitor (statin) addresses this patient's profile the best. The patient has abnormally elevated TC and LDL-C levels and the ratio of TC to HDL-C is 6.5; for men, an acceptable ratio is 4.5 or lower. In addition, his triglyceride level is markedly elevated. Statins reduce TC and LDL-C levels as well as triglyceride levels, and they elevate HDL-C. Metformin is an excellent drug for reducing insulin resistance and, as such, improves lipids in the face of insulin resistance. However, it is not established that this patient has insulin resistance. In any event, metformin's effect is modest compared with that of the statin drugs in this type of case.

3. The answer is A. The only risk factor known to this patient is obesity in his parents. The fact that neither parent has diabetes may mean that his parents both had hip–thigh obesity rather than the central obesity that is associated with the metabolic syndrome. Obesity is defined as a weight 20% above ideal. This patient's weight of 180 lb (81.5 kg) at a height of 70 in. (1.78 m) is calculated as a BMI of 25.8, which is overweight but not obese (top normal limit for men is 24 kg/m^2). Because his lipids are within normal limits for a man (TC to HDLC ratio is 4.5), there is no evidence that his overweight status is in his case a risk factor. Thus, the diet, although well designed for weight loss, is not clinically indicated, and certainly the radical VLCD is not. Sibutramine (Meridia) is an appetite suppressant and by definition of limited value for long-range control of weight.

4. The answer is C. Obesity in early childhood conveys a risk of obesity in adulthood with all the attendant risks of diabetes, hypertension, dyslipidemia, and vascular disease, as well as osteoarthritis. In addition, there is an association between childhood obesity not only with the adult organic health risks mentioned but also with poor psychological health and decreased economic well-being. In order for a child to be neurologically equipped for participation in a weight-loss program, he or she must have attained the age of 2 years.

5. The answer is E. The most well known of commercial programs is Weight Watchers. This is a good program for a patient who appears to need social support. Nevertheless, weight regain is common if patients are followed for years after a commercial program was instituted. Nutritional assessment and program modifications can be done by the physician, trained nursing staff, or a dietitian. Patients typically lose 11 to 22 pounds, but attrition is high. Commercial programs tend to be very expensive. Over Eaters Anonymous is one of the group self-help programs and is not commercial. They do not appear to achieve as much weight loss and they exhibit a high attrition rate. Reassurance is inappropriate because the patient is moderately obese. VLCDs and pharmacotherapy such as fluoxetine are not to be applied until these more conservative measures have been tried.

6. The answer is C, chronic obstructive pulmonary disease. Obesity is associated with an increased incidence of sleep apnea and restrictive lung disease, but not chronic obstructive pulmonary disease. Obesity is a risk for breast cancer and uterine cancer, perhaps based on the storage of estrogens in adipose tissue. Breast and uterine tissues are responsive to circulating estrogen. Osteoarthritis of the knees and hips are in greater incidence in obesity as a result of the increased load bearing required of the joints. Gall stones, especially cholesterol stones, occur in greater incidence in obesity, most likely because of the higher cholesterol levels found in obesity; for uterine cancer the risk is for unknown reasons.

7. The answer is C. The ideal weight for a man in pounds is 106 lb + 6 lb for each inch above 5 ft (1.52 m). For a woman the rule in pounds is 100 lb + 5 lb for each inch over 5 ft (1.52 m). For this patient the ideal weight at a height of 70 in. (1.78 m) is 106 + (6 × 10) = 166 lb (75.2 kg). Therefore, this patient is 44.6% overweight. Obesity is defined as 20% over ideal weight, moderate obesity is defined as 40% to 100% above ideal weight, and severe (sometimes called morbid) obesity is defined as ≥100% over ideal weight. This rule of thumb is very useful but must be adjusted for people who have done significant degrees of isometric exercise (i.e., weight lifting), whereby body mass is increased without a commensurate increase in body fat. Women have argued that this rule of estimation reckons female ideal weight to be proportionately low as compared with male ideal weight. Insofar as female body fat is defined as a higher percentage than male body fat, they make a good argument.

8. The answer is C. BMI is defined as weight in kilograms divided by height in meters squared. This man's body mass index is 34, because 240 lb/(2.2 kg/lb) = 109 kg; 70 in. × 2.54 cm = 178 cm, or 1.78 m; and 109 kg/(1.78 m)^2 = 34. A BMI above 24 is considered overweight. Above 27, health problems begin to accumulate in proportion to the degree that the individual is overweight.

9. The answer is B. About 30% of patients with moderate or severe obesity have a binge-eating disorder. Obese people consume more calories than needed for maintenance of a stable body weight but the amount is typically less than that found in age-, height-, and sex-comparable nonobese controls. (That generalization does not apply to bulimic, nonpurging, nonemesis-inducing individuals.) Physical activity and energy expenditure are lower than in nonobese patients, but caloric consumption is not on average higher. Psychological problems associated with obesity are a complicated area to consider. Most adults who succeed in weight-loss programs experience an increase in self-esteem, although relapses are frequent and with relapses, a greater possibility of reversal of self-esteem.

10. The answer is B. Combining niacin with a statin drug may increase HDL-C and certainly adds its effect to lower LDL-C. Atorvastatin is already at the maximum allowable dosage. Addition of gemfibrozil is contraindicated while a statin is in place because of the increased risk of myolysis, a known side effect of the statins. Changing to the bile sequestrant colestipol is a valid option but does not hold any particular promise in the present situation.

11. The answer is A. The 35-year-old female nonsmoker with mild hypertension and a TC-to-HDLC ratio of 250:30 (8:1) and a family history of cardiovascular disease, although at near ideal weight, is a strong candidate for drug therapy to correct dyslipidemia. Any further attempts at change in lifestyle or specifically diet would seem to be futile, given the foregoing information. She exhibits dyslipidemia at a young age and the apparent inheritance of genetically determined dyslipemia. Bile acid sequestrants have a relatively weak effect in raising HDL-C levels. Thus, niacin or the statins are more favorable choices. Measuring another lipid panel in 6 to 12 months offers no realistic expectation. Encouraging alcohol intake is unconventional and potentially dangerous, though it is true that people who drink moderately have more favorable lipid profiles than do nondrinkers.

12. The answer is C. Gemfibrozil (Lopid) is very effective in raising HDL-C and reducing triglyceride levels. The statins (i.e., here, simvastatin and atorvastatin) are effective in both these areas but not as effective as fibric acid derivatives such as gemfibrozil in raising HDL-C levels. Nicotinic acid is effective in reducing triglycerides but not in raising HDL-C. Bile sequestrants are most effective in reducing TC and LDL-C.

13. The answer is E. The stronger LDL lowering effect is warranted here, given the patient's high levels and documented coronary artery disease. The therapeutic diet has proven to be insufficient. Colestipol, niacin, and gemfibrozil, although good alternatives, would be neither as effective nor as well tolerated as statin drugs.

14. The answer is B. TC is 230 mg/dL, which is mildly elevated, but HDL-C is 30, significantly low. The triglyceride level of 1,000 mg/dL is in the monogenic category of dyslipidemia (i.e., Fredrickson type IV), assuming the blood specimen does not show the triglycerides as chylomicrons. Gemfibrozil does raise HDL and has a dramatic effect to lower triglyceride levels. The best candidate would be a patient with only modest TC elevations, but low HDL-C and a marked hypertriglyceridemia.

15. The answer is A. The definition of obesity requires that the patient be 20% overweight. At 148 lb (67 kg) she is 18 lb (5.89 kg) or <14% over ideal body weight, and thus she is not an appropriate candidate for pharmacotherapy, in particular because she is female. Her weight of 148 lb or 67 kg corresponds to a BMI of 24, which is quite in the acceptable range. As stated earlier, BMI is calculated by the formula of weight in kilograms divided by height in meters squared. By body mass criteria, moderate obesity for women is defined as 30 to 40; severe obesity as ≥40. A diet of 1,300 calories, with 175 g of carbohydrate,

50 g of fat, and 50 g of protein, would be a well-designed modest weight-reduction diet; 1,300 calories meets a guideline for the maintenance needs of a 130-lb (59 kg) woman; 175 g of carbohydrate approximates 55% of total calories, and 50 g of fat provides less than 30% of the total calories. This meets American Heart recommendations and would satisfy the requirements for managing diabetes. A VLCD is defined as 800 calories and is normally reserved for more severe cases, such as morbid obesity (100% above ideal weight). Fluoxetine, likewise, is reserved for severe cases (e.g., ≥40% above ideal weight).

16. The answer is E. Indications for bariatric surgery include being 100 lb (45 kg) overweight; having a BMI ≥40; or having a BMI of 35 to 40 in the presence of sleep apnea, Pickwickian syndrome, obesity-related cardiomyopathy, severe diabetes mellitus, and obesity-induced physical problems that are interfering with lifestyle (e.g., precluding or severely interfering with employment, family function, and ambulation). Osteoporosis is not associated with obesity as being overweight is in fact a protective factor against osteoporosis. Thus, it does not enter into the decision for bariatric surgery.

References

American Society of Bariatric Surgery Web site: www.asbs.org/html/rationale/rationale.html

Smith PO, Noble SL, Johnson WG. Obesity and dyslipidemias. In: Rudy DR, Kurowski K, eds. *Family Medicine: House Officer Series*. Baltimore: Williams & Wilkins; 1997:637–648.

chapter **38**

Smoking Cessation and Dangers of Smoking

1 A 25-year-old woman in her first trimester of pregnancy is seeing you for a prenatal visit. She smokes one pack of cigarettes per day. In advising her to stop smoking, you tell her that her baby will be at increased risk for which of the following, if she continues to smoke?

(A) Preterm birth

(B) Macrosomia

(C) Transient tachypnea of newborn

(D) Spinal cord defects

(E) Neonatal hypoglycemia

2 You are designing a program for your office to encourage patients to stop smoking. Which of the following is correct with respect to physician office efforts to encourage smoking cessation?

(A) It may be assumed that smokers have already been told of the adverse effects of smoking if they have seen other physicians recently.

(B) Smoking in the physician's office should only be allowed in partitioned, ventilated smoking areas.

(C) Counseling to cease smoking should await a time when a detailed, lengthier discussion of smoking cessation can occur.

(D) Smoking should be listed on the problem list of anyone who smokes and on the child's chart of any child in a smoking household.

(E) If the dangers of smoking are pointed out vigorously, cessation can usually be accomplished in one office visit.

3 A family consisting of mother, father, a 1-year-old boy, and a 3 1/2-year-old girl are under your care. Both parents smoke. The incidence of which of the following childhood diseases is increased in households with smokers present?

(A) Reactive airway disease

(B) Epiglotitis

(C) Sudden infant death syndrome

(D) Lymphatic leukemia

(E) Wilms tumor

4 A 33-year-old man who has smoked a pack per day for 15 years since his first year in college (15 pack years) has discovered that his uncle who smoked 30 pack years has been diagnosed with lung cancer. He is seriously considering quitting but asks your advice as to whether it is too late to reduce his risk of lung cancer. Which of the following is the best response to this patient in answer to the question?

(A) It is too late to reduce his risk of lung cancer, as the cumulative maximum smoking volume for reversibility of the odds for lung cancer is 10 pack years of smoking.

(B) It is too late for practical purposes because one must quit smoking for at least 40 years before the risk of lung cancer is significantly reduced.

(C) Actually, the risk of lung cancer begins to subside significantly at 10 years after cessation of smoking, and the vast majority of lung cancer patients have smoked for more than 20 years before contracting the disease.

(D) One must quit for 20 years and have smoked for fewer than 15 years in order to benefit from cessation to reduce risk of lung cancer.

(E) If the man stops smoking, he need not fear lung cancer after a period of 5 years.

5 You are counseling a 50-year-old man who has been smoking for 20 years. He has decided he wants to quit. In which of the following situations would he be the best candidate to benefit from a nicotine patch for smoking cessation?

(A) He has his first cigarette before breakfast.

(B) He smokes approximately a half-pack, in social situations such as while at clubs or parties, once or twice per week and not at other times.

(C) He smokes for solice or reward, usually at work, but seldom on weekends.

(D) He relapsed after being exposed to a situation that made him want to smoke.

(E) He clearly has a psychological but not a physiological addiction.

6 Which of the following represents a contraindication to the use of a nicotine patch in this patient?

(A) He would sometimes note pruritus at the patch site when he tried the patches 5 years ago.

(B) He has a history of hypertension and poorly controlled diabetes mellitus.

(C) He is currently being treated with oral sustained-release buproprion for smoking cessation.

(D) He had some erythema at patch sites when he used the patches 5 years ago.

(E) He suffered a myocardial infarction 2 weeks ago.

7 A 45-year-old man is a pack per day smoker who tends to smoke most heavily at his office, where he is a senior architect. His first cigarette of the day is usually mid-morning, after he has completed a phase of a design and is ready to present it to colleagues (or after he becomes discouraged and must start again at a different point in a project). On weekends he relaxes by playing golf or fishing at a local river, during which times he seldom smokes more than 10 cigarettes per day. He wishes to quit. Because you consider him not to be addicted, you discuss with him foregoing nicotine replacement therapy in favor of buproprion therapy. Which of the following would constitute a contraindication to bupropion in this patient?

(A) History of symptomatic coronary insufficiency

(B) History of asthma

(C) History of chronic obstructive pulmonary disease

(D) History of seizures

(E) History of peptic ulcer disease

8 A heavily smoking 45-year-old woman stops smoking and starts on the nicotine patches. She is applying a new patch each day. How long must she wait before she reuses a skin site where she had previously applied a patch?

(A) 1 day

(B) 2 days

(C) 3 days

(D) 1 week

(E) 2 weeks

9 Which of the following best describes the appropriate use of nicotine gum?

(A) Patients gradually taper their smoking after starting on the gum.

(B) The gum is usually placed next to the buccal mucosa for 30 minutes and chewed when the patient has an urge to smoke.

(C) The maximum dose is 50 pieces per day.

(D) The gum is more effective if used with coffee.

(E) Patients can use the gum as a cigarette substitute, which allows them to smoke fewer cigarettes per day.

10 A 25-year-old woman is seeing you for her yearly gynecologic examination. She smokes 1.5 packs per day and has done this since age 19. She has no complaints. She is on birth control pills and has no plans to have children in the near future. She has not considered stopping smoking and has never set a stop date. Which of the following is the most appropriate intervention?

(A) Avoid the topic of smoking and smoking cessation completely, as she may not be receptive to it

(B) Briefly discuss adverse health effects and give her smoking-cessation literature and mention your availability to pursue it further with her when she is interested

(C) Insist that she pick a start date and quit "on her own"

(D) Prescribe sustained-release buproprion

(E) Recommend a nicotine patch

Examination Answers

1. The answer is A, preterm birth. Smoking during pregnancy is associated with smaller, premature newborns, but not with tachypnea, specific birth defects, hypoglycemia, or macrosomia.

2. The answer is D. Smoking should be listed on the problem list of anyone who smokes and on the child's chart of any child in a smoking household. Surveys may demonstrate to patients how important the physician views the impact of smoking on their health and quantifies the habit. Some smokers say that their physicians never told them to quit and some will respond to brief interventions, but almost never in one session. Smokefree offices are necessary without exception. One need not wait for a "propitious" or adequate length of time for initiating conversation about the desirability of smoking cessation. Even 5 minutes devoted to the subject has been shown statistically to have eventual long-term success, compared with never mentioning smoking dangers and the wisdom of cessation at all.

3. The answer is A. Reactive airway disease and exacerbations of known asthma are more likely in children of households with smokers living in the abode than those without smokers. Ear and upper respiratory infections decrease if the smoking is stopped. Although cigarette smoking by the parents is not known to cause childhood asthma, the smoke can serve as a respiratory irritant that precipitates the asthma. In addition, otitis media is more likely in smoking households. No causal relationship between parental cigarette smoking and sudden infant death syndrome or childhood malignancies has been established.

4. The answer is C. The risk of lung cancer begins to subside significantly at 10 years after cessation of smoking, and it approaches the expected risk of nonsmokers by about 13 years. The vast majority of lung cancer patients have smoked heavily (one or more packs per day) for more than 20 years before contracting the disease.

5. The answer is A, he has his first cigarette before breakfast (i.e., "before his feet hit the floor"). This patient is among the 30% or so of smokers who are truly addicted, as opposed to those whose impulses to smoke occur in certain situations, rather than "on the clock."

6. The answer is E. If he suffered a myocardial infarction 2 weeks ago, the vasoconstrictive effects of nicotine are a clear danger. Recent myocardial infarction, unstable angina, cardiac dysrhythmia, or true hypersensitivity reaction to the patch (not just local erythema or pruritus) are the only real contraindications. The length of the critical period after a myocardial infarction is generally not given in the literature. However, following perioperative guidelines for elective surgery, and allowing for somewhat more leeway for smoking versus an assumed compelling case for even elective surgery, 3 months would be a good estimate.

7. The answer is D. Bupropion, most suitable in situations where the compulsion to smoke appears to be psychological rather addictive, is contraindicated in the presence of a history of seizures, bulimia, presence of monoamine oxidase inhibitors, headache, nausea, or recent head trauma.

8. The answer is D, 1 week. The 1-week delay before reusing a site in rotation is recommended so that contact irritation can be avoided.

9. The answer is B. The gum is usually placed next to the buccal mucosa for 30 minutes and chewed when the patient has an urge to smoke. Patients must stop smoking when they start any of the nicotine products. It should not be used as a cigarette substitute. The free alkaloid form of nicotine polacrilex is best absorbed through the oral mucosa. Acidic coffee or juices taken less than 15 minutes before chewing interfere with absorption.

10. The answer is B. Briefly discuss adverse health effects and give her smoking-cessation literature and mention your availability to pursue it further with her when she is interested. She is unlikely to be sufficiently motivated at this time to stop. Oral agents and nicotine patches or gums are unlikely to be successful when the patient's personal commitment is not set. Smokers should be advised of health risks of the habit and at least periodically be reminded of these risks and the opportunities for help.

References

Bope ET. Smoking cessation. In: Rudy DR, Kurowski K, eds. *Family Medicine: House Officer Series.* Baltimore: Williams & Wilkins; 1997:649–656.

Okoyemi KIS, Nollen ML, Ahluwahlia JS. Interventions to facilitate smoking cessation. *Am Fam Physician.* 2006; 74:262–271, 276.

chapter 39

Exercise and Health

1 Which of the following is the definition of basal energy expenditure (BEE)?

(A) The amount of energy expended per unit time by a person at rest, who has not eaten for 2 hours

(B) The amount of energy expended per unit time by a person at rest, who has not eaten for 12 hours

(C) The amount of energy expended by a person doing normal wakeful activity, not involving pulse-raising exercise

(D) The amount of energy expended per unit time by a person during sleep

(E) The amount of energy expended by a person in performing basic activities of daily living

2 A 55-year-old man with a 20% stenosis of his right coronary artery and a 30% stenosis of his left anterior descending is asymptomatic and wants to start an exercise program. Which of the following expresses the correct perspective with respect to exercise and coronary artery disease (CAD) risk factors?

(A) Exercise aggravates hypertension and should not be embarked upon until the blood pressure has been controlled to <140/90.

(B) The CAD risk factor of hypercholesterolemia is more prevalent in the United States than the risk factor of sedentary lifestyle.

(C) This patient's total and high-density lipoprotein cholesterol levels would be expected to decrease with exercise.

(D) The risk of developing CAD is five times greater in physically inactive individuals.

(E) The incidence of cardiac arrest is lower in those individuals who exercise than it is in those who do not.

3 A 45-year-man weighs 240 lb (109 kg) at a height of 5 feet 10 inches (1.77 m) and is now seriously contemplating weight loss. You feel you can exploit this teaching moment. How much time for exercise can you tell the patient is recommended for American adults by the Center for Disease Control and Prevention?

(A) 15 minutes of mild-intensity physical activity 3 days a week

(B) 15 minutes of moderate-intensity physical activity 3 days a week

(C) 15 minutes of moderate-intensity physical activity 5 to 7 days a week

(D) 30 minutes of moderate-intensity physical activity 3 days a week

(E) 30 minutes of moderate-intensity physical activity 5 to 7 days a week

4 Regarding the patient in Question 3, in helping the patient to recognize moderate exercise in his individual case, what pulse rate would this 45-year-old patient need to achieve to be reaching at least moderate physical activity?

(A) 70 beats per minute

(B) 104 beats per minute

(C) 122 beats per minute

(D) 154 beats per minute

(E) 170 beats per minute

5 Regarding the patient in Question 3, you tell the patient that each of the following benefits accrue to a person who exercises, except for which one?

(A) Prevention and control of diabetes type II are improved in regular exercise, even controlling for weight.

(B) Osteoporosis of aged individuals is retarded or prevented by regular exercise.

(C) Risk of colon cancer is lessened by regular exercise.

(D) Blood pressure control in hypertension is facilitated by regular exercise.

(E) Risk of rectal cancer is reduced by regular exercise.

6 A 35-year-old man weighs 210 lb (95 kg). His height is 5 ft, 10 in., or 70 in. (1.78 m). Thus, his ideal weight, 106 lb plus 6 lb for each inch over 5 ft, is 166 lb (75.2 kg). You point out that he is 44 lb or about 20 kg overweight. You advise him to begin walking 1 mile every day. How many kilocalories will he burn, regardless of his pace or pulse rate while walking?

(A) 50 kcal

(B) 100 kcal

(C) 140 kcal

(D) 200 kcal

(E) 240 kcal

7 The patient in Question 6 takes your advice and begins a walking program. In walking, he takes 20 minutes to move a mile and maintains a pulse of 100 while walking at that pace. How many calories will he burn if he is doing cycling for 1 hour, maintaining a pulse rate of 150 beats per minute?

(A) 110 cal

(B) 210 cal

(C) 320 cal

(D) 430 cal

(E) 630 cal

8 Regarding the patient in Questions 6 and 7, after safely embarking on a walking program, he says he would like to get back in athletic condition, with jogging and perhaps sports. He has heard about runners having lower pulses than the average person and wonders how long increased aerobic exercise must proceed before the pulse begins to be lowered. What is your answer?

(A) As soon as he begins exercising

(B) After 2 to 3 weeks of a regular program

(C) After 4 to 6 weeks of a regular program

(D) After 8 to 10 weeks of a regular program

(E) This type of exercise will not produce a change in the resting pulse rate.

9 Which of the following best applies to the "cooldown period" component of an exercise program?

(A) During this component there is a net clearing of lactic acid from the muscles.

(B) It has four characteristics described by the mnemonic FITT (frequency, intensity, type, and time).

(C) It is only necessary for patients in vigorous-intensity programs.

(D) It represents the aerobic phase of the workout.

(E) It increases peripheral blood pooling in muscles.

10 Which of the following is a valid reason to terminate an exercise session?

(A) The systolic blood pressure rises and the diastolic pressure falls during strenuous exercise.

(B) The pulse rate doubles during strenuous exercise.

(C) The patient experiences persistent headache during exercise.

(D) The patient is fatigued during strenuous exercise.

(E) Patient develops tachypnea.

Examination Answers

1. The answer is B. BEE is the amount of energy expended per unit time by a person at rest, who has not eaten for 12 hours. The basis of the 12-hour fast is that food intake adds energy consumption attached to it (i.e., the thermic effect of food). The third factor in energy consumption, of course, is that attendant to physical activity. For practical purposes it is too difficult to obtain subjects in a 12-hour fasting state. Therefore, a compromise is usually accepted for standardization, which is measurement of energy expenditure during a 2-hour fast. This adds about 10% to the BEE.

2. The answer is E. Individuals who exercise are less likely to experience cardiac arrest. The CAD risk factor of sedentary lifestyle is more prevalent than hypertension, smoking, or hypercholesterolemia, and the relative risk of CAD for sedentary lifestyle is 2 versus 2.5 for smoking, 2.1 for hypertension, and 2.4 for hypercholesterolemia. Total cholesterol tends to decrease, but high-density lipoprotein cholesterol increases with exercise. Physically inactive patients are about two times more likely to develop CAD than physically active patients. There is no basis for a mild to moderate hypertensive patient to delay exercise programs until perfect control of blood pressure is attained, assuming the patient has no symptoms of uncontrolled hypertension, such as headache, and does not have malignant hypertension. Exercise has a therapeutic effect on hypertension.

3. The answer is E, 30 minutes of moderately intense physical activity 5 to 7 days a week, preferably 7 days per week.

4. The answer is C, 122 beats per minute. Moderate activity produces about 70% of the predicted maximum pulse; thus, a functional definition of moderate exercise is that which produces a heart rate equal to 70% of the predicted maximum, in a patient with no heart disease. The maximum pulse is 220 minus the age, in this case 45 years. Thus, 220 minus 45 = 175; then, 175 $\times$ 0.7 (or 70%) $\geq$ 122 beats per minute.

5. The answer is E. The risk of rectal cancer is *not* reduced by regular exercise, in contrast to colon cancer. All the other statements regarding the benefits of exercise are true.

6. The answer is C; 140 kcal is the estimated caloric consumption for the 210-lb (95-kg) person in walking 1 mile at any pace. This is based on a rule of thumb that is easy to memorize: Weight in pounds multiplied by two-thirds.

7. The answer is E, 630 cal. It is assumed that calories consumed in exercise are directly proportional to the pulse during such exercise and to the time involved in such exercise, using as a baseline the calories consumed in walking 1 mile and the pulse in beats per minute during the normal walking pace:

$Cx = Cw \times (Px/Pw) \times (Tx/Tw)$,

where

Cw is the calories consumed in locomotion of 1 mile at any pace

Px is the pulse during exercise

Pw is the pulse during a 1-mile walk

Tx is the time spent at new exercise

Tw is the time spent walking 1 mile

$140 \times (150/100) \times (60/20)$

Thus, Cx = $140 \times (150/100) \times (60/20)$ = 630 kcal for this individual to peddle a bicycle for 1 hour, raising his pulse to 150 bpm. Thus, it is shown how to calculate a pulse-raising activity.

8. The answer is C, after 4 to 6 weeks of a regular program. Help with weight control and stress reduction may be noticed immediately, but improved muscle strength takes 2 to 3 weeks and cardiorespiratory improvement such as the diminished pulse takes 4 to 6 weeks. This does not negate the rough relationship between resting pulse, exercising pulse, and calorie consumption referred to in Question 7. This is because both the resting and the exercising pulse are readjusted downward proportionately.

9. The answer is A. The cooldown period is the voluntary deceleration of the exercise activity over several seconds to 1 minute. During this component, there is a net clearing of lactic acid from the muscles as a result of resumption of normal venous return. Lactic acid contributes to muscle soreness during the early phase of conditioning; the cooldown period decreases the peripheral blood pooling in muscles. This return to normal venous circulation serves also to minimize light-headedness and nausea as circulation returns to the head and to the splanchnic bed. The FITT mnemonic refers to the defining characteristics of an exercise program: frequency, intensity, type of activity, and time invested in the activity. The aerobic phase applies to the activity phase of the workout, not the cooldown period.

10. The answer is C. Headache consistently during exercise may be indicative of a metabolic abnormality or anemia; in any event, it is not a desirable concomitant of exercise. Doubling the heart rate is within normal limits for stress testing. Rising systolic and falling diastolic pressure during exercise is a physiological response. A rising diastolic pressure may be a sign of a pathological cardiovascular response to exercise.

References

Baron RB: Nutrition. In: Tierney LM, McPhee SJ, Papadakis MA, eds. *Current Medical Diagnosis and Treatment.* 45th ed. New York: McGraw-Hill/Appleton & Lange; 2006:1253–1285.

Coleman MT. Exercise and health. In: Rudy DR, Kurowski K, eds. *Family Medicine: House Officer Series.* Baltimore: Williams & Wilkins; 1997:657–668.

Pignone M, McPhee SJ. Approach to the patient and health maintenance. In: Tierney LM, McPhee SJ, Papadakis MA, eds. *Current Medical Diagnosis and Treatment.* 45th ed. New York: McGraw-Hill/Appleton & Lange; 2006:1–19.

chapter 40

Preventive Care and Triage of Newborns and Infants (Birth to 1 Year)

Examination questions: Unless instructed otherwise, choose the ONE lettered answer or completion that is BEST in each case.

1 Each of the following statements regarding routine circumcision of the male newborn is true except for which one?

(A) Circumcised males have fewer urinary tract infections.

(B) Phimosis is prevented.

(C) Circumcision reduces the chances of carcinoma of the cervix in future female partners.

(D) Circumcision is contraindicated in the presence of hypospadias.

(E) Circumcision reduces the lifetime risk of penile cancer.

2 A healthy newborn boy, weighing 7 lb 6 oz (3.34 kg), has been accepted for well baby care. In regard to hydration and renal function, which of the following is an accepted indication of adequate urine output in the first 24 hours of life?

(A) Moist mucosae

(B) Good skin turgor

(C) Nonsunken eyeballs

(D) One wet diaper

(E) Normal pasty stools

3 A full-term newborn boy was born to a gravida 3, para 3 woman who had not committed to regular prenatal care. There is a history of neonatal jaundice in her second baby caused by a minor blood group

incompatibility. Assuming this baby exhibits jaundice in the first few days of life, which of the following cut-off points is satisfactory for alerting the primary care physician to the likely need for phototherapy?

(A) Bilirubin level ≥15 mg/dL at 10 hours of age

(B) Bilirubin level ≥10 mg/dL at <12 hours of age

(C) Bilirubin level ≤15 mg/dL at 18 hours of age

(D) Onset of clinical jaundice

(E) Bilirubin level at ≥18 mg/dL at ≤48 hours of age

4 What is the average caloric requirement for a newborn infant?

(A) 50 kcal/kg/day

(B) 120 kcal/kg/day

(C) 150 kcal/kg/day

(D) 500 kcal/day

(E) 700 kcal/day

5 Each of the following is a risk factor for sudden infant death syndrome (SIDS) in the United States, except for which one?

(A) Low socioeconomic status

(B) Minority ethnicity

(C) Maternal smoking

(D) Sleeping in the prone position

(E) Family history of atopic disease

6 During which of the following age groups is SIDS most likely to occur?

(A) 0 to 2 months

(B) 2 to 4 months

(C) 4 to 6 months

(D) 6 to 8 months

(E) 1 to 2 years

7 Which of the following immunizations should be given in the newborn period?

(A) Diphtheria, tetanus, pertussis (DTaP), first dose

(B) *Hemophilus influenzae* type B (Hib), first dose

(C) Inactivated polio vaccine (IPV), first dose

(D) Pneumococcal vaccine (PCV), first dose

(E) Hepatitis B (HepB), first dose

8 At birth, a full-term female infant has received silver nitrate ointment 1%. Five days later she exhibits conjunctivitis. Which of the following is the most significant likely possible etiologic origin?

(A) *Staphylococcus aureus*

(B) Group A beta-hemolytic streptococci

(C) Gonococcus

(D) *Chlamydia trachomatis*

(E) *H. influenzae*

9 In counseling a first-time mother regarding normal growth and development of her baby, which of the following do you outline as the normal course of developmental milestones?

(A) Head up and controlled at 2 weeks, sit unsupported at 3 months, crawl at 6 months, and walk at 9 months

(B) Head up and controlled at 2 months, sit unsupported at 4 months, crawl at 6 months, and walk at 9 months

(C) Head up and controlled at 3 months, sit unsupported at 6 months, crawl at 9 months, and walk at 12 months

(D) Head up and controlled at 4 months, sit unsupported at 8 months, crawl at 10 months, and walk at 14 months

(E) Head up and controlled at 6 months, sit unsupported at 10 months, crawl at 12 months, and walk at 18 months

10 In advising the mother referred to in Question 9, which of the following rules of thumb do you suggest regarding body weight for her infant?

(A) The child should weigh 15 lb (6.8 kg) by 6 months and 22 lb (10 kg) by 1 year.

(B) The child should weigh 10 lb (4.5 kg) by 6 months and 15 lb (6.8 kg) by 1 year.

(C) The child should double the birth weight by the age of 6 months and increase it three times by the age of 1 year.

(D) The child should double the birth weight by 6 months and triple it by 1 year.

(E) Weight does not matter as long as the child has a normal appetite.

11 You are counseling an expectant couple regarding the many benefits of breast feeding. Which of the following is a recognized beneficial effect?

(A) It decreases neonatal jaundice.

(B) It increases weight gain in the infant relative to those who are fed formula.

(C) Breast milk supplies IgG antibodies.

(D) The uterus returns to normal size faster in mothers who breast feed.

(E) Term babies who are breast fed do not need fluoride supplementation.

12 Besides prematurity, certain situations predispose a child to iron deficiency. Which of the following children may have this problem?

(A) An infant who is breast fed

(B) An infant born at term, now 4 months old, who has been on Enfamil formula

(C) A postdate newborn, now 3 months old, who has been on Isomil formula

(D) A 10-month-old infant who has an allergy to cow's milk protein

(E) An infant started after 6 months on solid foods that are rich in vitamin C

Examination Answers

1. The answer is C. The incorrect statement is that circumcision reduces the chances of carcinoma of the cervix in future female partners. However, the presence of the foreskin does appear to be associated with a greater risk of penile cancer. It is true that uncircumcised males have a greater risk of urinary tract infections, compared with circumcised males; circumcision is contraindicated in newborns with hypospadias because the foreskin may be invaluable in plastic repair of the deformity, most specifically to reconstruct the urethral orifice. Obviously, phimosis is not possible in the absence of a foreskin.

2. The answer is D. One wet diaper in the first 24 hours should be adequate to ensure normal hydration and kidney function. Normal alimentation is not sensitive enough, whereas all the other signs listed, that is, waiting for dry mucosae, poor skin turgor, and sunken eyeballs, which are quite valid for clinical dehydration, are later in development than optimum care dictates. By day 2 there should be a wet diaper two to three times per 24 hours, and by day 5 there should be a wet diaper six to eight times per 24 hours.

3. The answer is B. A bilirubin level ≥10 mg/dL at <12 hours of age is an appropriate signal that the indirect-acting bilirubin may reach the level of 20 mg/dL by the third or fourth day, setting the stage for kernicterus. Other cutoff points are bilirubin levels of ≥14 mg/dL between 12 and 24 hours and ≥15 mg/dL at >24 hours of age. Jaundice that is due to a pathological as opposed to a physiological cause appears on the first day of life, and bilirubin levels can rise by more than 5 mg/dL/day. Peak bilirubin levels in physiologic jaundice rarely exceed 12 mg/dL but pathologic jaundice peaks at a much higher level, as stated. Exchange transfusion may be necessary if phototherapy does not obviate that need.

4. The answer is B; 120 kcal/kg/day is the average caloric requirement for a newborn infant. Obviously, this is calculated on weight and does not apply across all weights.

5. The answer is E. Family history of atopic disease is not mentioned the literature as a risk factor for SIDS. The two strongest (and remediable) risk factors are a smoking mother and prone sleeping position. Minority ethnicity and low socioeconomic status are risk factors but are not specific enough to be helpful.

6. The answer is B; 2 to 4 months is the peak period of SIDS incidence. The vast majority of cases occur when an infant is between a few weeks and 6 months of age.

7. The answer is E. HepB (hepatitis B) is the only routine immunization recommended for infants in the newborn period (≤1 month of age) and should be given at birth. It may await the first or second month if the mother is negative to hepatitis B surface antigen. DTaP, Hib, IPV, and PCV are each given at 2, 4, and 6 months.

8. The answer is D, *C. trachomatis.* The two most significant causes of neonatal conjunctivitis (ophthalmia neonatorium) are gonorrhea and *C. trachomatis.* Gonorrheal conjunctivitis is prevented by routine neonatal treatment with silver nitrate. Presently the approach to chlamydial conjunctivitis is diagnosis by culture or rapid antigen detection followed by treatment with erythromycin.

9. The answer is C. The timing is head up and controlled at 3 months, sit unsupported at 6 months, crawl at 9 months, and walk at 12 months. These are good screening guidelines and serve the family doctor or pediatrician well, not only in educating parents but also in reviewing to establish a database for a new pediatric patient. Many children, especially those from families of higher socioeconomic status, will walk before 1 year and some as early as 6 months. Also, children may take longer than 6 months to sit unsupported. If only one of these mile markers is a departure from the normal rules of thumb, it may be explained by factors unique to the child's personality or family living status. Nevertheless, such a departure should trigger a more detailed examination for development. Delay in walking may be based on neurological, orthopedic, or cerebral development. Such refinements of developmental evaluation include grasp progressing from ulnar palm to radial, including the thumb at 3 to 4 months; using the thumb in opposition to pick up objects at 7 months.

10. The answer is C. The child should double the birth weight by the age of 3 months and increase four times by the age of 1 year. Choice A is virtually the same rule for a child of average birth weight. Many children will exceed this rate of growth, which is acceptable as long as the child is not becoming obese (i.e., simply growing bigger and faster is alright). Obesity should be addressed when it appears and prescribed for by the age of 2.

11. The answer is D. The uterus returns to normal size more rapidly in mothers who breast feed. Breast-fed babies also have decreased weights relative to formula-fed babies during the initial months, but this does not affect their final stature or weight. Breast milk supplies secretory IgA and macrophages but not IgG. One disadvantage of breast feeding is that some infants develop jaundice. The neonatal jaundice produced by breast feeding is felt to be benign and is not believed to produce kernicterus.

12. The answer is D, a 10-month-old who has an allergy to cow's milk protein. The reaction to the ingested protein causes inflammation in the intestine and resultant chronic low-grade gastrointestinal blood loss, which predisposes to iron deficiency. The iron in breast milk, though not high in concentration, is very well absorbed because of the effect of lactoferrin in breast milk to enhance absorption. Vitamin C increases intestinal iron absorption. Term and postdate babies are not at increased risk, as even "standard" formulas are iron fortified.

References

Gegas BG. Preventive care and triage of the infant and newborn. In Rudy DR, Kurowski K, eds. *Family Medicine: House Officer Series.* Baltimore: Williams & Wilkins; 1997:669–688.

Thilo EH, Rosenberg AA. The newborn infant. In: Hay WW Jr, Levin MJ, Sondheimer JM, et al. eds. *Current Pediatric Diagnosis and Treatment.* 17th ed., New York: McGraw-Hill; 2005:1–65.

chapter **41**

Preventive Care of the Preschool Child (Ages 1 to 5 Years)

Examination questions: Unless instructed otherwise, choose the ONE lettered answer or completion that is BEST in each case.

1 You are counseling first-time parents of a 15-month-old child. The subject of language development arises. At what age do you alert the parents to expect the child to begin to speak in sentences of 2 to 3 words with a 50-word vocabulary?

(A) 15 to 18 months

(B) 18 to 26 months

(C) 2 to 3 years

(D) 3 to 4 years

(E) 4 to 5 years

2 A first-time mother brings her 18-month-old male child in for routine well care. His birth weight was 7 lb 8 oz (3.4 kg). His weight at 1 year was 22 lb 6 oz (10.13 kg). Today's weight is 25 lb 8 oz (11.55 kg). The boy walked at 11 months and is able to make known two "wants" and occasional two-word sentences. The mother is concerned regarding his apparent cessation in growth and notes that he eats less now than he had been eating at the age of 1 year. Your response is appropriately which of the following?

(A) Plan to track calorie intake for 30-days and re-evaluate

(B) Draw blood for thyroid functions tests

(C) Place the child on a high-calorie diet

(D) Draw blood for growth hormone and testosterone levels

(E) No action needed at this time; reassure the parent that the child is growing normally

3 A child should have at least four of each of the following immunizations by the age of 5 years, except for which one?

(A) Diphtheria, tetanus, pertussis (DTaP)

(B) Pneumococcal vaccine (PCV)

(C) Varicella

(D) *Hemophilus influenzae* type B (Hib)

(E) Inactivated polio vaccine (IPV)

4 Which of the following patients, according to opinions among the American Academy of Pediatrics (AAP), the American Academy of Family Physicians (AAFP), and the Advisory Committee on Immunization Practices (ACIP), should receive influenza vaccine on an annual basis?

(A) Infants from birth to 1 year of age

(B) Children from 1 to 5 years of age

(C) Children from 5 to 12 years of age

(D) All persons older than 6 months of age

(E) All adults only

5 Well examination of a 5-year-old child reveals that he speaks only six-word sentences but they are intelligible. The parents are concerned. Which of the following responses is most appropriate?

(A) Refer the child for specialized evaluation of growth and development

(B) Arrange a conference with the child's teacher

(C) Order a magnetic resonance image of the child's brain

(D) Reassure the parents that the child is developing within normal limits

(E) Review the milestones of growth and development in this child

6 Which of the following measures is the most effective to prevent drowning among children who are between 1 and 5 years of age?

(A) Providing consistent discipline in teaching children safety policies

(B) Teaching children to swim at the earliest possible age before allowing them to swim in private pools

(C) Requiring children to play in pairs (i.e., the "buddy system")

(D) Using high (4 ft or 1.8 m) fences with self-latching gates around swimming pools

(E) Outlawing private swimming pools

7 A 4-year-old girl is brought to a family doctor for her preschool checkup. She has had unremarkable growth and development. The family members are Italian-American (father) and Anglo-American (mother) and were born in the United States; the father is a worker in a factory that manufactures batteries, and the family lives in a house built in 1945. Which of the following has the highest priority as to routine testing at this point?

(A) Blood lead level

(B) Thyroid-stimulating hormone

(C) Tuberculosis skin testing

(D) Complete blood cell count

(E) Urinalysis for protein and sugar

8 Which of the following is the upper limit of tolerance for blood lead levels in children?

(A) <10 μg/dL

(B) <20 μg/dL

(C) <30 to 40 μg/dL

(D) <60 to 80 μg/dL

(E) <100 μg/dL

9 Which of the following accounts for the largest number of deaths in children?

(A) Motor vehicle accidents

(B) Infectious diseases

(C) Acute abdominal emergencies

(D) Violence (gunshots, knife wounds, strangulation)

(E) Drowning

10 You are evaluating a 1-year-old child who is short (less than fifth percentile on growth curves), even when you correct for midparental height. There are multiple potential causes for short stature. Which of the following is *not* among them?

(A) Parental deprivation

(B) Intrauterine growth retardation

(C) Human immunodeficiency virus (HIV) infection

(D) Klinefelter syndrome

(E) Familial short stature

Examination Answers

1. The answer is B, 18 to 26 months. That is, at about 2 years of age the normal child has achieved this level of language development and is progressing rapidly. The simplest two-word sentences are often managed by the age of 18 months.

2. The answer is E. No action is needed at this time; reassure the parent that the child is growing normally. Although babies should double the birth weight by 6 months and many babies triple their birth weights by the age of 1 year, growth rate decelerates rapidly after the first year. The average boy gains about 5 lb (2.26 kg) during the period from 1 year to 2 years of age. In this situation, there is neither indication for endocrinological testing nor for force feeding.

3. The answer is C. Varicella vaccine requires only one dose, when the child is between 12 and 25 months of age. It may be given at any time through the years of youth to anyone who has not received it. The child receives DTaP at 2, 4, 6, and 12 to 15 months, and then a booster at 4 to 6 years. PCV is given at 2, 4, 6, and 12 to 15 months. Hib vaccine is given at 2, 4, 6, and 12 to 15 months. IPV is given at 2, 4, and 6 to 15 months and at 4 to 6 years.

4. The answer is D. All persons older than 6 months of age should receive the influenza vaccine on an annual basis. The AAP and AAFP agree that all children between the ages of 6 months and 18 years should receive the vaccine, and the ACIP states that all adults should receive influenza vaccine yearly.

5. The answer is D. Reassure the parents that the child is developing within normal limits. A fair rule of thumb in evaluating language development is two-word sentences at age 2; four-word sentences at age 3; five-word sentences at age 4; and six- or seven-word sentences at age 5. Review of growth and development milestones is not a matter reserved for addressing a genuine concern. It is something that should take place at each well child visit.

6. The answer is D, high (4 ft or 1.8 m) fences with self-latching gates around swimming pools. Each of the other choices merits attention and would be an effective supplement to fencing the swimming pools, but the choices are unproven in effectiveness to prevent drowning. Choice E, outlawing private swimming pools, has not been tried and tested; such a law would not likely be passed in any community.

7. The answer is A. Lead-based paint was used in houses built before 1960. Nearby industry that places children at high risk includes lead smelting and battery manufacturing. Routine screening starts when the child reaches the age of 1 year, with checks at 6 months only for those children at high risk. Some physicians apply a written questionnaire for risk factors instead of automatic level checks in neighborhoods where lead toxicity is rare. Children should be checked with serum lead levels at any age if they have symptoms of lead poisoning or exhibit a lot of hand-to-mouth activity.

8. The answer is A, <10 µg/dL. Even exposures to levels in the range from 10 µg/dL to 15 µg/dL, if prolonged, can produce behavioral and cognitive effects. Ongoing studies have resulted in the steady reduction of lead-level cutoff points over the past 30 years.

9. The answer is A, motor vehicle accidents. Motor vehicle accidents (with children as a vehicle occupant or pedestrian) account for about 47% of injury deaths in children. In 1998, 57% of children 15 years of age and younger who died in motor vehicle accidents were unrestrained.

10. The answer is D, Klinefelter syndrome. Klinefelter syndrome is associated with tall stature with disproportional increases in long bones. All the other mentioned diseases result in growth retardation of a child. Parental deprivation leads to starvation, sometimes through anorexia; intrauterine growth retardation, by definition, is characterized by the child's starting life in a growth-retarded state; HIV infection exerts a nonspecific affect of failure to thrive; familial short stature has its effects from birth and could account for short stature in a 1-year-old child.

References

Goldson E, Reynolds A. Child development and behavior. In: Hay WW Jr, Levin MJ, Sondheimer JM, et al., eds. *Current Pediatric Diagnosis and Treatment.* 17th ed. New York: McGraw-Hill; 2005:1–66.

Kurowski K. Preventive care of the preschool child (1–5 years). In: Rudy DR, Kurowski K, eds. *Family Medicine: House Officer Series.* Baltimore: Williams & Wilkins; 1997:689–702.

US Preventive Services Task Force. The periodic health examination. In: *Guide to Clinical Preventive Services.* Baltimore: Williams & Wilkins; 1996:lvii–lxxi.

chapter 42

Preventive Care of the Child through the Latent Years (Ages 6 to 12 Years)

Examination questions: Unless instructed otherwise, choose the ONE lettered answer or completion that is BEST in each case.

1 A conscientious couple, a 25-year-old mother and 26-year-old father of three children, wish to discuss preventive health care for their eldest, a 6-year-old boy. Which of the following, against the background of current preventive measures already in place, is the area that presents the greatest opportunity of saving him from an earlier than average death?

(A) Practice safety in automobile travel

(B) Take measures to prevent fires

(C) Screen for lipids

(D) Teach proper care of firearms

(E) Enforce pneumonia vaccination

2 In 2001, there were 400,000 Americans injured in bicycle accidents; two-thirds of the victims were children. What percentage of children injured in bicycle accidents sustained head injuries?

(A) 15%

(B) 25%

(C) 50%

(D) 85%

(E) 95%

3 A 30-year-old mother brings her 12-year-old son for a routine well child visit. He has had four doses of diphtheria, tetanus, and pertussis (DTaP), four of *Hemophilus influenzae* type B (Hib), four of inactivated

polio vaccine (IPV), and two of varicella vaccine. Which of the following immunizations is specially indicated at this time?

(A) Varicella

(B) DTaP

(C) IPV

(D) Booster of tetanus toxoid and a smaller dose of diphtheria toxoid (Td)

(E) Hib

4 Children who have had significant social contact with people with acquired immunodeficiency syndrome (AIDS), who are human immunodeficiency virus (HIV) positive, or are prisoners, migrant farm workers, or illicit drug users are considered at risk for which of the following diseases?

(A) HIV disease

(B) Hepatitis B

(C) Infectious mononucleosis

(D) Syphilis

(E) Tuberculosis

5 Which of the following forms of hypertension is found in children in a lesser proportion of hypertensive cases than in adults?

(A) Essential hypertension

(B) Pheochromocytoma

(C) Coarctation of the aorta

(D) Renal artery stenosis

(E) Chronic renal failure

6 Which of the following is the accepted mode for screening for tuberculosis in a child?

(A) Tuberculosis tine test

(B) Chest x-ray

(C) Mantoux test

(D) Pulmonary sputum culture

(E) Throat culture

7 Parents, both 30 years old, are together in a family physician's office to support their 6-year-old boy at his well child visit. They ask what rate of growth can be expected over the years, between now and the boy's adolescence. What is the general rate of growth they can anticipate throughout this period?

(A) 0.5 to 1 in. (1.27 to 2.54 cm) per year

(B) 1 to 2 in. (2.54 to 5.08 cm) per year

(C) 2 to 2.5 in. (5.08 to 6.35 cm) per year

(D) 3 to 3.5 in. (7.62 to 8.89 cm) per year

(E) 4 to 5 in. (10.16 to 12.70 cm) per year

8 A 19-year-old young woman exhibits scoliosis of 20 degrees in the thoracic spine (convexity) with compensating lumbar curvature. What is the best approach for following this patient?

(A) Follow with x-rays for the next several years

(B) Refer to a spine surgeon

(C) Evaluate for bracing

(D) Evaluate for spinal fusion

(E) Reassure the patient that the degree of curvature is benign and bears no further attention

9 Which of the following may be constitutionally associated with scoliosis (part of the primary syndrome as opposed to being secondary to the disease)?

(A) Cerebral palsy

(B) Poliomyelitis

(C) Slipped femoral capital epiphysis

(D) Neurofibromatosis

(E) Constrictive lung disease

10 A 10-year-old boy is found to be falling behind in school. It develops that he has had trouble seeing the chalk board in the classroom for the past 3 months. Visual acuity is 20/75, both eyes, at 20 ft (6.09 m). However, he is able to read a written page at 7 in. (17.8 cm) in both eyes. The boy has a normal appetite and no complaints except for his visual problem in school. Conjunctivae and sclerae are normal to inspection. Funduscopy is negative for fields of vision by opacities in the refractive media, and papilledema and his confrontation are normal. The cover–uncover test discloses an exophoria. Which of the following is the appropriate approach to his problem?

(A) Check blood sugar

(B) Refer to an ophthalmologist for muscle alignment surgery

(C) Refer to an optometrist

(D) Advise observation for 3 months followed by re-examination

(E) Refer for psychological testing to determine intelligence

Examination Answers

1. The answer is A. Motor vehicle accidents are the leading cause of death in children. Assuming that the parents maintain recommended immunizations in the first 5 years of life and the required immunization schedules after the age of school matriculation, the best thing they could do for this child is to protect him from automobile accidents, the chief cause of mortality in children of all ages. Fires and burns are in second place.

2. The answer is D; 85% of injuries sustained by children in bicycle accidents involve head injuries. Therefore, bicycle helmets worn by children (and adults) should be routine practice.

3. The answer is D, Td vaccine. The other vaccines mentioned here have been completed by the time the child reaches the age of 5 to 6 years (see chapter 41). From the age of 12, all individuals should receive the Td vaccine every 10 years for the remainder of life.

4. The answer is E. Tuberculosis is contagious through close social contact and has a high prevalence in the groups mentioned, that is, people with HIV, prisoners, migrant farm workers, and illicit drug users, as well as people from countries with highly endemic tuberculosis. All the other choices in the question are diseases that require closer association than social (i.e., airborne) contact, except for infectious mononucleosis. The latter is not particularly contagious and is not particularly prevalent in the groups mentioned.

5. The answer is A, essential hypertension. Although hypertension in children is defined the same as in adults (i.e., blood pressure consistently in the 95th percentile or higher), the causes are more likely to be secondary rather than primary in children as compared to the distribution of hypertension in adults; 28% in children, whereas in adults only about 5% of hypertension falls into that category.

6. The answer is C, the Mantoux test, the intradermal injection of 5 units of purified protein derivative, followed by inspection for palpable induration in 48 to 73 hours.

The tine test should not be used because it is lacking in sensitivity. A chest x-ray is not practical from the cost standpoint. The sputum culture is not ordered except in symptomatic cases.

7. The answer is C, 2 to 2.5 in. (5.08 to 6.35 cm) per year. The period begins with a growth rate of 2.5 in. or 6.35 cm per year and subsides to about 2 in. or 5.08 cm per year by the time the child reaches the age of 10, prior to the growth spurt that occurs at puberty.

8. The answer is A, observe for the next several years, following with plain x-rays. Twenty percent of curvature is nearly always asymptomatic and most cases will not progress. The longer the patient manifests no progression of the curvature, the less likely it will ultimately require correction. The male-to-female ration is 1:4 for affliction with scoliosis. This disorder has its onset when the child is between 8 and 10 years of age. The most serious degrees of scoliosis will occur before the child reaches the age of 16 (i.e., before the closure of the epiphyses). Only with progression should consultation be resorted to, with consideration of aggressive methods of prevention. At 40 to 60 degrees of curvature, bracing is indicated. At 60 degrees, fusion may be indicated to prevent respiratory deficiency in the future. However, the latter is a very serious undertaking and entails the better part of a year of nearly total disability in the patient.

9. The answer is D. Neurofibromatosis may be constitutionally associated with scoliosis. Cerebral palsy, poliomyelitis, and muscular dystrophy may predispose the patient to scoliosis on the basis of asymmetrical forces bearing on the spinal column. Constrictive lung disease may occur secondary to the scoliosis because of impedance of expansion of the lung fields. Slipped femoral capital epiphysis is not known to be associated with scoliosis.

10. The answer is C. Refer the patient to an optometrist; the point is that the patient has a refractory error, not a medical or surgical problem. Hence, though an ophthalmologist would be a good referral, it would not be with muscle-imbalance surgery in mind. The patient has myopia, which, in the extreme, causes exotropia from the first year of life as a result of the attempts at relaxation of accommodation for distance that produces divergence of gaze beyond parallel; a strabismus of the exotropic type results. Suppression amblyopia occurs if this is not corrected by the time the child reaches the age of 7 years. A cosmetically significant exotropia becomes permanent unless surgery on the extraocular muscles is carried out to correct the malalignment. In milder cases such as the one in the vignette, amblyopia may have been avoided by using alternating suppression of the individual eyes. The cover–uncover test may show a falling to the outside of the covered eye, which is then seen to recover to the original gaze when the blocking cover is switched to the opposite eye (thus esotropia). Although diabetes changes refractory density of the light-conducting media, a 10-year-old child would have type I diabetes, a disease that does not remain asymptomatic for more than a matter of weeks.

References

Goldson E, Reynolds A. Child development and behavior. In: Hay WW Jr, Levin MJ, Sondheimer JM, et al., eds. *Current Pediatric Diagnosis and Treatment.* 17th ed. New York: McGraw-Hill; 2005:1–65.

Welker MJ. Preventive care of the child through the latent years (5–12). In: Rudy DR, Kurowski K, eds. *Family Medicine: House Officer Series.* Baltimore: Williams & Wilkins; 1997: 703–712.

chapter 43

Preventive Care through Adolescence (Ages 12 to 20 Years)

Examination questions: *Unless instructed otherwise, choose the ONE lettered answer or completion that is BEST in each case.*

1 Members of which of the following groups are most likely to *attempt* suicide (without succeeding)?

(A) Black men who are 20 to 30 years old

(B) White boys or men who are 15 to 24 years old

(C) White girls or women who are 15 to 24 years old

(D) Black women who are 20 to 30 years old

(E) White women who are 20 to 30 years old

2 Members of which of the following groups are most likely to *commit* suicide?

(A) Black men who are 20 to 30 years old

(B) White boys or men who are 15 to 24 years old

(C) White girls or women who are 15 to 24 years old

(D) Black women who are 20 to 30 years old

(E) White women who are 20 to 30 years old

3 You are examining an 18-year-old young man for employment. His growth and development have been normal. In interviewing him, which of the following would you most expect by way of change since your last examination, done for routine school qualification 3 years ago?

(A) He is expressing more desire for independence from his parents.

(B) He has become more concerned about intimate relationships and careers.

(C) He has been participating in more risk-taking behaviors.

(D) He becomes more concerned with peer-group acceptance.

(E) He has become more involved in drinking and promiscuous sexual activity and delinquency.

4 Parents of a 13-year-old boy believe their son, who is demonstrating a growth spurt, is not drinking enough milk and ask you about calcium-intake requirements. What do you tell them are the current daily recommendations for calcium intake?

(A) Between 300 and 500 mg/day

(B) Between 600 and 1,000 mg/day

(C) Between 1,200 and 1,500 mg/day

(D) Between 1,500 and 2,000 mg/day

(E) Between 2,000 and 2,500 mg/day

5 Regarding the patient in Question 4, which of the following diets would ensure the boy of minimally adequate calcium intake at this time of life?

(A) Two exchanges of dairy products; two exchanges of meat; three exchanges of fruit; eight exchanges of grain

(B) Four exchanges of dairy products; two exchanges of meat; six exchanges of fruit; eight exchanges of grain

(C) Three exchanges of dairy products; two exchanges of meat; three exchanges of fruit; six exchanges of grain

(D) Six exchanges of dairy products; four exchanges of meat; six exchanges of fruit; eight exchanges of grain

(E) Two exchanges of dairy products; one exchange of meat; six exchanges of fruit; eight exchanges of grain

6 You are deciding on preventive screening for a young woman who began menarche at age 13. Her cycles are every 30 days, with 4 days of moderate flow. Her last menstrual period was 2 weeks ago. She denies ever being sexually active. She denies any vaginal discharge or pelvic area pain. At what age should Pap smears be performed on her?

(A) At age 13

(B) At age 15

(C) At age 20

(D) At the age of first sexual activity

(E) At the age of regular sexual activity

7 Which of the following contraceptive methods is acceptable in sexually active nulliparous adolescents?

(A) Intrauterine device

(B) Diaphragm

(C) Withdrawal

(D) Cervical cap

(E) Contraceptive pill (birth control pill, or BCP)

8 A 19-year-old sexually active female college student has recently married and has been taking oral contraceptive medication for 3 months. She complains of headaches since starting "the pill." Her blood pressure is 132/78; she weighs 120 lb (54.4 kg) at a height of 5 ft, 4 in. (1.63 m). Which of the following alterations in her regimen would be the most appropriate?

(A) Reduce the estrogen component of her BCP

(B) Reduce the progestational component of her BCP

(C) Investigate the androgenic effects of her BCP

(D) Prescribe a 5-hydroxytryptamine agonist (e.g., sumatriptan)

(E) Discontinue the BCP

9 Regarding the tolerability of oral contraceptive medications, each of the following is a side effect of the estrogenic component of BCPs, except which one?

(A) Increased breast size

(B) Enlargement of leiomyomas

(C) Hepatocellular adenomas

(D) Cyclic weight gain

(E) Oily skin

10 A 16-year-old female patient visits her family doctor for treatment of a viral upper respiratory tract infection. She appears to have lost weight since the last visit of 6 months ago. The doctor inquires regarding her menstrual history, and finds she has missed the last two periods. Pregnancy testing is negative. Suspecting anorexia, the doctor checks her weight against the ideal for her age and sex. Which of the following weight criteria satisfy the minimal definition of anorexia nervosa?

(A) Weight <100 lb (45 kg) in a female individual

(B) Weight <100 lb plus 5 lb for every inch over 60 in. (5 ft, or 1.52 m)

(C) Ideal body weight (IBW) <60th percentile for age and sex

(D) Weight <85% of IBW

(E) Caloric intake <500 kcal/day

11 You are seeing a 14-year-old girl for a school physical and decide to use some of the interaction time to discourage her from starting smoking. Which is the correct percentage that you can quote to her regarding the chance that a teenager will become a regular smoker if she or he smokes just two cigarettes completely?

(A) 25%

(B) 50%

(C) 60%

(D) 70%

(E) 85%

12 A 16-year-old is undergoing a routine health maintenance examination. He has had five immunizations of diphtheria, tetanus, and pertussis (DTaP; three in the first year, one at 2 years, and one at 5 years); four shots of *Hemophilus influenzae* type B (Hib); four shots of inactivated polio vaccine (IPV); two shots of measles, mumps, and rubella (MMR) vaccine; a varicella vaccine; three shots of pneumococcal vaccine (PCV); three doses of hepatitis B vaccine (HBV); and yearly influenza vaccines. Besides the yearly influenza vaccine, which of the following vaccines is due at this time?

(A) DTaP, sixth dose

(B) MMR, third dose

(C) Diphtheria and tetanus booster (Td)

(D) IPV, fifth dose

(E) Varicella, second dose

Examination Answers

1. The answer is C. White female individuals who are between 15 and 24 years of age attempt suicide at a rate three times that of male individuals in the same age group. For all groups, the ratio between suicide threats to attempts and successful suicide ranges from 50:1 to 100:1.

2. The answer is B. White male individuals who are between 15 and 24 years of age, which is a high-risk age group, are five times as likely to commit suicide as women. This age group produces the greatest number of both attempts and completed suicides. Problems underlying suicide are depression that is due to pathologic grief or to perceived inability to meet demands, such as grades in school (which matches, perhaps, the perceived expectations of the parents). The third category is psychosis. The physician must be alert to depression and ready to ask the patient directly regarding depression and indirectly regarding suicidal ideation. If the latter is present, then the doctor asks if a method of suicide has been considered or chosen. The method of suicide is firearms in 67% of cases of both male and female individuals.

3. The answer is B. He has become more concerned about intimate relationships and career. Choices C and E are abnormal patterns. Risk taking, including sexual activity and delinquency, should have abated. Struggle for independence from the parents would have occurred earlier. The patient should be less concerned with peer approval now than he was in early adolescence.

4. The answer is C, between 1,200 and 1,500 mg/day. The new adolescent recommendations are close to the 1,500 mg/day recommended for adults to help prevent osteoporosis.

5. The answer is B. Four exchanges of dairy products; two exchanges of meat; six exchanges of fruit; and eight exchanges of grain supply the calcium needed to support adolescent growth. This diet also supplies the other nutrients required for that group (i.e., protein, vitamins, fiber, and energy). As to supporting bone growth, of course it is the dairy exchanges that "carry the ball." Dairy unit equivalents are 1 cup of milk or yogurt, 1½ slices of cheddar cheese, 1 cup of pudding, 1¾ cups of ice cream, or 2 cups of cottage cheese. By comparison, a child should have 3 dairies, 2 meats, fruits or vegetables, and 6 to 11 grains. Adults require the same as children except for needing only two dairy exchanges. Pregnant women require the same as teenagers except for needing 3 meats instead of 2. Lactating women require the same as teenaged adolescents. (These nutritional recommendations are taken from chapter 43, by Speer and Felmar, of Rakel's *Textbook of Family Practice*.)

6. The answer is D, at the age of first sexual activity. Officially, most authorities maintain that Pap smears should begin when sexual activity starts but, in any event, no later than at age 18.

7. The answer is E. The BCP is reasonably safe in female adolescents. The intrauterine device, the diaphragm, and the cervical cap require skill for insertion and are perceived as arduous; hence they are unpopular with teenagers. Teenagers should be taught that withdrawal is unsafe as a preventative of pregnancy.

8. The answer is B. Reduce the progestational component of her BCP. Progestational agents in BCPs may cause side effects consisting of breast tenderness, hypertension, headaches, and, rarely, myocardial infarction (the latter presumably related to the androgenic effects of progestational agents that include reduced high-density lipoprotein cholesterol and elevated low-density lipoprotein cholesterol and increased insulin resistance). This patient's blood pressure appears to be elevated for her age. Although it is true that many people experience migraine headaches when they begin oral birth control medications, manipulating the progesterone agent may address both the headaches and the possible hypertension lurking in the wings with this patient, although hypertension may be caused by the estrogenic effects as well.

9. The answer is E. Oily skin as a change in someone who has started the BCP is caused by androgenic effects, which are due to the progestational agent. Related to that is exacerbation of acne, depression, and fatigue. The other effects mentioned among the distracters are due to estrogenic effects, in addition to which are thromboembolic phenomena (rare), cervical ectasia (cervical ectopy), and rise in biliary cholesterol.

10. The answer is D, weight <85% of IBW. This corresponds approximately to the definition of malnutrition, which is less than fifth percentile for body mass index. Use of percentile and percent of ideal may cause confusion: 85% of ideal weight refers to the spectrum of people who are living at less than ideal weight, only 5% of whom would be expected to weigh less than 85% of ideal. Thus, the choice of 60% of ideal weight may hardly exist in a living person, except in a prison camp situation. A weight of <100 lb (45 kg) in a female individual may well be within normal limits for a small person. There is no direct relationship between caloric intake and anorexia. However, anorectics may take in as little as 100 to 200 kcal/day. The formula of 100 lb plus 5 lb for every inch of height over 60 in. is simply a rough formula for *ideal* weight estimation. There are two forms of anorexia: The "classic" is the type wherein the individual, ostensibly in unreasonable fear of weight gain, simply overrides her appetite and refuses to take in more than a minimal amount of food. The other form applies to those who vomit or purge following food intake, often prodigious amounts (i.e., bulimia). These people often experience deterioration of teeth, particularly the upper incisors, from frequent vomiting. In both cases, amenorrhea occurs after a critical level of weight loss, which is the result of homeostatic mechanisms that result in hypothalamic hypofunction in response to malnutrition, especially when it occurs in association with stress. This can be thought of as a redirecting of energy resources in favor of survival.

11. The answer is E, 85%. If a teenager smokes two cigarettes, she or he stands an 85% chance of becoming a regular smoker. Surveys also show that most people (virtually all people, by the time they reach middle adulthood) are sorry they started.

12. The answer is C. Vaccines of Td, a tetanus booster with an attenuated dose of diphtheria, should be administered every 10 years, starting when the child reaches the age of 11 or 12. Each of the other choices mentioned is up to date and completed at this point.

References

Centers for Disease Control. Childhood and adolescent vaccine schedules. Endorsed by the Advisory Committee on Immunization Practices, the American Academy of Pediatrics, and the American Academy of Family Physicians.

Centers for Disease Control. Adult immunization schedules. Endorsed by the Advisory Committee on Immunization Practices, the American Academy of Pediatrics, and the American Academy of Family Physicians.

Kaplan DW, Love-Osborne K. Adolescence. In: Hay WW Jr, Levin MJ, Sondheimer JM, et al., eds. *Current Pediatric Diagnosis and Treatment.* 17th ed. New York: McGraw-Hill; 2005:102–146.

Rakel RE. *Textbook of Family Practice.* 6th ed. Philadelphia: WB Saunders; 2001.

Sigel EJ. Eating disorders. In: Hay WW Jr, Levin MJ, Sondheimer JM, et al., eds. *Current Pediatric Diagnosis and Treatment.* 17th ed. New York: McGraw-Hill; 2005:00–00.

Sternback M, Lipsky MS. Preventive care of the adolescent (12–20 years). In: Rudy DR, Kurowski K, eds. *Family Medicine: House Officer Series.* Baltimore: Williams & Wilkins; 1997:713–720.

chapter 44

Preventive Care of the Young Adult (Ages 20 to 40 Years)

Examination questions: *Unless instructed otherwise, choose the ONE lettered answer or completion that is BEST in each case.*

1 What category among the following accounts for the largest proportion of deaths in the age group of 25 to 40 years?

(A) Homicide

(B) Accidental injuries

(C) Cancer

(D) Suicide

(E) Human immunodeficiency virus (HIV) infection

2 A 25-year-old man purchases a new midsized automobile. What is the chance that he will attach his seatbelt when driving?

(A) 1/10

(B) 1/4

(C) 1/3

(D) 1/2

(E) 2/3

3 Cancers are the third leading cause of death in the age group of 25 to 44 years. In this age group, which cancer is the leading cause of cancer death?

(A) Lung

(B) Breast

(C) Prostate

(D) Colorectal

(E) Cervix

4 A 30-year-old man who weighs 170 lb (77 kg) at a height of 5 ft, 10.5 in. (1.79 m) has a repeatable blood pressure level in the 110 to 130/70 to 75 range. His family history reveals only that his parents are living and well at 50 and 55 years of age. He wishes to know when he should be screened for cholesterol. You reply that, according to the U.S. Preventive Services Task Force (USPSTF), screening should begin at what age?

(A) 25 years

(B) 30 years

(C) 35 years

(D) 45 years

(E) 50 years

5 A 35-year-old woman is sent for a pre-employment physical examination but had all scheduled immunizations to the age of 20. She has not seen a doctor or other health care professionals for 15 years. Which of the following immunizations should she have, assuming no special occupational risk factors and compliance with recommendations for immunizations at earlier ages?

(A) Measles, mumps, rubella (MMR) vaccine

(B) Pneumococcal vaccine

(C) Influenza vaccine

(D) Tetanus booster

(E) Hepatitis B vaccine

6 Which of the following is the least statistically important condition for which to screen in a 30-year-old woman who has no known special risk factors or family history and presents for an annual physical examination?

(A) Breast cancer

(B) Papanicolaou smear

(C) Blood pressure

(D) Complete blood cell count

(E) Presence of a smoke detector in the home

7 What is the leading category of causes of death in the United States for the age group of 25 to 34 years?

(A) Cardiovascular diseases

(B) Homicide

(C) Suicide

(D) Malignant neoplasms

(E) Accidents

8 What are the three leading causes of death in the age group of 35 to 44 years?

(A) Malignant neoplasms, heart disease, accidents

(B) Suicide, homicide, accidents

(C) Acute lower respiratory disease, liver disease

(D) Kidney diseases, diabetes mellitus, chronic lung disease

(E) Cerebrovascular disease, influenza, chronic lung disease

9 Suicide and suicide attempts may take many turns. Which of the following statements is not true regarding suicide, the fifth-leading cause of death in the age group of 25 to 44 years and the third-leading cause of death in the age group of 25 to 34 years?

(A) Victims have often been in contact with medical services in the period just prior to suicide.

(B) Firearms are a significantly prevalent method in male individuals, young adults, and adolescents.

(C) Persons who have histories of previous suicidal "gestures," often dramatic, are at low risk for suicide.

(D) HIV infection and acquired immunodeficiency syndrome (AIDS) constitute significant risk status.

(E) Suicidal persons often leave subtle hints of their intentions.

For Questions 8 through 12, match the numbered immunization with the lettered condition under which it should be offered. A choice may be correct for more than one item.

10 Tetanus booster, in combination with an attenuated dose of diphtheria (Td)

11 MMR vaccine

12 Hepatitis B vaccine

13 Pneumococcal vaccine

14 Influenza vaccine

(A) Those with chronic medical conditions

(B) Those individuals born after 1956 who lack evidence of immunity

(C) Health care workers, or recipients of blood products

(D) All adults every 10 years

(E) One dose per year for ≥50 years

Examination Answers

1. The answer is B. Accidental injuries as a category is the most common cause of death in the age group of <45 years.

2. The answer is E. About two-thirds of American motorists wear seatbelts when driving. This is unfortunate, because seatbelts are 60% effective in preventing automobile-accident fatalities.

3. The answer is B. Breast cancer is the leading cause of cancer death in the age group of 25 to 44 years. This is astounding because the statistic applies to both sexes. In fact, for all ages, breast and prostate cancers are virtually tied for third-ranking causes of death in causation, well behind lung cancer and the second cause, colorectal cancer. Be that as it may, the ages of onsets of the four most incident cancers in the U.S. population lend a perspective. Lung cancer is the greatest killer but, although the cause of that cancer is laid down in the period when a person is between 16 and 40 years of age, the cancer does not generally strike until the person reaches his or her 50s and 60s. Colorectal cancer is the second-leading cause of cancer deaths and, like lung cancer, strikes nearly equally each sex but not until the person's 50s or later, except in unusual cases. Prostate cancer also does not strike until a person's 50s in the most aggressive cases, and most often when a person is well into the 60s and 70s.

4. The answer is D. Assuming no more than one cardiovascular risk factor (age >45 years, maleness, previous heart disease, hypertension, or diabetes), the USPSTF recommends "periodic" cholesterol measurement in men beginning at age 45 and in women at age 55. Most practitioners consider this to be overly conservative and would most likely favor obtaining a baseline set of lipids in the early adult years before setting out a recommended frequency of testing for each patient individually. Nevertheless, the student must know what the authoritative organizations say.

5. The answer is D. A tetanus booster, usually given as a Td vaccine, should be administered every 10 years.

6. The answer is A. Breast cancer is the least likely among the listed screenings to be positive in a 30-year-old woman with no particular personal or familial risk factors. Breast cancer, though the second-ranking cancer killer of women, is not screened routinely until a woman reaches the age of 40, or at an age 10 years younger than a first-degree relative who has or has had breast cancer. The perspective of this question is a matter of intuition to an experienced practitioner but has not been posed in the literature in this manner. The Pap smear is, of course, recommended annually in a woman who is sexually active, reduced in frequency to every 3 years after three negative smears. Blood pressure is recommended by the USPSTF for all patients at all visits. A complete blood count has a higher chance of revealing an iron-deficiency anemia in a menstruating female than discovery of breast cancer at this age. Physicians are expected to become involved in the inquiring of environmental risk factors; thus, the choice of the presence of a smoke detector was given in the question. The same might be said of carbon monoxide detectors in a home that heats by gas. Some physicians, particularly some psychiatrists and pediatricians, feel patients should be asked about guns being kept in the home and how they might be stored safely. Drug or alcohol abuse should also be explored in all adult patients.

7. The answer is E. Accidents accounted for 29.6 deaths per 100,000 over the 3 years from 1999 to 2001, which is nearly twice the rate of the second and third causes; homicide averaged 11.3 and suicide 12.5 over the same 3-year period.

8. The answer is A. Malignant neoplasms, heart disease, and accidents easily comprise the ranking causes of death in the decade of life from 35 to 44, averaging 36.8, 31, and 29.7, respectively, over the 3 years of 1999, 2000, and 2001. These data present a stark contrast to those of the previous decade and portend a significant change in the risks of life over that 10-year period. In fourth place is homicide at 14 deaths per 100,000. Thus, cancer and vascular disease virtually burst upon the scene, whereas accidents remain significant, but markedly decreased, as causes of death.

9. The answer is C. The incorrect statement is that those who have made previous ostensible attempts are at no more risk for suicide than the population at large. Although the suicidal "gesture" has become notorious in emergency rooms, anyone who makes such a gesture or attempt falls along a spectrum of attention getting at one end and determination at the other. Virtually no one in that group who has gone so far as to "rehearse" the act is without a level of intent or serious consideration for suicide.

MATCHING THE NUMBERED IMMUNIZATIONS WITH THE LETTERED CONDITIONS

10. Td booster: **The answer is D,** all adults every 10 years.

11. MMR vaccine: **The answer is B,** those born after 1956 who lack evidence of immunity.

12. Hepatitis B vaccine: **The answer is C,** health care workers, or recipients of blood products.

13. Pneumococcal vaccine: **The answer is A,** those with chronic medical conditions.

14. Influenza vaccine: **The answer is E,** one dose per year for ≥50 years.

References

Arias E, Anderson RN, Kung H-C. Deaths: Final data for 2001. Centers for Disease Control. *Natl Vital Stat Rep.* 2003; 52(3): 1–116.

Ferrante JM. Preventive care of the young adult (20–40 years). In: Rudy DR, Kurowski K, eds. *Family Medicine: House Officer Series.* Baltimore: Williams & Wilkins; 1997:721–728.

U.S. Preventive Services Task Force. Screening for high blood cholesterol and other lipid abnormalities. In: *Guide to Clinical Preventive Services: Report of the U.S. Preventive Services Task Force.* Baltimore: Williams & Wilkins; 1996:39–53.

chapter 45

Preventive Care of the Middle-Aged Adult (Ages 40 to 65 Years)

Examination questions: *Unless instructed otherwise, choose the ONE lettered answer or completion that is BEST in each case*

1 You are consulting with a 50-year-old man at the time of his first comprehensive physical examination in 15 years. You have on hand a baseline electrocardiogram (EKG) taken when he had his last examination 15 years ago, read as normal (another was unchanged during an emergency department visit for atypical chest pain 1 year ago). He expresses a desire to begin preventive health care under your guidance. Along the way you elicit information that he smokes one package of cigarettes per day, weighs 208 lb (94.2 kg) at a height of 5 ft 10 in. (1.78 m), and has a history of "high cholesterol." Which of the following is the most appropriate combination of screening tests for this person, in addition to routine physical examination?

(A) EKG, complete blood cell (CBC) count, and lipid screen

(B) EKG stress test, CBC count, and liver and kidney function studies

(C) Chest x-ray, EKG, and comprehensive chemical profile

(D) Prostate-specific antigen (PSA) test, lipid screen, fecal occult blood test (FOBT), and blood sugar test

(E) Chest x-ray, pulmonary function studies, lipid screen and routine chemistries, and CBC count

2 A 45-year-old white woman returns to you for routine preventive care, having not seen you except for episodic problems for the past 6 years. Her family history is unremarkable except for the mention of colon polyps in her sister, who is 10 years older than she is. Her weight is 120 lb (54.4 kg) at a height of 5 ft 5 in. (1.65 m). She is a nonsmoker. Which of the following, in addition to a routine physical examination, is the most appropriate combination of screening tests for this patient?

(A) EKG stress test, CBC count, and liver and kidney function studies

(B) Papanicolaou smear (Pap smear), mammogram, colorectal cancer (CRC) screening, CBC count, and comprehensive chemical profile

(C) Chest x-ray, Pap smear, EKG, and comprehensive chemical profile

(D) Lipid screen, FOBT, mammogram, and blood sugar

(E) Chest x-ray, pulmonary function studies, lipid screen and routine chemistries, and CBC count

3 The patient in Question 3 returns for her routine examination on schedule for the following 2 years. Her Pap smears have all been normal and adequate for evaluation. She is in a monogamous relationship. She asks how frequently she should have Pap smears in the future. What is your answer?

(A) Every 6 months

(B) Annually

(C) Every 2 years

(D) Every 3 years

(E) Every 5 years

4 A 55-year-old woman is being followed for her type II diabetes. She takes 500 mg of metformin three times per day and 4 mg of pioglitasone daily, and the diabetes control has been fair. Her glycohemoglobin level was 7.1 on her last visit 2 weeks ago. Each of the following is recommended by the American Diabetes Association (ADA) in monitoring this diabetic's progress, except for which one?

(A) Annual examination by an ophthalmologist

(B) Glycohemoglobin level check every 3 months

(C) Annual electrocardiogram

(D) Annual check of blood urea nitrogen and creatinine levels

(E) Examination of the feet on each visit

5 A 55-year-old man with diabetes, obesity, and hypertension has just completed his examination and relevant laboratory tests have been ordered. Assuming they were due or overdue, which of the following combinations of immunizations should you order at this time?

(A) Tetanus toxoid and an attenuated dose of diphtheria toxoid (Td) vaccine, influenza vaccine, pneumococcal vaccine

(B) Smallpox revaccination, influenza vaccine

(C) Hepatitis B vaccine, Td vaccine, pneumococcal vaccine

(D) Td vaccine, influenza vaccine, *Hemophilus influenzae* type B, hepatitis B vaccine, pneumococcal vaccine

(E) Influenza and the pneumococcal vaccinations

6 A 48-year-old male municipal bus driver is 40 lb (18 kg) overweight. In counseling him to lose weight, you allude to all of the following problems as aggravated by obesity except for which one?

(A) Coronary heart disease

(B) Diabetes

(C) Osteoporosis

(D) Osteoarthritis

(E) Hypertension

7 A 41-year-old black man comes to you for his first comprehensive physical examination. Of the following, which screening procedures merit attention not accorded to white men, otherwise matched for age, weight, and other risk factors?

(A) Prostate cancer and glaucoma

(B) CRC and lung cancer

(C) Diabetes and dyslipidemia

(D) Coronary artery disease and mitral valve prolapse

(E) Hypertrophic cardiomyopathy

8 In selecting out special guidelines for management of certain diseases in certain ethnic groups, in which of the following groups should you adjust therapeutic targets to tighter control of hypertension and diabetes?

(A) Mexican Americans

(B) Ashkenazi Jews

(C) South Asians (Indians and Pakistani)

(D) Chinese Americans

(E) African Americans

9 A 30-year-old woman has had a negative professional breast examination. She has a family history of breast cancer in her mother, who contracted the disease at the age of 48. At what age should she commence having routine screening mammograms?

(A) 30 years

(B) 38 years

(C) 48 years

(D) 55 years

(E) 60 years

10 A 45-year-old man, a new patient, visits the office for a complete physical examination. You discover while eliciting the family history that his father died of colon cancer, contracted at the age of 60. He has no other first-degree relatives with colon cancer. On the basis of the American Cancer Society recommendations, you recommend that this patient have CRC screening by what modalities?

(A) Digital rectal examination (DRE), FOBT, and flexible sigmoidoscopy every 2 years

(B) DRE and FOBT annually

(C) DRE and colonoscopy now and every 3 years if negative

(D) Colonoscopy annually

(E) Flexible sigmoidoscopy and barium enema every 5 years

Examination Answers

1. The answer is D, PSA, lipid screen, FOBT, blood sugar. This smoking, overweight man first should have certain screening examinations that begin at the age of 50 years in individuals of average health risk status. These include prostate cancer screening (which, in addition to the PSA, requires a digital rectal examination for prostate cancer) and CRC screening. The minimal level of CRC screening is the FOBT (two sites on each of three random stools, annually). In addition, a lipid screen should be obtained (at the least, total cholesterol level, but ideally the total spectrum of total, high-density lipoprotein, and low-density lipoprotein cholesterol levels, as well as serum triglyceride level). Comprehensive chemistries including hepatic and renal function studies serve a commonsense purpose in a 50-year-old man who has not had a complete examination in years; however, the U.S. Preventive Services Task Force, an ultraconservative organization, is not assertive on this issue. An EKG, especially in light of two previous baseline traces, has limited value and is not recommended on a routine basis, though often done in consultation with the patient. Chest x-ray in an asymptomatic patient has no screening value, even in a smoker, as lung cancers diagnosed on x-ray are at too advanced a stage for cure. Pulmonary function studies and EKG stress testing are also not recommended for routine screening.

2. The answer is B, Pap smear, mammogram, CRC screening, CBC count, and comprehensive chemical profile. There are three critical points to be made here. First, a Pap smear is essential in a sexually active woman. Second, a mammogram should be performed annually, beginning when the woman reaches the age of 40 years. Third, CRC screening, starting at 50 years of age in people of average risk, should begin annually in a person's 40s when there is a first-degree family history of either adenomatous polyps or CRC. The CBC count and chemical profile are reasonable in a patient who has not had a comprehensive examination for 6 years. Chest x-ray has no place as a screening tool. The EKG is not important but has some value to provide a baseline datum.

3. The answer is D. Pap smears can be performed at the reduced frequency of every 3 years after three consecutive benign readings (i.e., no precancerous or malignant changes), provided the patient has no significant risk factors. This is in accord with most medical organizations,

with the possible exception of the American College of Obstetrics and Gynecology. Although the Pap smear has a mediocre sensitivity (60%), its specificity is excellent. Thus, together, three consecutive negative tests confer a sensitivity of 94%.

4. The answer is C. An annual EKG is not one of the recommendations of the ADA. Each of the other parameters should be checked according to the ADA in the frequencies noted. In addition, lipids should be checked annually; home blood sugars should be recorded upon every visit, along with blood sugar levels at the times of visits with the physician; and, of course, blood pressure and weight should be recorded at each visit as well. An annual ophthalmologic examination is done in order to diagnose early retinopathy of the proliferative type that extends into the vitreous body, which is treatable by laser. Renal function deteriorates at an accelerated pace in the face of poor blood sugar (and blood pressure) control. Thus, in addition to blood urea nitrogen and creatinine, urine for microalbumen should be investigated annually as well. Feet should be examined for light touch, sharp and dull perception, skin nutrition, and pulses, as well as for non-healing ulcers and other sores.

5. The answer is A, Td, influenza, and pneumococcal vaccinations. As a person with diabetes, this patient should have the pneumococcal vaccination primary series of two doses if he has not already had it; otherwise, he should have a single dose after the age of 50; being older than 50 years of age and diabetic, he should have influenza vaccine yearly; assuming he has not had it in 10 years or more, he should have the Td vaccine.

6. The answer is C. Osteoporosis is the least aggravated by obesity among those conditions listed. Sedentary lifestyle predisposes one to all the others listed. Sedentary life style is characterized by a tendency for obesity that may precipitate diabetes, aggravate hypertension, increase total cholesterol, and decrease high-density lipoprotein cholesterol. In addition, through an increase in weight bearing, obesity promotes osteoblastic in excess of osteoclastic activity (thus protecting against osteoporosis). All but osteoporosis and osteoarthritis are in turn risk factors for coronary artery disease.

7. The answer is A. Prostate cancer and glaucoma are two conditions that merit screening at the age of 40 in black men, whereas in the rest of the male population, otherwise matched for weight, family history, and other risk factors, these conditions are not addressed until the age of 50. Although diabetes is more prevalent in African Americans, it is not so when matched for weight and age with white individuals. The same can be said for coronary heart disease and dyslipidemia. Mitral valve prolapse and hypertrophic cardiomyopathy are not discussed meaningfully in epidemiologic terms.

8. The answer is E. African Americans with hypertension suffer earlier onset and a greater incidence of cerebrovascular disease (strokes) and renal failure as complications than do other group with matched levels of average blood pressure. Therefore, the therapeutic target for control of hypertension is set at 125/75 rather than simply settling it for statistically normal blood pressure, ≤140/≤90. Similarly, diabetes mellitus exacts a greater price in accelerated decremental renal failure for given levels of blood sugar control. Although Mexican Americans and indigenous Americans have a far greater risk of diabetes for a given body mass index, their complication rates are not out of proportion to their levels of blood sugar control.

9. The answer is B; 38 years, the age that would be 10 years younger than that at which her mother devel-

oped breast cancer, is the age this patient should have her first mammogram and annually thereafter. If this rule of thumb works out to place the patient in her early 30s, the breast tissue may be too dense to obtain an adequate reading. Magnetic imaging is now coming to the field of breast cancer screening for patients such as the one mentioned here. However, third parties, as of this writing, are not hurrying to cover that cost.

10. The answer is C, colonoscopy now and every 3 years if negative. A family history of colon cancer in a first-degree relative (father at age 60) multiplies the lifetime risk of colon cancer, normally about 2.5%, times 3, so this patient now has a 7.5% chance of colon cancer. Most of the risk in this circumstance is telescoped into the decades of the 50s and above. Thus, this patient's chances are higher than 7.5%. Colonoscopy, if negative, need not be repeated for 3 years because of the long "dwell time" for that cancer.

References

Kerlikowske K, Grady D, Barclay J, et al. Effects of age, breast density, and family history on the sensitivity of first screening mammography. *JAMA.* 1996; 276:33–38.

Marwick C. Other voices weigh in on mammography decision. *JAMA.* 1997; 277:1027–1028.

Miller KE. Preventive care of the middle-aged adult (40–65 years). In: Rudy DR, Kurowski K, eds. *Family Medicine: House Officer Series.* Baltimore: Williams & Wilkins; 1997:729–740.

chapter 46

Preventive Care of the Older Adult (Ages 65 Years and Older)

Examination questions: Unless instructed otherwise, choose the ONE lettered answer or completion that is BEST in each case.

1 A 78-year-old woman has seemed difficult to follow in conversation. In interviewing her, the doctor sometimes wonders if his mind had wandered because he cannot discern a coherent message in her conversation. Otherwise she manifests no neurological symptoms or signs. A comprehensive metabolic profile reveals both alanine aminotransferase and aspartate aminotransferase levels to be elevated by about 50% of their normal values. Suspecting alcoholism, you contemplate which strategy you should use to confirm this fact. Which of the following would be the most sensitive?

(A) Ask the patient how much she drinks

(B) Check the patient's cerebellar function on physical exam

(C) Ask the patient standardized screening questions for alcoholism, such as those from the CAGE questionnaire

(D) Palpate for ascites

(E) Look for spider angiomas on the patient's skin

2 A 65-year-old woman is being seen for a general physical examination. She is active and without complaints. She had a complete hysterectomy 20 years ago for benign uterine fibroids. She has not had a Pap smear since then. She had a screening flexible sigmoidoscopy 2 years ago, which showed normal results; this was followed by fecal occult blood tests (FOBTs), two sites on each of three random stools, per year since then. She has no family history of colorectal cancer. She had a flu vaccination 2 months ago and a pneumonia vaccination 5 years ago. She had a normal mammogram last year. She had a normal cholesterol level 2 years ago. Her physical examination is unremarkable. Her lungs are clear. Her breasts have no masses. There are no abdominal masses. Her rectal examination shows no masses and is negative. She is concerned regarding costs accruing to her, as she is $1,000 short of meeting her $2,000 annual deductible insurance expense. Which of the following preventive measures is clearly indicated for her?

(A) Repeat pneumonia vaccination

(B) Colonoscopy

(C) Mammogram

(D) Pap smear

(E) Lipid profile

3 A 55-year-old female of mixed English and Scottish descent is undergoing her annual pelvic examination, Pap smear, and breast examination. The subject of her cigarette smoking comes up, as it does each year. Again the doctor takes time to point out the dangers of smoking, hoping for the "teachable moment." For each of the following items, smoking is a significant risk, except for which one?

(A) Bladder cancer

(B) Obesity and metabolic syndrome

(C) Hip fracture

(D) Lung cancer

(E) Peptic ulcer disease

4 Of the following persons, who is most likely to be an abuser of an elderly individual in the United States?

(A) A spouse

(B) A hired caretaker

(C) A son

(D) A daughter

(E) A stranger who has broken into the home

5 Which of the following hypertensive blood pressure readings is most likely to be found particularly in a patient over the age of 65 years?

(A) 210/110

(B) 190/100

(C) 120/95

(D) 150/80

(E) 140/90

6 In isolated systolic hypertension (ISH) in an elderly patient, which of the following single drug-agent categories is most likely to be effective?

(A) Calcium channel blockers

(B) Beta-adrenergic blockers

(C) Vasodilators

(D) Ganglionic blockers

(E) Thiazide diuretics

7 A 75-year-old man is in good health and mentally competent to care for himself. He underwent a complete examination 5 years ago that included a normal screening colonoscopy, and he has submitted FOBTs in the intervening years. He lives alone and wishes to undergo a routine health maintenance examination. Which of the following would be least fruitful as a screening test?

(A) Flexible sigmoidoscopy and FOBTs

(B) Thyroid-stimulating hormone test

(C) Urinalysis

(D) Blood pressure reading

(E) "Up-and-go test"

8 A 50-year-old patient brings in her dependent mother, aged 81. The elderly woman has been forgetting things recently, but she is able to subtract sevens from 100 (she is a retired math teacher). She is well groomed and socially adept. The daughter wishes for her to be screened for Alzheimer's disease (AD). Which of the following would be the most relevant reason for screening for early diagnosis of AD?

(A) Improve the intelligence quotient of the patient

(B) Stop the progression of AD

(C) Reverse the course of AD

(D) Prepare caregiver(s) and family for management and socioeconomic issues

(E) Prevent strokes

9 In the case presented in Question 8, the family doctor chooses to screen for Alzheimer's disease with the Folstein Mini-Mental State Examination, of which the sensitivity is known to be 87%. What approximate percentage of those individuals tested will exhibit a false-positive result?

(A) 10%

(B) 20%

(C) 40%

(D) 50%

(E) 60%

10 Each of the following statements regarding falls in "older elderly" persons (>75 years of age) is true, except for which one?

(A) Most falls occur outside of the home environment.

(B) The risk of falls is directly related to the number of medications the elderly patient is taking.

(C) Alcohol is a contributing risk factor for falls.

(D) The most common injuries incurred in falls among elderly individuals are wrist, hip, and vertebral fractures.

(E) Falls often occur in mentally competent elderly people.

11 An elderly couple ask several questions about living wills while you are updating their health history. Which of the following statements is correct with respect to living wills?

(A) They are not usually honored by courts.

(B) They are only appropriate for the terminally ill individual to communicate desires regarding specific life-support measures.

(C) The wishes of immediate family members take legal precedence over the living will of the individual.

(D) They allow the individual to communicate desires for or against specific life-support measures toward the time when health status makes him or her unable to do so.

(E) They must be prepared by attorneys.

Examination Answers

1. The answer is C, ask standardized screening questions for alcoholism such as the CAGE questionnaire. Sets of standardized alcoholic screening questions are a more sensitive indicator than just asking about alcohol consumption. Cerebellar function impairments may be subtle and only manifest with acute intoxication. Patients vary in their propensities to develop alcoholic hepatitis and telangiectasias, even for a given amount and duration of alcohol consumption. An elevated aspartate aminotransferase level is a nonspecific indicator of hepatocellular damage, which is not necessarily present in alcoholism. The other choices yield positive results but at a much later stage of alcoholism than the CAGE questionnaire, assuming it is done with a low threshold for suspicion. (CAGE is an acronym taken from the following items: C, cutting down; A, annoyed by criticism of others; G, guilty about drinking; E, (need) eye opener.)

2. The answer is C. A mammogram should be done yearly, beginning when the woman reaches the age of 40 years and continuing until she reaches at least the age of 70. (In fact, the incidence of breast cancer increases with each year, although its aggressiveness diminishes.) It is due for this patient. The Pneumovax vaccine is effective for at least 6 or 7 years in immunocompetent individuals. Colonoscopy is not necessary because the combination of flexible sigmoidoscopy every 5 years and annual FOBT as described in the vignette is one of five methods acceptable to the American Gastroenterology Association, which suggests that this process begin when a person reaches the age of 50 years. This screening (along with colonoscopies every 3 years) begins at age 40 if the patient has ulcerative colitis or a family history of familial polyposis. The patient's hysterectomy was for benign disease and she does not need a Pap smear. A favorable lipid profile on a postmenopausal woman need not be repeated frequently unless there has been material change in the patient's living style and weight.

3. The answer is B. Obesity and metabolic syndrome is not a sequela of smoking. Actually, part of the addiction, if it occurs at all, is due to a stimulant effect of nicotine. This results in an amphetaminelike effect so that one of the complications of *smoking cessation* is weight gain. All the other diseases mentioned in the choices occur at significantly greater incidence in smokers than in nonsmokers.

For the slender postmenopausal woman of Celtic origin, osteoporosis is a significant risk, multiplied 1.5-fold to twofold in a cigarette smoker.

4. The answer is A, a spouse. Relatives, especially spouses, are most likely to be the abusers. They may be actively or passively abusive.

5. The answer is D; 150/80 is most characteristic of ISH. This is more likely in the older age group.

6. The answer is E. Thiazide diuretics are most effective in salt- or water-retention conditions, namely the low-renin end of the hypertensive spectrum. Implied is that ISH is a low-renin state. It is well known that if beta-adrenergic blocking agents are used in the oldest age group, then a greater dosage is required; that is, being antirenin agents, they are less effective because renin played a less significant part in ISH as compared with the broad spectrum of the remainder of hypertension types. Conversely, vasodilator and ganglionic blocking agents are most effective against peripheral resistance-driven hypertension (i.e., vasoconstricted physiological states). Calcium channel blocking agents are in the neutral zone of effectiveness on the continuum of volume versus peripheral resistance.

7. The answer is A. Flexible sigmoidoscopy and FOBTs are the least likely to prevent disease in a patient who has a life expectancy of 5 to 10 years. Blood pressure control can prevent strokes; thyroid-stimulating hormone can unearth hypothyroidism in the absence of typical symptoms, especially in an elderly person; urinalysis can reveal subclinical urinary tract infection. The up-and-go test can rule out the possibility that the patient may be physically unable to care for himself alone. The test consists of asking the patient to arise from a sitting position without the use of his or her hands, walk 10 ft (3 m), and return to the originally sitting site and position. If the patient can perform this satisfactorily in ≤10 seconds, then he or she is assumed to be physically able. If the activity requires more than 30 seconds, then the patient very likely will require physical assistance at home.

8. The answer is D. Preparing caregiver(s) and the family for management and socioeconomic issues for a patient with imminent AD is worthwhile in the view of most clinicians. Early diagnosis of AD alerts the primary care physician to avoid anticholinergic medications, as these are agents that worsen dementia. Although there was originally great hope for the reversible acetycholinesterase inhibitors (e.g., donepezil), improvement in cognition in early AD from this medication has been incremental and temporary. Further, later in the course of AD, improvement that is due to donepezil (Aricept) has been unmeasurable. Although theories of causation of AD include microinfarctions and atherosclerosis risk factors appear to be risk factors for AD as well, prevention of strokes would seem to be already in play in the management of any elderly patient (i.e., through control of blood pressure, blood sugar in diabetics, and platelet deaggregation). Among the serious mental illnesses to be found in elderly individuals, dementia is the most prevalent, with the others being depression, delirium, schizophrenia, and bipolar disorder. Another good reason for early diagnosis of dementia is the unearthing of reversible causes of dementia in elderly persons, such as anemia, urinary tract infection, chronic pain, and, sometimes, simply radical change of environment.

9. The answer is C, 40%. Actually, the official figure for the false-positive rate in the Folstein Mini-Mental State Examination is 39.4%. Somewhere in the range of 30% to 50% of elderly persons older than the age of 85 years suffer from a degree of dementia, but the vast majority do not qualify for a diagnosis of AD. This should lend a note of sobriety to the administration of the Folstein test. Elderly persons may fail the test because of fatigue, motivation, or anxiety. Dementia, of which AD is the most common form among elderly individuals, involves (a) at least one language-impairment problem (word finding, later difficulty following a conversation, or mutism); (b) apraxia (inability to perform certain previously learned manual tasks, such as cutting a loaf of bread by using both hands despite manifesting no sensory or motor abnormalities); and (c) impaired organization (sometimes called executive ability), such as poor mental flexibility, planning, and judgment. Subsets in screening regarding the foregoing categories are in play. In the verbal category, including attention and concentration, the patient may be asked to recite name, address, and phone numbers; to recall three unrelated words such as "tulip, umbrella, scar" or parts of objects such as lapel and cuff; and follow a mildly complex command such as "point to the ceiling before you point to the floor." A corollary to praxis functioning is visuospatial organization, such as

drawing a clock with a prescribed time indicated. Regarding organizational ability, there may be questions involving logic, such as "how is a peach like a pear?"

10. The answer is A. The incorrect statement is that most falls among elderly persons occur outside of the home environment. Thus, most falls among elderly persons occur in or around the home. Falls in the home may be indirectly caused by conditions that would be viewed as relatively benign for agile and mentally competent people, such as slippery or warped floors, shag carpet, or thick rugs, that present opportunities for elderly individuals to trip. Risk of falls is directly related to the number of medications the elderly patient is taking, obviously especially those involving sedatives, antihypertensives, alcohol, antidepressants, or neuroleptics, or overdosage with beta-adrenergic blocking agents. The most common injuries incurred in falls among elderly individuals are wrist, hip, and vertebral fractures. Hip fractures will occur in one-third of women and one-sixth of men in the "old elderly" age group. Hip fractures carry a 20% first-year mortality rate. Another significant risk from trauma in elderly individuals is subdural hematoma. Falls often occur in mentally competent elderly people. These are the frail elderly, often victims of osteoporosis or malnutrition, the former more often among women and the latter among men.

11. The answer is D. They allow the individual to communicate the desire for or against specific life-support measures in the event that the individual's health status at some point makes him or her unable to do so. Living wills have been honored by courts and do not require the use of an attorney. Catastrophic illness, which leaves the individual unable to communicate wishes, can occur with anyone, but particularly with elderly persons. Living wills give them a mechanism to convey their wishes.

References

Bross MH, Tryon AF. Preventive care of the older adult (>65 years). In: Rudy DR, Kurowski K, eds. *Family Medicine: House Officer Series.* Baltimore: Williams & Wilkins; 1997:741–750.

Dickman R. Care of the elderly. In: Rakel RE, ed. *Textbook of Family Practice.* 6th ed. Philadelphia: WB Saunders; 2001:88–130.

Johnston CB, Harper GM, Landefeld CS. Geriatric medicine. In: Tierney LM, McPhee SJ, Papadakis MA, eds. *Current Medical Diagnosis and Treatment.* 45th ed. New York: McGraw-Hill/Appleton & Lange; 2006:49–66.

Rudy DR. Endocrinology. In: Rakel RE, ed. *Textbook of Family Practice.* 6th ed. Philadelphia: WB Saunders; 2001:1027–1106.

chapter 47

Travel Medicine

Examination questions: Unless instructed otherwise, choose the ONE lettered answer or completion that is BEST in each case.

1 Which of the following diseases is encountered most commonly among travelers?

(A) Diarrhea

(B) Pneumonia

(C) Malaria

(D) Skin rashes

(E) Viral hepatitis

2 Which of the following is the most significant (i.e., serious as well as frequent) medical problem of those related to travel?

(A) Diarrhea

(B) Pneumonia

(C) Sunburn

(D) Skin rashes

(E) Viral hepatitis

3 Which of the following drugs is the first choice for malaria prophylaxis in an area of the world in which the plasmodium is known to be resistant to chloroquine?

(A) Hydroxychloroquine

(B) Doxycycline

(C) Halofantrine

(D) Mefloquine

(E) Pyrimethamine

4 Your patient, a 25-year-old married woman who is pregnant, solicits your opinion as to advisability of travel. Which of the following statements is true regarding travel during pregnancy?

(A) Travel is best done in the first trimester.

(B) Most airlines require a physician's permission for air travel by a pregnant woman.

(C) Travel to areas of high risk for malaria should be avoided.

(D) For treatment of upper respiratory tract infections in the first trimester, for example, in covering symptoms as well as the possibility of beta-hemolytic streptococcal disease, ampicillin may be used, along with astemizole (Hismanal) or terfenadine (Seldane).

(E) For diarrhea during the first or second trimester, sulfamethoxazole, erythromycin, and loperamide (Imodium) should be avoided.

5 Traveler's diarrhea is caused by bacteria in 80% of cases, mostly Escherichia coli, but also Shigella, Salmonella, and Campylobacter organisms. Which of the following statements about traveler's diarrhea is true?

(A) Prophylactic antibiotics are generally recommended routinely before travel to areas where potability of water is questionable, regardless of length of stay in the area.

(B) Bismuth subsalicylate tablets, 262 mg each, two to four times per day while in the endemic area, is a safe prophylactic measure under all circumstances.

(C) Bismuth subsalicylate, two to four times per day while in the endemic area, is virtually 100% effective in preventing traveler's diarrhea.

(D) For travel to South Asia, in special circumstances in which antibacterial prophylaxis is employed, trimethoprim/sulfamethoxazole is used routinely.

(E) Antibiotic or antibacterial prophylaxis is best employed in anticipation of short stays, or the presence of diabetes or chronic diarrhea; in those situations, it is 90% successful in prevention of disease.

6 Alveolar PO_2, normally about 100 mm Hg in a healthy person at sea level, falls to what level at an altitude of 10,000 ft (3,048 m)?

(A) 47 mm Hg

(B) 79 mm Hg

(C) 61 mm Hg

(D) 46 mm Hg

(E) 88% saturation

7 A 25-year-old male patient is mountain climbing. On the second day he develops nausea, headache, inability to concentrate, and 1 to 2+ ankle edema. What is the altitude above which, it can be said, these symptoms begin to occur in significant numbers of travelers who have not accommodated to altitude in advance?

(A) 2,000 ft (610 m)

(B) 6,500 ft (1,981 m)

(C) 8,000 ft (2,438 m)

(D) 12,500 ft (3,810 m)

(E) 15,000 ft (4,572 m)

8 Regarding the patient in Question 7, which of the following measures would be most reasonable and beneficial, assuming descent is not a practical solution and relief seems necessary at this time?

(A) Acetazolamide (Diamox) administration

(B) Dexamethasone in a tapering course

(C) Oxygen administration

(D) Pressure tent

(E) Diltiazem

9 The most serious symptoms that may occur with high-altitude sickness (HAI) are pulmonary edema, that is, high-altitude pulmonary edema (HAPE), and cerebral edema, that is, high-altitude cerebral edema (HACE). At what altitude do they become significant possibilities for travelers who are unaccommodated to altitude?

(A) 2,000 ft (610 m)

(B) 6,500 ft (1,981 m)

(C) 8,000 ft (2,438 m)

(D) 12,500 ft (3,810 m)

(E) 15,000 ft (4,572 m)

10 An 18-year-old man, who lives on the east coast, flies to Cuzco, Peru (11,152 ft, or 3,399 m) and immediately pursues his plan to hike to 2,000 ft (610 m) above the town, joining a group of high-altitude hikers. On the morning of the second day, the group has reached 12,000 ft (3,658 m) of altitude en route to the Fortress of Sacsayhuaman. He begins to complain of coughing and shortness of breath, eventually producing a frothy pink sputum. Each of the following would be appropriate except for (which) one?

(A) Rapid descent of 500 ft (152 m), if possible

(B) Furosemide

(C) Oxygen 1 to 2 L/minute

(D) Acetazolamide

(E) Hyperbaric tent

11 A 45-year-old female patient reveals that a friend has offered to take her on a transcontinental flight in his private unpressurized aircraft. The patient has a history of HAI at 13,500 ft (4,114 m) during a mountain hiking expedition. She has had numerous benign experiences at altitudes of 10,000 ft (3,048 m) or lower. Otherwise she is healthy. Which of the following is appropriate advice for her regarding the prospective flight and her health?

(A) She should not make the flight because of her history of HAI.

(B) She should postpone the trip until she has undergone blood gas studies.

(C) She may take the trip and will require no special preparations or treatments compared with other people on the plane.

(D) She is safe but should undergo electrocardiogram testing before making the final decision.

(E) She may go on the trip as long as she takes oxygen throughout the flight.

12 What cabin altitudes (terrestrial altitudes equivalent in atmospheric pressure to pressures in cabins of pressurized aircraft) would the patient in Question 11 expect to encounter in pressurized commercial jet aircraft?

(A) Sea level (cabin pressure encountered at sea level)

(B) 500 ft (152 m)

(C) 2,000 ft (610 m)

(D) Up to 5,000 ft (1,524 m)

(E) Up to 10,000 ft (3,048 m)

13 Which one of the following conditions is a contraindication to air travel?

(A) Status of 3 months after acute myocardial infarction (stable)

(B) Chronic obstructive lung disease with PCO_2 of 55 mm Hg; PaO_2 of 60 mm Hg

(C) Diabetes mellitus without symptoms of hypoglycemia or acidosis

(D) Chronic renal failure on renal dialysis

(E) Uncomplicated pregnancy

14 Many immunizations are recommended before travel simply for the general principle of the traveler remaining current for all routine immunizations. Others are recommended for reasons more specific to the country to be visited. Which of the following immunizations is recommended in the period of 1 to 3 months before travel to any developing country?

(A) A tetanus booster with an attenuated dose of diphtheria (Td)

(B) Influenza

(C) Polio

(D) Rabies

(E) Japanese encephalitis

15 A 36-year-old woman with a history of atopic diseases consisting of seasonal rhinitis (in the spring and fall), but without asthma, consults you in August after a week of rhinitis symptoms because she is planning a trip by commercial air travel to Nova Scotia. Once, while recovering from a cold, she had suffered severe ear pain. Which of the following statements is true regarding secretory otitis media of flight ("barotitis" or "aerotitis")?

(A) It occurs most frequently during ascent in flight.

(B) The most frequent bacterial organism causing barotitis media is *Streptococcus pneumoniae*.

(C) It can be prevented if the patient is able to force air into the middle ears through the Eustachian tube during descent by means of the modified Valsalva maneuver.

(D) The physical evidence of this form of secretory otitis media is a bulging tympanic membrane seen at otoscopy.

(E) The same problem may occur during scuba diving, requiring the diver to delay ascent in order to control symptoms and to "clear the ears."

16 Your patient consults you regarding travel abroad. Eventually you introduce the topic of typhoid because you know he is planning a trip into a country for which typhoid vaccination is recommended. To which of the following regions is he planning to travel?

(A) Canada

(B) Israel

(C) Europe

(D) Australia

(E) New Zealand

17 Which of the following is true regarding "jet lag"?

(A) Rapid west-to-east travel across time zones often results in somnolence that is inappropriate to local time at the destination.

(B) Rapid east-to-west travel often results in difficulty in sleep onset relative to local time at the destination.

(C) Antijetlag diets have proven effective in preventing jetlag symptoms.

(D) Paradoxical hypovolemia in the face of fluid retention plays a significant part in the pathophysiology of jetlag.

(E) Cabin altitudes of 5,000 ft (1,524 m) play a significant part in the pathophysiology of jetlag.

18 An emerging concept in travel medicine is that of posttravel evaluation. Which of the following would be checked for logically in an *asymptomatic* returning traveler who had been to a tropical location?

(A) Giardiasis

(B) Tuberculosis skin testing

(C) Hepatitis screen

(D) Sigmoidoscopy for schistosomiasis

(E) Malarial smear

19 Which of the following patients should be denied medical approval for travel?

(A) A 55-year-old white man with stable angina pectoris

(B) A 62-year-old African American man with nocturnal dyspnea and orthopnea

(C) A 58-year-old white woman whose status is 5 weeks after uncomplicated myocardial infarction

(D) A 57-year-old man with chronic lung disease who is unable to climb two flights of stairs or to walk for two blocks

(E) A 35-year-old woman who is 7 months into an uncomplicated pregnancy

1. The answer is A. Diarrhea is the most common medical problem in travelers. It is possible that other problems are more common in travel but do not come to the attention of the medical professions. Of 30 million travelers from the United States to other countries, only slightly more than one-quarter of them go to developed countries. This has significant implications for health among travelers. Those who spend at least 1 month in the other country face a 60% chance of becoming ill and a 1% chance of being admitted to a hospital.

2. The answer is E. Viral hepatitis, of those mentioned in the question, is the most serious common medical problem encountered in travel. Not only is it commonly encountered, but it is also likely to be particularly disabling to a traveler. Unless the traveler has participated in parenteral illicit drug use or risky sexual practices, any hepatitis encountered will be hepatitides A or E, contracted from water or uncooked raw vegetables in an underdeveloped country.

3. The answer is D. Mefloquine is the first choice for malaria prophylaxis in areas known to harbor chloroquine- and hydroxychloroquine-resistant organisms. Halofantrine and Pyrimethamine are considered only in highly resistant areas, such as Thailand. Halofantrine is another alternative choice but is associated with cardiac toxicity and is contraindicated in the presence of prolonged QT interval and in pregnancy.

4. The answer is C. Travel during pregnancy to areas of high risk for malaria should be avoided, especially in areas noted for chloroquine resistance. Malaria has a more malignant course in pregnancy and the alternative therapies in event of chloroquine resistance are more toxic, even in nonpregnant patients. Travel is best done in the *second* trimester. Most airlines require a physician's permission for air travel by a pregnant woman only after she has reached 35 or 36 weeks of gestation. Although ampicillin is safe in pregnancy, astemizole and terfenadine should not be used in the first trimester. For diarrhea during pregnancy, trimethoprim/sulfamethoxazole, erythromycin, and loperamide are safe to use.

5. The answer is E. Antibiotic or antibacterial prophylaxis against traveler's diarrhea is best employed in anticipation of short stays, or the presence of diabetes or chronic diarrhea; in those situations, it is 90% successful. Prophylactic antibiotics are generally *not* recommended except in the aforementioned situation. Bismuth subsalicylate is not necessarily a safe prophylactic measure under all circumstances. Because it is a salicylate, care must be taken to avoid its use in the presence of influenza or varicella in order to avoid Reye's syndrome. Bismuth subsalicylate is about 65% effective in preventing traveler's diarrhea. Because relatively large volumes of bismuth subsalicylate or other bismuth preparations are required, this modality may present a degree of inconvenience for air travel. For travel to South Asia, the best regimen is a quinolone, such as norfloxacin 400 mg/day, ciprofloxacin 500 mg/day, or ofloxacin 200 mg/day.

6. The answer is C; 61 mm Hg is the *alveolar* PO_2 at an altitude of 10,000 ft (3,048 m). Remember, the alveolar PO_2 is, at best, the ambient PO_2 minus the partial pressure of alveolar CO_2 and H_2O, the latter constant at 47 mm Hg; 47 mm Hg is the constant partial pressure of water vapor at all *ambient* pressures. Note that 79 mm Hg is the *ambient* PO_2 at 18,000 ft (5,486 m), the altitude beneath which lies half the atmosphere; 46 mm Hg is the *alveolar* PO_2 at an altitude of 15,000 ft (4,572 m); 88% represents the arterial blood saturation, normally 95%, in a healthy person at 7,500 ft (2,286 m).

7. The answer is B; 6,500 ft (1,981 m) is the altitude above which it can be said that symptoms of mountain sickness occur in 25% of travelers. This degree of illness is called acute mountain sickness. The incidence increases to 50% as altitude rises to 10,000 ft (3,048 m). These symptoms are likely to be classified as mild, consisting of headache, dysphoria, nausea, peripheral edema, unexpected sighing, and nocturnal Cheyne-Stokes breathing. Nearly always, resting at altitude for 1 to 2 days will result in abatement of mild symptoms of altitude sickness. Wrong advice would be to exercise strenuously during the first 2 days at altitude in order to prevent altitude sickness. All others are correct. The saying is "climb high, sleep low," especially at higher altitudes, in order to avoid HAPE and HACE.

8. The answer is A. Acetazolamide (Diamox) administration, one 750 mg tablet, perhaps repeated, or 250 mg every 6 hours, will probably be enough to treat the symptoms in the scenario presented. The other measures are generally not needed for acute mountain sickness.

9. The answer is D, 12,500 ft (3,810 m). Pulmonary HAPE and cerebral HACE are the most serious symptoms that may occur with mountain sickness. Both are emergencies. HAPE symptoms, which are more likely and worse if ascent is rapid, consist of tachycardia, tachypnea, severe dyspnea, frothy or blood-tinged sputum, and weakness. HACE symptoms and signs consist of undue drowsiness, unsteadiness, irritability, hallucinations, and neurologic focal symptoms and signs.

10. The answer is B. Furosemide would not be appropriate in this patient who has HAPE. The pulmonary edema is not due to passive congestion as in congestive heart failure with significant hypervolemia. Rather it is caused by porosity of the alveolar capillary bed, caused by relative hypoxia. The man lives at sea level and should have taken a day or more to accommodate to 11,000 ft (3,353 m) of altitude before embarking and physically exerting on a hike to yet a higher altitude. His youth in itself is not an advantage in the avoidance of HAI. Not only would remaining at 11,000 ft or 3,353 m have allowed him to acclimatize, but the resting period of a day would also in itself make him more resistant to altitude sickness. Acetazolamide is a first-line drug; rapid descent is always a good idea, if it is possible; if it is not possible, then oxygen therapy and a hyperbaric tent is effective, if available, and if all else fails and the situation becomes urgent.

11. The answer is C; 10,000 ft (3,048 m) is the altitude limit for normal passenger conveyance in unpressurized aircraft, a safe altitude for this patient. Above that level, oxygen supplementation must be supplied. However, this patient need not have oxygen throughout the trip unconditionally any more than any other person. Above 10,000 ft or 3,048 m, oxygen should be supplemented at increasing concentrations for all passengers and for the pilot. At 20,000 ft (6,096 m), supplemental oxygen must be given at 100% concentration. At 40,000 ft (12,192 m) oxygen must be applied under pressure exceeding the atmosphere. In commercial travel the foregoing are effected by cabin pressurization.

12. The answer is D. Up to 5,000 ft (1,524 m) is supposedly the maximum cabin pressure encountered in commercial pressurized aircraft. In practice, some probably will go as high as 8,000 ft (2,438 m; equivalent to that found at Macchu Picchu) but never more.

13. The answer is B. Hypercapnia is a contraindication to air travel, as are other conditions characterized by compromised oxygen exchange, such as PaO_2 <50 mm and diffusing capacity <50% of predicted value. All other conditions named, assuming no complications, are safe with which to travel by commercial air.

14. The answer is B. Influenza vaccination is recommended in the period of 1 to 3 months before travel to every developing country. Td immunization is also recommended to be *current* before travel to these countries, but one may be current for up to 10 years before travel, as long as the person has not had a skin wound in the country when the Td booster was last given more than 5 years previously.

15. The answer is C. Secretory otitis media of flight (aerotitis media) can be prevented if the patient is able to force air into the middle ears through the Eustachian tube ("clear the ears") during descent by the modified Valsalva maneuver. Naturally, this presupposes that the underlying cause (e.g., viral upper respiratory tract infection or atopic symptoms) is not so severe as to preclude this preventive measure, wherein the Eustachian tube may be so obstructed even before descent in flight that it cannot be opened. Thus, barotitis in flight occurs most frequently during *descent*. Bacterial organisms are not involved in barotitis media. The physical evidence of this form of secretory otitis media is a retracted tympanic membrane seen at otoscopy. This entity occurs during scuba diving, likewise during descent, but the definitive treatment is simply to return to the surface, along with clearing the ears.

16. The answer is B. Israel, surprisingly and perhaps unnecessarily, is the one region mentioned among the choices where typhoid vaccination is recommended. In contrast, Canada, Europe, Australia, and New Zealand are among the very few regions of travel for which typhoid vaccination is not recommended. Examples of other countries that present significant risk of typhoid fever are all of Latin America, all of Africa, and all of Asia and India; in short, all countries except for all of western Europe, the United States, Canada, Australia, and New Zealand.

17. The answer is D. Paradoxical hypovolemia in the face of fluid retention plays a significant part in the pathophysiology of jetlag. Rapid east-to-west travel often results in difficulty in staying awake appropriate to the local time, whereas west-to-east travel results in sleep onset relative to the local time at destination (the opposite to the statements as presented in the question). Antijetlag diets have not proven effective in preventing jetlag symptoms. Cabin altitudes of 8,000 ft (2,438 m) for prolonged periods may play a significant part in the pathophysiology. Resting in a seat at 5,000 ft (1,524 m), the altitude of Denver, has little effect on healthy persons.

18. The answer is E. Only a malarial smear, among those items mentioned, should be checked for in an asymptomatic returning traveler who had been to a tropical location. All the others are aimed at symptomatic conditions, except for tuberculosis. In the latter case, though conversion may occur without symptoms, we recommend skin testing only in symptomatic cases. The only hepatitides to be acquired in travel are A and E, neither of which causes chronic disease and need not be screened for in the absence of symptoms.

19. The answer is B, a 62-year-old African American man with nocturnal dyspnea and orthopnea. The latter symptoms, as do symptoms of congestive heart failure,

would warrant disapproval. Allow the 55-year-old white man with stable angina pectoris to travel. If the angina is unstable, the patient should not travel. Approve the 58-year-old white woman whose status is 5 weeks after an uncomplicated myocardial infarction—but do not approve such a person if ≤4 weeks have passed since the event. Approve the 57-year-old man with chronic lung disease, unable to climb two flights of stairs or to walk for two blocks, as long as he can climb one flight of stairs and walk one block. Approve the 35-year-old woman who is 7 months into an uncomplicated pregnancy. The only squeamishness by the commercial airlines is that they prefer that women do not fly with them near their due dates. The other caveat is that pregnant women should not travel to areas where the risk of malaria is significant.

References

Gross Z, Rudy DR. Travel medicine. In: Rudy DR, Kurowski K, eds. *Family Medicine: House Officer Series.* Baltimore: Williams & Wilkins; 1997:751–770.

SECTION XV

Behavior and Psychology in Primary Care

chapter 48

Depression

Examination questions: *Unless instructed otherwise, choose the ONE lettered answer or completion that is BEST in each case.*

1 The highest incidence of depression occurs in which of the following age groups?

(A) 5 to 14 years

(B) 15 to 24 years

(C) 25 to 34 years

(D) 35 to 55 years

(E) >65 years

2 A 28-year-old woman reports feeling depressed after her 18-year-old younger sister died after an illicit drug overdose 1 month earlier. She does not feel like participating in her usual social activities, but she has continued to work and take care of her family without difficulty. She has unintentionally lost 5 lb (2.27 kg) over the last month and admits that she has had a relatively depressed appetite. She expresses guilt that maybe if she had been spending more time watching her sister, her death could have been avoided. She has had some difficulty initially falling to sleep, but once she does she sleeps through the night. She has not noted episodes of inflated self-esteem and has not been going on spending sprees. She has been on no medication (including no street drugs), and she has no medical condition to explain these symptoms. She denies suicidal ideation, hallucinations, or delusions. She has no personal or family history of psychiatric illness. How would you best classify her symptoms according to the criteria listed in the fourth edition of the *Diagnostic and Statistical Manual of Mental Disorders*?

(A) Mixed episode

(B) Dysrhymic disorder

(C) Major depressive episode

(D) Cyclothymic disorder

(E) Adjustment disorder with depressed mood or bereavement

3 A 55-year-old woman complains of inability to sleep through the night, though she falls off to sleep relatively easily. You note that you have seen her for several falls at home leading to contusions, and on one occasion for a laceration of the scalp requiring sutures in repair. She admits that she has lost the ability to enjoy occasions that, in the past, were fulfilling to her. You notice vascular ectasias about the face and upper trunk anteriorly. Laboratory studies show elevated serum glutamic pyruvate transaminase and gamma-glutamyl transpeptidase levels. You suspect she is alcoholic and also that she is depressed. Which of the following is the wisest strategic approach to this patient?

(A) Because she is female, the chances of her being both depressed and alcoholic are slight. Therefore you should choose one or the other and treat accordingly.

(B) Alcoholic depressed patients fail at abstinence unless the depression is treated first.

(C) The alcoholism should be arrested before the depression is treated.

(D) Suicide is of low probability because patients with the two diagnoses are less likely to attempt suicide.

(E) Antidepressants are to be avoided in alcoholics, even if their depression persists after months of abstinence.

4 A 35-year-old woman has suffered from rheumatoid arthritis for 3 years and exhibits symptoms of Sjogren syndrome as well. She visits monthly and more frequently when she runs through pain medication, which is oxycodone, ahead of schedule. Rarely has she pressed for increased dosage and frequency but complains of dysphoria and sleep problems that don't

357

always appear to be related to her nocturnal pain. What are the odds that this patient suffers from depression?

(A) About one in five

(B) About one in four

(C) About one in three

(D) About two in three

(E) About three in four

5 Patients with which of the following chronic medical diseases have the highest suicide rate?

(A) Diabetes mellitus

(B) Acquired immunodeficiency syndrome (AIDS)

(C) Chronic obstructive pulmonary disease

(D) Rheumatoid arthritis

(E) Lupus erythematosus

6 To which category of antidepressant medications does each of the following belong: citalopram, escitalopram, and enantiomeer?

(A) Tricyclic antidepressants (TCAs)

(B) Selective serotonin reuptake inhibitors (SSRIs)

(C) Central nervous system stimulants

(D) Monoamine oxidase inhibitors (MAOIs)

(E) Atypical antidepressants

7 Which of the following categories of antidepressants is associated with the side effects of headache, nausea, tinnitus, insomnia, and akisthesia?

(A) TCAs

(B) SSRIs

(C) Central nervous system stimulants

(D) MAOIs

(E) Atypical antidepressants

8 Which of the following classes of antidepressants are associated with the side effects of anticholinergic effects, including cardiac dysrhythmias, sedation, and orthostatic hypotension?

(A) TCAs

(B) SSRIs

(C) Central nervous system stimulants

(D) MAOIs

(E) Atypical antidepressants

9 Which of the following classes of antidepressants are associated with hypertensive crises when combined with certain sympathomimetic drugs and meperidine

and dextromethorphan when followed by foods with tyramine?

(A) TCAs

(B) SSRIs

(C) Central nervous system stimulants

(D) MAOIs

(E) Atypical antidepressants

10 With respect to postpartum depression, which of the following statements is correct?

(A) It lasts on average as long as major depressive episodes not occurring in association with childbirth.

(B) It affects about 3% of new mothers.

(C) It takes longer for a spontaneous remission to occur than in major depressive episodes not associated with childbirth.

(D) The depression is more severe and suicide attempts are more common in postpartum depression.

(E) It is sometimes considered an adjustment disorder with depressed mood.

11 A 45-year-old male patient unknown to you has been brought in by his sister's family, whom he has been visiting from out of town. He was observed to have what was described as a grand mal seizure. In inquiring about his medications, you find he has been treated with a medication for depression, the identity of which the patient cannot recall. He has history of neither head trauma nor seizure disorder in the past. Which of the following is the most likely antidepressant drug he has been taking?

(A) Fluoxetine (Prozac)

(B) Amitriptyline (Elavil)

(C) Trazodone (Desyrel)

(D) Buproprion (Wellbutrin)

(E) Phenelzine (Nardil)

12 You are selecting an antidepressant for a 35-year-old man. Which of the following antidepressants carries the highest incidence of the side effect of priapism?

(A) Trazodone

(B) Nefazodone

(C) Escitalopram

(D) Sertraline

(E) Fluoxetine

13 Venlafaxine (Effexor), a relatively new antidepressant, is of the class that operates through both SSRI and norepinephrine reuptake inhibition. Which of the following side effects is especially associated with this drug?

(A) Dry mouth

(B) Insomnia

(C) Constipation

(D) Abnormal ejaculation and orgasm

(E) Blurred vision

14 You are concerned about the potential for suicide in an 18-year-old patient you are treating for depression. Which of the following increases this patient's risk for suicide?

(A) The patient is felt to have dysrhythmic disorder.

(B) The patient has a moderate bout of depression that improves after the patient has been on SSRIs for 1 month.

(C) The patient fulfills criteria for a major depressive episode.

(D) The patient is an African American living in an inner-city environment.

(E) The patient is frequently asked if he has suicidal thoughts or plans.

15 A 45-year-old man has been successfully treated for depression twice before, 10 years ago and 3 years ago; the first bout lasted 9 months and the second lasted 1 year. He responded to desipramine (Norpramin, a TCA) on the first occasion and to sertraline (Zoloft, an SSRI) the second time. On neither occasion was there evidence of mania. Which of the following strategies would be the most appropriate for this patient, who is currently depressed?

(A) Refer for electroshock therapy

(B) Refer for deep analytic psychotherapy

(C) Repeat a 9-month course of a TCA

(D) Commit the patient to lifelong maintenance on either the TCA or sertraline

(E) Start lithium therapy

16 Venlafaxine (Effexor) and duloxetine (Cymbalta) are both serotonin and norepinephrine reuptake inhibitors. Which of the following possible advantages does duloxetine have over other SSRIs and other antidepressants in general?

(A) In addition to antidepressant activity, it is anxiolytic.

(B) It is, in addition, an antipsychotic drug.

(C) It possesses analgesic properties.

(D) It possesses nonselective beta-blocking properties.

(E) It has antidiabetic properties.

17 A 48-year-old depressed patient, during an interview by his family doctor, reveals that his mood has been precipitated by his interpretation of his situation at work. He assumes that an impending change in his job description is a sign of his failure in his sales ability. Thus, he feels he has hopelessly lost out in his chosen field and feels it impossible to start over in a new direction at his age. Since finding out about the coming change, he has had difficulty in falling to sleep and is prone to frequent awakening; he is ultimately unable to complete a night's sleep. The physician engages him in a realistic discussion of the company's changing fortunes and helps him to conclude that, if anything, the change in job description within the company may be a vote of confidence in him, because he has not been asked to resign; that, in fact, the patient's interpretation of events has given rise to a negative value judgment. Which of the following therapeutic methods is being brought into play?

(A) Cognitive therapy

(B) Deep psychoanalytic therapy

(C) Reike therapy

(D) Supportive therapy

(E) Corporate engagement therapy

Examination Answers

1. **The answer is C,** 25 to 34 years. Depression remains a common diagnosis at all ages, however. Note that the peak age group for suicide (white boys or men, predominantly) and suicide attempts (white girls or women, predominately) is 15 to 24 (see chapter 43).

2. **The answer is E,** adjustment disorder with depressed mood or bereavement. Although this patient has some symptoms of a major depressive episode, they are temporally related to the recent loss of a loved one. Note also that she is basically functioning well and without impairment. She has had no manic or euphoric episodes to suggest a mixed disorder. Dysrhythmic and cyclothymic disorders are both characterized by a long term (>2 years) with mild mood alterations but without sustained remissions. In the former, patients have a chronically depressed mood of varying but milder intensity. In the latter, episodes of elevated mood alternate with periods of depression.

3. **The answer is C.** Alcoholism should be treated first if the two diagnoses exist, if one assumes that the suicide risk is assessed and accounted for. In many cases the depression will abate after the patient has abstained from alcohol for a significant period. However, the depression is also treated if it persists after 1 month of alcohol abstinence. When the two diagnoses coexist, there is an increase in the incidence of attempted and successful suicides. Both alcoholic men and women have an increased incidence of depression.

4. **The answer is C.** About one-third of patients with chronic disease suffer from depression in roughly direct proportion to the length of time with the disease. The cause of this is not known, but contributing factors might include catecholamine depletion from chronic stress. It may be situational, based on a philosophically reasonable sense of defeat or discouragement (i.e., an adjustment disorder with depressed mood).

5. **The answer is B,** AIDS. There is approximately a 66-fold increased risk of suicide in AIDS patients. This may be changing, as newly developed treatments have increased the survival time for AIDS patients.

6. **The answer is B.** Each of the drugs mentioned is an SSRI, albeit less well known than fluoxetine, sertraline, paroxetine, and fluvoxamine.

7. **The answer is B.** SSRIs are known to cause headache, nausea, tinnitus, insomnia, and akisthesia. Paroxetine (Paxil) also causes dry mouth. The greatest advantages of this class are the relative rapidity of onset and, the foregoing notwithstanding, the relative paucity of side effects.

8. **The answer is A.** TCAs are well known to cause anticholinergic effects, including cardiac dyrhythmias, sedation, and orthostatic hypotension. In regard to significant side effects that can lead to necessarily discontinuing the drug, this class has a narrow therapeutic window in comparison with the SSRIs.

9. **The answer is D,** MAOIs. The management of MAOIs is complicated, and most primary care doctors (including the author) avoid them because of severe dietary restrictions that include most cheeses, fermented aged meats, broad bean pods, meat and yeast extracts, red wine and many other alcoholic beverages, soy sauce, and sauerkraut. These foods contain tyramine, which, when MAO has been exhausted, may result in a hypertensive crisis. The latter occurs not only through effects of the MAO inhibiting medications but especially when much MAO has been depleted by prior exposure to phenylpropanolamine, phenylephrine, and the other drugs listed in the question. Thus, MAOIs are third-line drugs but nevertheless applicable for refractory panic disorder and depression.

10. **The answer is E.** Postpartum depression is sometimes considered an adjustment disorder with depressed mood. Postpartum depression tends to be milder with a shorter time period for spontaneous remission and less likely to be characterized by suicidal attempts. It affects about 10% of new mothers, though a less severe form, sometimes called the "postpartum blues," occurs in as many as 80% of new mothers. The foregoing is at odds with the sensational image given the illness by the mainstream media.

11. **The answer is D,** buproprion (Wellbutrin). Although tricyclic antidepressants have rarely been associated with seizures, as have SSRI agents, buproprion is associated with seizures in about 0.4% of those individuals who take the drug. Taking a higher dosage or having a history of seizures or central nervous system tumor or head trauma further increases the risk.

12. **The answer is A.** Trazodone, a heterocyclic antidepressant, has priapism among its side effects, according to its literature. Nefazodone might be a better heterocyclic alternative, especially in a male patient. Further, it does not tend to produce the orthostatic hypotension as does trazodone, but both are sedating. Among the others, escitalopram (Lexapro), an SSRI, carries no similar caveat and has no other sexual side effects. Sertraline (the SSRI trade named Zoloft) may cause ejaculation failure; fluoxetine (the SSRI Prozac) may cause decreased libido.

13. **The answer is D.** Abnormal ejaculation and orgasm are mentioned among the side effects of this drug but not so with the tricyclics, heterocyclics, or SSRIs without norepinephrine reuptake inhibition. The other side effects mentioned among the distracters are common to many other antidepressants and apply across several classes. One way to remember the connection between this side effect and venlafaxine is to consider that norepinephrine reuptake inhibition conveys a relative sympathomimetic effect and would be expected to mimic the sexual effect of mild anxiety so that erection may be attainable but ejaculation premature. This accounts also for the side of effect of excessive perspiration.

14. **The answer is C.** The patient fulfills criteria for a major depressive episode. Patients with a major depression are more likely to commit suicide than those with more moderate depressions or other related diagnoses such as dysrhythmic disorder or adjustment disorder with depressed mood. The criteria for diagnosis of major depression are, aside from depressed mood, as follows: social withdrawal; anhedonia (inability to enjoy formerly enjoyable activities); and feelings of guilt. One aspect of suicidality not adequately emphasized in training of nonpsychiatrists is a state of frantic, catastrophyzing agitation, with obsessive preoccupation with issues seemingly beyond reason. Asking the patient about suicidal ideation and plans is important to determine risk and does not increase the patient's rate of suicide.

15. **The answer is D,** commit the patient to lifelong maintenance on either the TCA or sertraline. Anyone 40 years of age or older who has a third bout of depression or anyone 50 years of age or older with a second bout should be maintained on an antidepressant for life. Electroshock therapy has been employed only rarely in the past 20 years. Psychotherapy is very useful as an adjunct and often improves outcomes or hastens a favorable outcome. However, depression is now felt to be caused ultimately by chemical imbalances addressed by the agents being discussed.

16. **The answer is C.** It possesses analgesic properties. This new antidepressant agent is being touted as having analgesic properties, a possible advantage when pain is part of the cognitive aspects of a depressive affect. The latter often occurs in association with diabetes when the complication of painful neuropathy occurs and, for example, in chronic musculoskeletal pain in which the patient has developed circular thinking.

17. **The answer is A.** Cognitive therapy is based on an Ellis and Harper model, developed further by Tosi. It is predicated on the fact that every emotional impulse is preceded by an interpretation of an event. Thus, event A is followed by an interpretation B, which may add an unnecessarily negative value to the process and is thus followed by an emotion or affect that may be anxiety or depression, for example. In many cases, counseling may relatively easily unearth an irrationally negative thought, and thus reverse the negative affect.

References

Bauman KA. Depression. In: Rudy DR, Kurowski K, eds. *Family Medicine: House Officer Series*. Baltimore: Williams & Wilkins; 1997:791–810.

Cobb C, Crichlow R. Duloxetine (Cymbalta) for treatment of depression. *Am Fam Physician*. 2006; 72:1099–1101.

Diagnostic and Statistical Manual of Mental Disorders. 4th ed. Washington, DC: American Psychiatric Association; 1994.

Eisendracht SJ, Lichtbacher JE. Psychiatric disorders. In: Tierney LM, McPhee SJ, Papadakis MA, eds. *Current Medical Diagnosis and Treatment*. 45th ed. New York: McGraw-Hill/Appleton & Lange; 2006:1038–1099.

Rupke SJ, Blecke D, Renfrow M. Cognitive therapy for depression. *Am Fam Physician*. 2006; 73:83–86, 93.

chapter 49

Anxiety and Phobias

Examination questions: *Unless instructed otherwise, choose the ONE lettered answer or completion that is BEST in each case.*

1 A 35-year-old female patient comes to your office complaining of bouts of palpitations, pounding heart, shortness of breath, and diaphoresis, along with feelings of impending doom. During an attack witnessed in the physician's office, the patient's blood pressure (BP) was 160/70 and her heart rate was 120 beats per minute and regular. The patient's face was flushed during the attack. After the attack passed over a period of 15 minutes, the BP had subsided to 110/75 and the heart rate to 80 beats per minute and regular. Which of the following would least resemble the clinical picture presented?

(A) Thyrotoxicosis

(B) Depression

(C) Carcinoid syndrome

(D) Pheochromocytoma

(E) Panic disorder

2 The patient in Question 1 is interviewed further. The onset of her symptoms coincided with a commercial airline flight. She is stably married with three children, is college educated, and stays at home to care for her children. During the attacks she feels that she is "losing (her) mind." Her affect is appropriate to the situation. Her vital signs, repeated, show BP is 115/75 and heart rate is 84 and regular. Along with counseling, which of the following would be the most appropriate for her acute attacks?

(A) Propranolol 20 mg by mouth (po)

(B) Diazepam 5 mg po

(C) Buspirone 10 mg po

(D) Lorazepam 0.5 mg, given sublingually

(E) Rebreathing exhaled air

3 Assume the patient is Question 1 had not developed any avoidance behavior. Although the acute attacks have been treated with some success, the question arises regarding prevention of attacks over time. Which of the following pharmacologic approaches would be most helpful as maintenance therapy?

(A) Sertraline (Zoloft) 25 to 50 mg daily

(B) Propranolol (Inderal) 20 to 40 mg daily

(C) Trazodone (Desyrel) 50 mg daily

(D) Divalproex (Depakote) 250 mg daily

(E) Chlorpromazine (Thorazine) 25 mg daily

4 Regarding the patient in Questions 1 to 3, she now has refused to accompany her husband on business trips if they involve flying. Further, she avoids crowds and fears visits to a supermarket to shop for food for her family. Which of the following is her diagnosis?

(A) Generalized anxiety disorder

(B) Panic disorder

(C) Phobic disorder

(D) Depression

(E) Adjustment disorder

5 Which of the following statements regarding anxiety and depression is true?

(A) They usually (i.e., in the majority of cases) occur as clearly defined entities, easily separated from each other.

(B) Anxiety disorders are seldom confounded with medical conditions.

(C) Mixed anxiety and depression is less disabling than pure cases of anxiety or depression.

(D) One important aid in managing mixed anxiety and depression is to delay diagnostic closure and disposition while observing the patient through several visits.

(E) Clear diagnosis of anxiety or depression usually obviates the need to further evaluate for organic disease.

6 A 52-year-old woman complains to her family physician of bouts of anxiety and depression, the latter often very deep but short lived (i.e., lasting <24 hours). Between such bouts she often feels "like I'm going to jump out of my skin." Her periods have changed within the past 6 months, becoming much less frequent but often heavy when they do occur. She denies suicidal ideation. She has difficulty sleeping through the night. Which of the following would be the most reasonable initial approach to this patient?

(A) Refer the patient to a psychiatrist

(B) Start a selective serotonin reuptake inhibitor (SSRI) for panic disorder

(C) Start a tricyclic antidepressant (TCA)

(D) Draw a follicle-stimulating hormone level and start an estrogenic agent

(E) Perform thyroid function studies

7 Regarding the patient in Question 6, after she has been treated empirically she is much improved except that she still feels empty and "at loose ends." She relates that her third and last child has just left home to attend college. Her husband feels similarly and his response is to throw himself into his work as an attorney. The family physician now addresses the psychosocial issues attendant to the change in the family dynamics. What is the expected likelihood that this phase should require the consultative assistance of a psychologist or psychiatrist?

(A) 1%

(B) 4% to 6%

(C) 10% to 15%

(D) 20%

(E) 30%

8 A 30-year-old woman complains of irritability, apprehension, anxiety, difficulty concentrating, and various somatic complaints that differ with each visit to the doctor. She has had difficulty falling off to sleep for the past 8 months, though once she is asleep she generally remains so for the night. Vital signs are within normal limits; menstrual periods are regular and unchanged for the past 10 years. Although she has between 1 and 3 "good days" per week, she notes the foregoing more often than not. She has not changed her patterns of living, remaining in her stable marriage and her job as a receptionist for a small business, neither of which appears to be a focus of difficulty. Which of the following is the presumptive diagnosis?

(A) Panic disorder

(B) Phobic reaction

(C) Chronic depression

(D) Generalized anxiety

(E) Adjustment disorder

9 Which of the following could logically constitute the mainstay for therapy for the patient in Question 8?

(A) Paroxetine (Paxil)

(B) Chloral hydrate (Noctec)

(C) Zolpidem (Ambien)

(D) Temazepam (Restoril)

(E) Diazepam (Valium)

10 A 45-year-old woman is disturbed over her propensity to wash her hands several times an hour and constantly check locks behind her numerous times after she has left her house to enter her automobile, delaying her departure. Her husband has complained and become impatient over this development. She admits that the behavior she exhibits is absurd. She functions well in her work as a bookkeeper. Which of the following classes of drugs is most likely to give her relief?

(A) SSRIs

(B) TCAs

(C) Heterocyclic antidepressants

(D) Barbiturate sedatives

(E) Major tranquillizers

11 A returning American soldier has recurring memories of scenes of his fellow soldiers being killed. He exhibits extreme reactions to sudden sounds, as well as insomnia, irritability, and avoidance of sights and sounds reminiscent of the precipitating event(s). Which of the following treatments have been shown to be of benefit to this condition?

(A) Antipsychotic agents

(B) Sedative–hypnotics

(C) SSRIs

(D) TCAs

(E) Major tranquilizers

12 What is the mean duration of posttraumatic stress disorder (PTSD) symptoms without treatment?

(A) Lifelong

(B) 10 years

(C) 64 months

(D) 32 months

(E) 24 months

13 Of the following benzodiazepine medications, which has the shortest half-life?

(A) Chlordiazepoxide (Librium)

(B) Diazepam (Valium)

(C) Clonazepam (Klonopin)

(D) Alprazolam (Xanax)

(E) Triazolam

Examination Answers

1. The answer is A. Thyrotoxicosis is unlikely because the cardiac rhythm and rate between attacks was normal. The typical BP and rate and rhythm in thyrotoxicosis are sinus tachycardia with systolic BP elevation. These persist until the condition is treated. Statistically, based on relative prevalence and incidence of attacks, panic disorder is the most likely basis for the picture portrayed, but the significant and threatening organic causes must first be ruled out. Furthermore, a significant portion of those individuals with panic disorder will prove to have an underlying depression. Carcinoid syndrome, a relative rarity in primary care practice, presents with attacks similar to that which is portrayed except that the BP is more likely to show a widened pulse pressure (systolic without diastolic elevation), as in the persistent pattern with thyrotoxicosis. Nearly all patients who present in the manner shown will be investigated for pheochromocytoma (and very few will prove out to have that syndrome). Pulmonary embolism presents in many ways, but acutely often with a picture similar to that in the vignette. However, such an acute attack would be unlikely to subside in such a short time. Acute angina may manifest the clinical picture shown, without chest pain, especially in a female patient; a similar situation may occur in the case of myocardial infarction.

2. The answer is D. Lorazepam 0.5 mg (0.5 to 1 mg) given sublingually acts rapidly enough to make a difference, even in such short-lived bouts of anxiety as occur with panic attacks, from which the patient in the vignette suffers. The other three medications mentioned do not act swiftly enough. Rebreathing exhaled air (e.g., breathing into a paper bag) may be beneficial if acute hyperventilation is a major manifestation of the panic attacks. In fact, often the first few attacks are accompanied by hyperventilation, which compounds the somatic manifestations of panic. However, in panic disorder, educating and training of the patient in understanding the physiology and avoidance of hyperventilation do not generally alleviate the panic attacks themselves. Panic disorder may lead to phobic responses. Panic disorder is more prevalent among female individuals (2:1 over male individuals) and the tendency is not entirely acquired, as there is a 50% concordance among twins and 18% among relatives.

3. The answer is A. Sertraline (Zoloft, an SSRI) 25 to 50 mg daily is effective in suppressing panic attacks in a majority of cases. Trazodone, a TCA, may be equally effective but has the disadvantage of all TCAs, which is that of a higher incidence of side effects than SSRIs. Propranolol, the nonselective beta-adrenergic blocking agent, has not been satisfactory in panic disorder, except for specific phobias, such as stage fright, in which it suppresses the visceral response to panic while not impeding motor responsiveness. Divalproex is an anticonvulsant. Chlorpromazine is a previously developed antipsychotic agent, seldom any longer in use.

4. The answer is C, phobic disorder. Panic attacks may lead to phobic reactions. It may be that such progression can be prevented by proactive counseling of the patient not to change his or her lifestyle because of the panic attacks. A rational approach goes something like this: "Imagine the worst that could occur during a panic attack. Embarrassment? It does not warrant changing your life." If phobias develop early in life, then intervention is obviously more difficult.

5. The answer is D. An important aid in managing mixed anxiety and depression is maintenance of "evenly hovering attention" and delay of diagnostic closure (assuming no evidence of suicidality). Mixed anxiety and depression is more common than either anxiety or depression alone. Anxiety is often confounded with medical conditions, such as diagnostically with pheochromocytoma and thyrotoxicosis, and further because it often occurs in conjunction with such conditions. Thus, while the psychiatric condition is being studied and defined, confounding medical conditions can be ruled out.

6. The answer is D. Draw a follicle-stimulating hormone level and start an estrogenic agent. If the hormone level is elevated, then the estrogen should be continued for a suitable period and the patient's psychological state observed. Of such patients, 70% will complain of paroxysmal hot flashes, making the diagnosis more readily apparent. The acute menopause syndrome is a great imitator of other organic diseases. Only after the acute symptoms of estrogen withdrawal have been addressed and treated should the elements of depression and anxiety be addressed, if symptoms have not dissipated during the empiric therapeutic trial.

7. The answer is B. Of patients with psychosocial problems seen in primary care, 4% to 6% are referred to psychiatrists or psychologists. Nearly half of patients in primary care have some degree of anxiety, depression, mixed anxiety and depression, or somatizing symptoms of psychological distress. Thus, it is imperative that the family doctor be trained and prepared in counseling techniques.

8. The answer is D. Generalized anxiety disorder is defined as the situation in which a person has symptoms of irritability, apprehension, anxiety, difficulty concentrating, somatic complaints, and insomnia on more days than he or she does not have them, over a period lasting at least 6 months. Panic attacks do not last all day, not to mention several days running. This patient has not changed her pattern of living to avoid symptoms; therefore, she does not have a phobic disorder. Her sleep patterns are not those usually encountered in depression (i.e., early and frequent awakening). Adjustment disorder does not fit the situation because nothing has changed materially in her life.

9. The answer is E. Diazepam (Valium), an intermediately long-acting benzodiazepine, is appropriate for generalized anxiety disorder. Not mentioned but quite acceptable and perhaps safer is buspirone for generalized anxiety. Paroxetine is an antidepressant (and in some cases psychiatrists are not beyond mixing an anxiolytic and an antidepressant). Chloral hydrate, zolpidem, and temazepam are all sedatives for facilitation of sleep. On occasion one of the latter group can be used adjunctively in generalized anxiety but are not the main aspect of therapy.

10. The answer is A. SSRIs are the first-line drugs of choice. This patient manifests, of course, obsessive compulsive disorder. In its pure form these patients are usually predictable, orderly, conscientious, and intelligent. Experts state that obsessive compulsive disorder may coexist and overlap with depression (even being a risk for major depression), tics, Tourette's syndrome, and eating disorders.

11. The answer is C. SSRIs have shown a 54% to 62% improvement in patients in 12-week trials, as opposed to 37% improvement in those who received placebo for PTSD. The diagnostic criteria for this entity are as follows: (a) the traumatizing event; (b) the recurrent re-experiencing of the event; (c) persistent avoidance of stimuli that remind the patient of the precipitating event; (d) persistent symptoms of increased arousal (e.g., the insomnia, irritability, and temper flare-ups); (e) duration of the symptoms for more than 1 month; and (f) significant resultant stress in social life.

12. The answer is C, 64 months. With treatment, the average duration of symptoms is reduced to 32 months. These data come from research and call for a skeptical eye in dealing with patients who promote PTSD as a way of life.

13. The answer is E. Triazolam has no active metabolites to prolong its pharmacologic effects and partly as a result of this has a half-life of 1 to 3 hours. For this reason it is promoted as a sleep-facilitating drug without significant morning "hangover." Its popular trade name is Halcion. All of the other drugs mentioned are employed as anxiolytic drugs, of which alprazolam has the shortest half-life (i.e., <24 hours); the remaining three benzodiazepines (chlordiazepoxide, diazepam, and clonazepam) each have a half-life >24 hours. Clonazepam is used as an anticonvulsant. Drugs with short half-lives, when used as anxiolytics, may give rise to rebound anxiety within a dosage cycle. Those with half-lives >24 hours should be used with caution in the aged population.

References

Eisendracht SJ, Lichtbacher JE. Psychiatric disorders. In: Tierney LM, McPhee SJ, Papadakis MA, eds. *Current Medical Diagnosis and Treatment.* 45th ed. New York: McGraw-Hill/Appleton & Lange; 2006:1038–1099.

Ronning GF. Anxiety, phobias, and the undifferentiated primary care syndrome. In: Rudy DR, Kurowski K, eds. *Family Medicine: House Officer Series.* Baltimore: Williams & Wilkins; 1997: 811–828.

chapter 50

Somatic Symptoms without Organic Basis

Examination questions: Unless instructed otherwise, choose the ONE lettered answer or completion that is BEST in each case.

1 A family physician sees 30 patients a day, 5 days per week. Included in his practice are both sexes and all age groups. What percentage of the symptoms given by these patients will have no biomedical basis of explanation?

(A) 5% to 10%

(B) 10% to 20%

(C) 20% to 40%

(D) 40% to 60%

(E) 60% to 80%

2 A 22-year-old woman has been brought home from a private college on a medical basis because of the occurrence of seizures that often occurred in her room in a women's dormitory and, as described, would seem to be grand mal seizures. She is hospitalized and her family doctor visits her at her hospital bed. He witnesses a seizure and suspects that they are not organically based; that is, they are "hysterical" or pseudoseizures. Each of the following would be evidence of a pseudoseizure, except for which one?

(A) The patient is found to be urine incontinent.

(B) Her limbs flail in an asynchronous manner.

(C) She resists when her nose and mouth are held closed.

(D) She remains conscious as evidenced by her directional gaze.

(E) She began to manifest the seizure as soon as the doctor entered her hospital room for the first time since her admission.

3 Which of the following somatoform disturbances is present in the patient featured in Question 2?

(A) Conversion disorder

(B) Somatization disorder

(C) Pain disorder

(D) Hypochondriasis

(E) Malingering

4 Regarding the case in Question 2, which of the following laboratory studies drawn during the seizure or shortly thereafter would be most helpful in determining the validity of the seizure?

(A) White blood cell count

(B) Blood sugar

(C) Lactic acid dehydrogenase

(D) Prolactin

(E) Alkaline phosphatase

5 You are seeing a 28-year-old woman, who has been your patient for the past 2 years, who complains to you that she has vague left chest pain, occasional feelings of shortness of breath, and fatigue. At other times she has complained of right flank and lower quadrant abdominal pain and difficulty concentrating. Two months ago she complained of left upper quadrant abdominal pains that were intermittent and "nondescript." Over the past year she has had complaints of urinary frequency and burning. She has no present or family history of coronary disease, hypertension, diabetes, or stroke, and she is not a smoker. Her chest pains are not associated with climbing stairs; she does not have bouts of nausea, light-headedness, or diaphoresis during these moments of discomfort. At other times this patient has had complaints of cramping abdominal pain, constipation, and diarrhea, as well as symptoms of vague difficulty in swallowing, none of which symptoms yielded diagnoses upon ancillary clinical evaluation. Today, the abdominal examination is negative for deep or rebound tenderness except for a probable exaggerated guarding response to deep palpation in the right lower quadrant. From which of the following somatoform disorders does this patient most likely suffer?

(A) Conversion disorder

(B) Somatization disorder

(C) Pain disorder

(D) Hypochondriasis

(E) Depression

6 A 45-year-old white man has sustained a cervical strain that prevents him from being able to manage the steering wheel to drive a truck as required on his job. Over a period of 6 months he has remained off work because his employer won't entertain the concept of "light duty." He has returned regularly looking haggard, complaining of ongoing pain in both the neck and the lumbar spine regions. There are no radicular signs in either the cervical or sciatic sectors of the physical examination. Electrical studies of both regions have returned negative results. Physical therapy modalities have failed to yield results satisfactory to the patient. From which of the following somatoform disorders does he suffer?

(A) Conversion disorder

(B) Somatization disorder

(C) Pain disorder

(D) Hypochondriasis

(E) Anxiety

7 A 35-year-old woman complains of vague abdominal sensations attributed to a hepatic cyst that has been diagnosed on a previous abdominal computed tomography scan. She has been followed for several years for "gastrointestinal dysautonomia." When she comes to the doctor's office, she invariably invokes a sensation with an anatomic attachment, not usually involving pain. In addition to the hepatic cyst, she has also cited a posterior lung field "cyst" attached to an otherwise vague right thoracic sensation. Which of the following somatoform syndromes does she display?

(A) Conversion disorder

(B) Somatization disorder

(C) Pain disorder

(D) Hypochondriasis

(E) Malingering

8 A 26-year-old man comes to the doctor with a complaint of low back pain radiating down the posterior left thigh to the midcalf. Deep tendon reflexes are difficult to evaluate and on occasion seem to anticipate the tap of the hammer. The straight-leg raising test is positive in that it results in a complaint of radiating pain in the same pattern as described in the chief complaint at 45 degrees. The doctor then has the patient sit up on the examining table and extends the knee to horizontal without resulting in a complaint or facial register of pain. Which of the following is the underlying condition?

(A) Herniated nucleus pulposus at L5 to S1

(B) Lumbosacral strain

(C) Pain disorder

(D) Hypochondriasis

(E) Malingering

9 A 45-year-old female patient has been seen three times for a left upper quadrant abdominal pain which has yielded no historical, physical, radiographic, or laboratory findings that suggest any disease of organic basis. She continues to worry that she has cancer of the stomach and cannot be dissuaded despite negative upper gastrointestinal x-rays and upper endoscopy. From which of the following somatoform disorders does this patient most likely suffer?

(A) Somatization disorder

(B) Conversion disorder

(C) Depression

(D) Hypochondriasis

(E) Anxiety

10 Regarding the patient in Question 9, if instead of *worrying* that she has cancer of the stomach, suppose she *insists* she has cancer despite the definitive negative studies. Which of the following fits the clinical picture best among the choices?

(A) Somatization disorder

(B) Factitious disorder

(C) Depression

(D) Hypochondriasis

(E) Body dysmorphic disorder

11 A 42-year-old lawyer makes an appointment for chest pains approximately 1 week after a 52-year-old associated suffered a myocardial infarction. His pain is intermittent, not severe, not associated with exertion, and more likely to occur while he is sitting and watching television in the evening. A resting electrocardiogram

(EKG) is normal, as is a subsequent EKG treadmill stress test. One week after the stress test the physician explains the results and the patient says the symptoms have disappeared. Which of the following is the best diagnosis?

(A) Somatization disorder

(B) Conversion disorder

(C) Depression

(D) Hypochondriasis

(E) Anxiety

12 A 34-year-old man complains of vague chest pain, more or less constant, though not severe, for the past 2 to 3 weeks. He cannot remember the date or time of onset. When asked whether he is concerned about the significance of the pain, he is vague in his answer while appearing sadly disturbed. He indicates the location of the pain with two fingers and a soft pressure over the left precordium. He has no family history of coronary artery disease; he has never smoked; and an EKG stress test showed a normal response. Which of the following is the diagnosis?

(A) Somatization disorder

(B) Conversion disorder

(C) Depression

(D) Hypochondriasis

(E) Angina pectorus

13 A 35-year-old woman complains of nervousness. Her heart rate is 120 and regular, repeated on several occasions. She exhibits a stare with widened palpebral fissures and moist, velvety skin to palpation. The thyroid gland is nonpalpable. Her free thyroxine (T_4) level is elevated above the normal range by 50%. The thyroid-stimulating hormone (TSH, or thyrotropin) level is suppressed. Which of the following is the diagnosis?

(A) Toxic nodular goiter

(B) Graves disease

(C) Factitious hyperthyroidism

(D) Anxiety reaction

(E) Sinus tachycardia

Examination Answers

1. The answer is D; 40% to 60% of symptoms given by patients in a primary care setting have no biomedical basis of explanation. Reasons for presenting with such symptoms vary from straightforward desire for information and alleviation of fears to somatization of anxiety, depression, and hysterical conversion as well as other defined somatization syndromes discussed in this unit.

2. The answer is A. If a patient who is having a seizure is found to be incontinent of urine, almost certainly the event is a genuine convulsion. Patients do not maintain consciousness as they enter into a grand mal seizure. In such a seizure, tonic–clonic movements tend to be symmetrical. The occurrence of a seizure just as soon as the doctor entered the room, taken from a real case, would be too coincidental to have happened by chance.

3. The answer is A, conversion disorder. This picture, taken from a real case, is fairly typical of that condition. The student had learned early that she could escape certain responsibilities by deflecting attention to herself in a sympathetic manner. She was treated in a manner that walked the tightrope between reinforcement of neurosis and cure by allowing her self-respect and suggesting, without being direct, that she knew what to do to get herself reinstated at the college.

4. The answer is D. The prolactin level rises abruptly in the postictal state after a grand mal seizure and not so during or after a pseudoseizure. An electroencephalogram tracing available during the seizure is, of course, a crucial tool in determining the credibility of a seizure.

5. The answer is B, somatization disorder. This patient satisfies the criteria of four symptoms, other than pain, in unrelated systems as well as four symptoms related to the gastrointestinal system, all of which have yielded no findings on clinical or ancillary evaluation. This disorder is most likely to have its onset prior to the time the individual reaches the age of 30 years, usually as early as adolescence, and occurs ten times as frequently in female individuals as in male individuals. It has been referred to as Briquette syndrome.

6. The answer is C, pain disorder. The criteria for this classification are that there is pain out of proportion to any anatomic evidence and that it coincides with certain psychological needs. In the present vignette the patient was probably obtaining an escape from the responsibilities of his job and the necessity of supporting his family. His management consisted of allowing the medical evaluation phase to run to completion; then suggesting that he would have no more or less pain by returning to his job than by staying home; and finally supporting him in prescriptions of noncontrolled analgesics so as to allow preservation of self-respect.

7. The answer is D, hypochondriasis. That which differentiates hypochondriasis from other somatoform syndromes, in particular, the chronic pain syndrome, is the patient's focus on a diagnosis rather than the pain itself. The patient may have her own "theory" of the pathophysiology, usually with an air of certainty, quaint though it may be.

8. The answer is E, malingering. This is a conscious effort by the patient to feign a positive straight-leg test, which, if genuine, would have been matched by a positive Lesegue test, extending the knee on the ostensibly symptomatic side while the patient was in the sitting position.

9. The answer is D, hypochondriasis. This patient has the definitive fixation on a single disease and a single persistent symptom.

10. The answer is C, depression. There is a subtle but definite line between persistent worry and insistence in the patient who resists reasonable evidence against her having the serious organic disease, cancer of the stomach in this case. In the case of insistence, especially when associated with agitation, there may be depression, bordering on psychotic depression or other psychotic illness. Such agitation, especially when attached to fixation on body image or an unreasonable life issue such as employment, may signal a suicide risk.

11. The answer is E, anxiety. One might well refer to this constellation as an anxiety somatic equivalent. As opposed to a patient with hypochondriasis, somatization disorder, conversion reaction, or depression, this patient has fears that are closely related to reality, amenable to reason, and subject to reassurance after presentation of the proof of testing and explanation.

12. **The answer is C,** depression. Some psychiatrists would refer to this syndrome as somatic depressive equivalent. Whereas most patients with chest pain are anxious about the possibility of coronary disease, this patient lacks that symbolism. In fact, the two-finger mild touch analogy is more symbolic of "pressure" – that is, depression.

13. **The answer is C,** factitious hyperthyroidism. If the patient had Graves disease, the TSH level would be elevated and there would virtually always be a goiter. If the TSH level is suppressed by an autonomous primary thyroid condition such as toxic thyroid nodule or toxic nodular goiter, then there should be a palpable goiter that would be nodular (sometimes not known to be such until scanning studies, but nevertheless palpable). Anxiety reaction is inappropriate as a diagnosis because it does not explain the T_4 and TSH findings. Sinus tachycardia is not a diagnosis in this vignette because it is obviously secondary to another condition as evidenced by the other clinical information.

References

Eisendracht SJ, Lichtbacher JE. Psychiatric disorders. In: Tierney LM, McPhee SJ, Papadakis MA, eds. *Current Medical Diagnosis and Treatment.* 45th ed. New York: McGraw-Hill/Appleton & Lange; 2006:1038–1099.

Margo KL. Psychological interventions for noncardiac chest pain (Cochrane for clinicians). *Am Fam Physician.* 2005; 72:1701.

Post DM, Rudy DR. Somatic symptoms without organic basis. In: Rudy DR, Kurowski K, eds. *Family Medicine: House Officer Series.* Baltimore: Williams & Wilkins; 1997:829–842.

SECTION **XVI**

Miscellaneous Areas of Clinical Practice

chapter 51

Dermatology

Examination questions: Unless instructed otherwise, choose the ONE lettered answer or completion that is BEST in each case.

1 A young mother comes to you with her 8-month-old formula-fed baby. She is concerned about a rash involving the facial cheeks and the tops of folds of skin over various parts of the body. On occasion the patches weep and form crusts. The baby does not seem to be bothered greatly by the rash. The parents are each healthy and without especially apparent inherited diseases, except that the mother has allergic rhinitis in the autumn months and the father had asthma as a child. Which of the following is the most likely diagnosis of the rash?

(A) Psoriasis

(B) Eczema

(C) Chafing caused by lip licking

(D) Candidiasis

(E) Cellulitis

2 Regarding the case in Question 1, which of the following would be least likely associated with the condition shown?

(A) Contact dermatitis

(B) Food allergies

(C) Allergic rhinitis at later ages

(D) Allergic asthma

(E) Drug allergies

3 For the patient in Question 1, which of the following would be the approach most fundamental toward addressing the causation of the rash?

(A) Triamcinolone ointment applied twice daily for 1 month and a follow-up visit at that time

(B) Systemic glucocorticoid course over a 2-week period

(C) Admission to the hospital for intravenous antibiotics

(D) Trial of change in formula from patient's cow-milk-based preparation to a soybean-based formula

(E) Application of topical antibiotic ointment

4 The 12-year-old brother of the patient in Question 1 is brought to you a month or so after you have treated the infant successfully, complaining of pruritic patches of dry, scaly skin at the antecubital fossae, the medial aspects of the ankles above the malleoli, and the popliteal spaces. Which of the following therapeutic modalities would be most appropriate and effective?

(A) Applications of lotion containing 1% hydrocortisone two to three times daily

(B) Ten-day course of tapering prednisone, beginning with 40 mg daily

(C) Prescription of hydroxyzine 25 mg per os every 4 hours as needed for pruritus

(D) Prescription of 2% hydrocortisone ointment to be applied four times daily to the pruritic patches as needed for itching

(E) Prescription of a food-elimination diet

5 A 35-year-old male type II diabetic patient comes to you with severe contact dermatitis caused by poison ivy, 2 days after he worked in his garden with short sleeves, for the first time in several years. The dorsal aspects of his forearms manifest weeping areas involving about two-thirds of the surfaces distributed in the midportions where there had been blebs that ruptured yesterday. The fluid has a serous appearance and there is no purulence and no red streaking. There is no extraordinary degree of pain in the affected areas. Which of the following treatments is the most rational approach to this condition at this time?

(A) Prednisone per os 40 mg/day, tapering over a 10-day period

(B) Hydrocortisone ointment applied two to three times daily under an occlusive dressing twice daily for the next 3 days, and a revisit at that time

(C) Application of 1% hydrocortisone in a lotion, applied under loose gauze until the dressing dries, repeated two to three times daily; revisit in 3 days

(D) Ten-day course of an antibiotic effective against both beta-hemolytic streptococci and staphylococci

(E) Desensitization with poison ivy antigen

6 A 28-year-old man notes the onset over the past few months of intensely pruritic vesicles distributed over the lateral aspects of the shoulders, buttocks, elbows, and knees. The axillae and interdigital web spaces are spared. The condition has not abated during this time and the patient has had to rely on systemic antipruritic prescriptions in order to get to sleep. You have put the patient on standard food-elimination diets with no alleviation of the symptoms. Topical ointments containing hydrocortisone have not been effective in controlling the itching. At the time of onset, the patient had been on no prescription or nonprescription drugs. On examination you see excoriations but no patch thickening. Which of the following diagnoses is most likely?

(A) Psoriasis

(B) Discoid lupus erythematosus

(C) Scabies

(D) Food allergy

(E) Dermatitis herpetiformis

7 A 55-year-old white female patient draws your attention to a pigmented 15-mm raised lesion on the posterolateral aspect of her left arm. Because she does not often see that part of her body, she is not certain how long it has been present and denies sensory irritation of any kind. She is concerned about the possibility of melanoma. On examination you find the lesion to be well demarcated both at the base and at the circumference of its shallowly raised (i.e., raised with a flat rather than a domed top), and flat surface that extends to a diameter that is slightly broader than the base. In addition you find three other similar lesions that are located on the back of the torso that range from 5 mm to 1.5 cm in diameter, none of which shows signs of inflammation or breakdown of the surface. Which of the following is the most likely diagnosis?

(A) Squamous cell carcinoma

(B) Malignant melanoma

(C) Basal cell carcinoma

(D) Seborrheic keratosis

(E) Actinic keratosis

8 A 28-year-old white male former college basketball player complains of intermittent arthralgias over the past 3 months, which involve the left ring finger proximal interphalangeal joint (PIP) and right index and middle finger distal interphalangeal (DIP) joints. He admits to morning stiffness. On examination you note dysplasia of the right index nail with some pitting. The remainder of the integument is within normal limits. Which of the following is the most likely diagnosis?

(A) Rheumatoid arthritis

(B) Psoriatic arthritis

(C) Osteoarthritis

(D) Gouty arthritis

(E) Traumatic arthritis

9 A 35-year-old man comes to you with the complaint of a rash virtually covering the anterior chest and abdomen to well below the beltline, and the upper half of his posterior trunk. The patient has taken neither prescription nor over-the-counter medications. Since onset the course has been steady, without waxing or waning in intensity. The lesions are papuloquamous and ovoid with their long axes oriented more or less horizontally, tilting downward and laterally. He has had the rash about 1 week and remembers a period of mild malaise and slight nausea 3 weeks ago. On closer examination you find neither vesiculation nor bulla formation. The patient says he has not changed soaps and wears cotton T shirts that are tucked outside of his underwear that is made of a synthetic fiber. You look for a larger patch that may have preceded the rash and find none. The patient is monogamous and shows neither oral nor palmar lesions. Which of the following is the most likely diagnosis?

(A) Pityriasis rosea

(B) Secondary syphilis

(C) Contact dermatitis

(D) Nummular eczema (neuroeczema)

(E) Food allergy

10 A blond mother of a red-headed daughter seeks information to fortify her in counseling her teenaged daughter not to pursue suntans during the summer months. Which of the following is the least protective of skin against skin cancer and aging?

(A) Avoidance of sun exposure between the hours of 10 AM and 2 PM

(B) Daily low-grade exposure to sunlight (e.g., experienced by people in outdoor occupations)

(C) Use of sunscreens that block ultraviolet B (UVB)

(D) Use of sunscreens that block UVB and ultraviolet A (UVA)

(E) Sunlight exposure to normally unexposed areas of the body only during special occasions such as trips to the beaches and winter vacations in tropical or semitropical latitudes

11 A 45-year-old black woman complains to you of hyperpigmented spotty areas on her lower legs, especially prominent just above the medial malleoli. She reminds you that, last month, you treated her successfully for itching patches in those areas that had been present for several weeks. She is concerned from the cosmetic point of view and worries as to the cause. You notice no fasciculations. Which of the following is the diagnosis of the condition?

(A) Hyperpigmentation caused by Addison disease

(B) Melanoma

(C) Acanthosis nigricans

(D) Hyperpigmentation secondary to inflammation

(E) Pigmented seborrheic keratosis

12 Your patient, a 45-year-old white woman, complains to you of having irregular menses, being overweight, and having hair on her upper lip. On examination, in addition to the foregoing, you notice a pigmented velvety thickening of the skin in 3- to 4-cm patches on her dorsal neck surface and deep in the axillae. Her palms and sublingual areas are unremarkable. Which of the following is the likely diagnosis?

(A) Addison disease

(B) Seborrheic keratoses

(C) Nummular eczema

(D) Epidermoid cysts

(E) Acanthosis nigricans

13 Regarding the patient in Question 12, to which of the following endocrine conditions should you be alert?

(A) Polycystic ovary syndrome (PCOS)

(B) Autoimmune thyroiditis

(C) Addison disease

(D) Graves disease

(E) Pregnancy

14 Regarding the patient in Question 12, aside from endocrine situations, which of the following should be ruled out in evaluating the case?

(A) Adrenocortical tumor

(B) Lymphoma

(C) Colorectal cancer

(D) Ovarian cancer

(E) Cerebellar hemangioblastoma

15 A 35-year-old woman complains that, for about a year, she has had a mysterious rash involving her face that is nonpruritic. She stopped using topical facial make-up preparations 6 months ago. In the past 2 months she has noticed muscle weakness of the neck, trunk, and limbs. You see on inspection that her eyes manifest a purple discoloration and discernible periorbital edema. Which of the following is the correct diagnosis?

(A) Lupus erythematosus

(B) Dermatomyositis

(C) Polymyositis

(D) Charcot–Marie–Tooth disease

(E) Contact dermatitis

16 Regarding the patient in Question 15, in addition to ordering confirmatory diagnostic studies and treating the patient's symptoms, which of the following actions would be most appropriate?

(A) Prescribe a drying cream for the facial rash and search for a contact allergen

(B) Prescribe a moistening ointment and search for a contact allergen

(C) Prescribe a muscle relaxant for the muscle weakness

(D) Perform blood, urine, and imaging screening for cancer

(E) Draw rheumatoid factor, sedimentation rate, and antinuclear antibodies

17 A 55-year-old man complains of stinging pain for 3 days in the facial area involving the right forehead from beneath the scalp anteriorly and as low as the level of the right eye, seemingly out of proportion to a red rash he notes that is appearing today. The area of erythema involves a band that matches the area of pain reported by the patient. Examination reveals 1- to 3-mm vesicles on the right cheek against the erythematous background. Which of the following is the most likely diagnosis?

(A) Herpes simplex

(B) Dermatitis herpetiformis

(C) Contact dermatitis

(D) Herpes zoster

(E) Nummular eczema

18 Regarding Question 17, which of the following findings would be most reassuring to you that the likelihood of involvement of the eye is low?

(A) Lack of involvement of the tip of the nose

(B) Lack of pain in the ipsilateral eye

(C) Small size of the area of involvement

(D) Lack of involvement of other areas on the body besides the face

(E) Equally sized and light-reactive pupils

19 A 24-year-old white woman has severe acne. You note that it is inflammatory and scarring, despite her denial of manipulating the lesions. Her previous physician had tried topical antibiotics and, for the past 2 months, systemic doxycycline maintenance therapy. She wishes to discuss trying isotretinoin (Accutane). You respond that the drug must be prescribed with great trepidation. This drug may be associated with each of the following side effects, except for which one?

(A) Teratogenicity

(B) Elevation of serum trigycerides to as high as 800 mg/dL

(C) Hepatitis

(D) Lupuslike autoimmune response

(E) Psychological symptoms

Examination Answers

1. The answer is B, infantile eczema. Psoriasis rarely occurs on the face and the mean age at onset is between 20 and 30 years. Compulsive licking followed by chafing the lips usually occurs during the juvenile years, and the lesions in this case are farther from the mouth than the reach of the tongue. Candidiasis affects the intertriginous areas, opposite from the rash in this case, which involves the tops of the folds of skin. Cellulitis is a serious bacterial infection that occurs in a focal area, not in separate distinct patches, and it would not manifest chronicity as the patient's illness would bring the affair to an early crisis. Finally, statistically, not only the greater prevalence of infantile eczema, but also the fact that this disorder is a manifestation of the heavily familial inherited group of atopic diseases, marks this as eczema. The other members of the group are allergic rhinitis and conjunctivitis ("hay fever") and asthma.

2. The answer is A. Eczema is one part of the atopic triad of infantile eczema, allergic rhinitis, and allergic asthma. These conditions are found together in individuals and in families; hence they have a strong genetic causation. In addition, atopic persons are more likely than people in the general population to have drug and food allergies. Susceptibility to contact dermatitis is not significantly associated with atopy.

3. The answer is D. Infantile eczema, though genetically determined, is often precipitated by a food allergy in the first year of life. For a baby on a common formula (as opposed to breast feeding, for example) the most likely causation is allergy to cow's milk. Later, after advancement of the feeding schedule beyond liquid formula, common offenders are egg whites and wheat. Often, a simple change of formula to one based on soy will result in total clearing of the eczema within 1 week. Systemic glucocorticoids would be a radical step for an infant who is not critically ill. Although topical glucocorticoids may be employed for infantile eczema, such preparations as triamcinolone are too potent and carry a high rate of complications of atrophy and scarring striae at the areas of application, particularly on infantile skin. Antibiotics, either systemic or topical, have no place in a noninfectious inflammatory process such as infantile eczema.

4. The answer is D. The sibling of the child with infantile eczema has a commonly evolved stage of eczema. Thus, as the patient enters into the years of youth and adulthood, he frequently develops the form referred to variously as neuroeczema, nummular eczema, and neurodermatitis. The skin is more sensitive and has a lowered threshold for itching. In the accessible areas referred to in the vignette, scratching and rubbing causes a thickening, which is called lichenification by dermatologists. Paradoxically, lichenification causes the threshold for pruritus to be further lowered, which leads to further rubbing and the vicious circle of itching and scratching. This cycle is effectively interrupted in the vast majority of cases by topical glucocorticoids. Systemic glucosteroids are not effective and systemic antipruritics such as hydroxyzine (e.g., Vistaril) are usually not needed. Although some allergists may try food elimination in intractable cases, food allergy is rarely a factor and usually the elimination diet is ineffective.

5. The answer is C. The most significant part of the treatment of a weeping lesion is to apply a drying agent. The most drying are the wettest upon application, such as saline or Burow solution, and the most moistening are occlusive agents such as petrolatum (Vaseline). Creams are positioned toward the moistening end of the spectrum and lotions toward the drying end. When the etiology is a noninfectious inflammatory process as in contact dermatitis, not as a part of a chronic connective tissue disease, glucocorticoids are a legitimate therapeutic modality. Systemic glucocorticoids are not as effective on the thicker parts of the dermal organ (as opposed to being more effective on the glabrous skin, e.g., volar forearm, face, and genitalia). In this case the presence of diabetes is relatively contraindicated because of predictable certain rocketing levels of blood sugar during their use. In the latter cases, topical glucocorticoids are not only more effective but are also fraught with complications involving skin atrophy and local striae formation if the preparation is too potent or used for too long a period of time. Thus, in this instance, the mild agent hydrocortisone at the low concentration of 1% is chosen rather than a potent preparation such as a fluorinated ointment.

6. The answer is E. Dermatitis herpetiformis is a vesiculating disease of the skin that makes its onset during the third and fourth decades and then is generally lifelong. The vesicles are approximately the size of those found in varicella and occur on the extensor surfaces of the body referred to in the vignette. The vesicles are often not present on examination because of the excoriations (which are due to the intense itching and scratching) that obliterate them. However, most patients readily describe the vesicles that recur and lead to the scratching. The disease is genetically transmitted, with a strong prevalence in people with human leukocyte antigen types HLA-B8 and HLA-DR3. Diagnosis requires an index of suspicion suggesting skin biopsy that shows immunoflourescently visible immunoglobulin A deposits at the tips of dermal papillae. Therapy with oral dapsone, given as 25 to 50 mg daily, is dramatically effective. An alternative, sulfapyridine, for those with allergy or intolerance to the foregoing, or colchicine, in usual dosages has been found to be effective. Neither psoriasis nor discoid lupus is pruritic. Discoid lupus occurs in isolated, usually single, plaques. Scabies, although pruritic to a degree rivaling dermatitis herpetiformis, does not produce vesicles and tends to affect the axillae and web spaces. Food allergy typically causes urticaria and virtually never vesicles.

7. The answer is D. Seborrheic keratosis is typically well demarcated, often pigmented and rough on the surface without inflammatory signs. It has been described by dermatologists as waxy and "stuck on" in appearance as if it could be peeled off. Squamous cell carcinoma nearly always displays an inflammatory appearance and an irregular buildup of keratin. Squamous cell carcinoma may be pigmented but occurs on sun-exposed parts of the body. Actinic keratosis occurs in the regions where squamous cell carcinoma is found, is less inflammatory, and is less likely to be pigmented. Melanoma also is likely to be irregular at the edges or early manifesting inflammatory foci centrally. Basal cell carcinoma displays a very slow progression, often pearly appearance, and sometimes central ulceration. In any of the foregoing situations, a biopsy is necessary for confirmation.

8. The answer is B. Psoriatic arthritis occurs in about 45% of patients with psoriasis and may precede the onset of dermal manifestations of psoriasis by varying amounts of time. As an inflammatory arthritis (psoriasis is an autoimmune disease), this arthritis exhibits morning stiffness and gelling after periods of inactivity. What differentiates psoriatic arthritis from rheumatoid arthritis is its asymmetrical involvement of hands and feet and that it includes the DIP as well as PIP joints and occasionally knees and hips. The pinpoint-type pitting of fingernails is a hallmark of psoriasis, occurring in 30% of patients. The DIP joints of the hands are involved

in osteoarthritis in people in their sixth and seventh decades (Heberden nodes). Traumatic arthritis is mentioned as a red herring, given the patient's history of basketball activity and presumed history of numerous stoving injuries. Traumatic arthritis is a form of osteoarthritis and thus is noninflammatory, manifesting no significant stiffness. Gout would not be seriously considered in this age group without more classic presentations such as great toe metatarsophalangeal joint involvement.

9. The answer is A. Pityriasis rosea occurs without a discernible herald patch in about 50% of cases. Secondary syphilis should be considered in all cases of pityriasis rosea but is unlikely in a monogamous man. (Nevertheless, the standard of care dictates a serologic test for syphilis in all cases.) Contact dermatitis is unlikely in a situation in which the affected areas of the skin are in contact with different fabrics. Nummular eczema will not occur in unreachable areas such as the upper back; classically, it affects the antecubital and popliteal fossae among other places. Food allergies follow a waxing–waning course, depending on meals and their times of ingestion.

10. The answer is E. Intermittent intense sun exposure constitutes a greater skin cancer risk than daily less intense exposure over a period of years. This is apparent to people who have experienced sunburns to the trunk and legs on numerous occasions during their youth and young adult years and daily but less intense exposure to the head, neck, and forearms. In the late middle years, actinic changes are to found to a much greater degree on the thighs and lower legs than in the head, neck, and forearms, the latter areas having received many more hours of sun exposure than the intermittently and more intensely exposed areas. The best prevention is total blockade and shade. Next would be sunscreens that block both UVA and UVB; next would be sunscreens that block UVB. Avoidance of the most direct hours of sunlight (10 AM to 4 PM, according to the U.S. Preventive Services Task Force) is advisable but does not confer secure protection against skin aging and cancer.

11. The answer is D. Dark-skinned people, be they of African, Southeast Asian, or other ethnic origin, manifest, as a result of the subacute phase of an inflammatory process, a muddy-looking hyperpigmentation locally. Inflammation that lasts much longer causes the opposite, that is, a loss of pigmentation. Both conditions will reverse after subsidence of the inflammatory process. Hyperpigmentation will reverse itself sooner than hypopigmentation.

12. The answer is E, acanthosis nigricans. This patient probably has polycystic ovary syndrome (PCOS) and thus stands a strong chance of being insulin resistant, hence prediabetic type II or clinically diabetic. Acanthosis nigricans accompanies such conditions in a minority but significant proportion of cases. The pigmentation of Addison disease tends to involve the creases of the palms, soles, and axillae (as opposed to the concavities), extensor joint surfaces, tongue, nails, and belt or bra lines. Seborrheic keratoses may be pigmented but they occur as "stuck on" 1 cm^2 lesions on the open areas of the skin. Nummular eczema is pruritic and pigmented only in dark-skinned people. Epidermoid cysts are not noted for dark coloration except at the punctum, where is found the sebaceous comedone.

13. The answer is A. PCOS is associated with irregular menses, obesity, hirsutism, and insulin resistance. Acanthosis nigricans is apparently connected with the insulin resistance of type II diabetes, both type A (PCOS) and type B (autoimmune). Addison disease does not fit the pattern of pigmentation (see discussion of Question 12). Thyroid diseases have no particular association with pigment abnormalities in humans. Pregnancy often manifests the "mask of pregnancy," involving the face.

14. The answer is C. Acanthosis nigricans in the age group of the 40s and 50s is often associated with the following cancers: nonsmall cell lung, breast, gastrointestinal, prostate, and myeloproliferative disease, as well as carcinoid. Among gastrointestinal cancers, colorectal cancer is by far the most incident and in fact is third in incidence of all cancers in each sex in the United States (after prostate, breast, and lung, respectively) and second for cancer mortality in females after lung cancer. The only dermatosis associated with any of the other choices is ovarian cancer, which is associated with dermatomyositis.

. lung
. prostate/breast
. GI
. myeloproliferative

15. The answer is B. Dermatomyositis in its classic presentation involves the purple discoloration of the eyelids and periorbital edema ("heliotrope eyes") and proximal muscle weakness. In 10% of patients the rash precedes myositis by up to 2 years. Lupus erythematosus causes a classic facial rash (seldom seen in primary care practice); polymyositis is generally assumed to be dermatomyositis without dermatitis. Charcot–Marie–Tooth disease is a demyelinating disease of the central nervous system involving the distal extremities, leading to the stork-leg deformity. Contact dermatitis seldom occurs on the face except in reaction to cosmetics and virtually always is pruritic.

A muscular atrophy of variable inheritance, beginning in the m. supplied by the peroneal & slowly & progressive to inv. m of hands + arms.

16. The answer is D. The patient has dermatomyositis, an autoimmune disease. The gold standard of diagnosis is muscle biopsy. Electrical studies are also diagnostic but not specific and rheumatologic studies are quite relevant. However, the question asks what is to be the next step beyond diagnostic confirmation and symptomatic treatment. There is a definite but not specific association of dermatomyositis with developing cancers, especially ovarian carcinoma. Contact dermatitis is unlikely in the given distribution. In any event, the choice of ointments versus lotions or creams would be determined by whether the rash is weeping, crusting, or dry (see Question 5).

17. The answer is D. Herpes zoster ("shingles") is characterized by a searing superficial-type pain associated with a varicelliform vesicular rash. The vesicles occur on an erythematous background. The rash occurs simultaneously or within 2 to 3 days after the onset of the pain and lasts about 10 days through phases of subsequent crusting, dark-colored eschar, and resolution, sometimes with scar formation. Shingles is seldom confused with herpes simplex because the vesicles of herpes simplex are distributed within an area of only a few centimeters whereas herpes zoster usually covers the majority of a complete dermatome or, as this case, a cranial nerve (i.e., the ophthalmic branch of cranial nerve V). Dermatitis herpetiformis, contact dermatitis, and eczema are all pruritic whereas herpes zoster is not, unless it is late in the healing phase.

18. The answer is A. There is a close correlation, when the ophthalmic branch of the trigeminal nerve is involved in herpes zoster, between involvement of the tip of the nose and involvement of the cornea. It is too early in the present vignette to be reassured by the lack of symptoms in the eye itself. There is no relationship between the size or number of the area(s) of involvement in herpes zoster and ophthalmic involvement.

19. The answer is D. Drug literature does not mention this side effect or associated condition with the taking of isotretinoin. Each of the other conditions presented has been reported, as have many others. The most critical effect is teratogenicity. For that reason the patient must not only have a negative pregnancy test before starting but also must be on a contraception program that must continue through the course of therapy and for 1 month thereafter. Psychological symptoms reported, though not necessarily proven by prospective study, include suicidality and behavioral manifestations including violent acting out.

References

Fitzgerald PA. Endocrinology. In: Tierney LM, McPhee SJ, Papadakis MA, eds. *Current Medical Diagnosis and Treatment.* 43rd ed. New York: McGraw-Hill/Appleton & Lange; 2004:1062–1145.

Habif TP. *Clinical Dermatology.* St. Louis: Mosby; 2004.

Jemal A, Tiwari RC, Murray T, et al. Cancer statistics 2004. *CA Cancer J Clin.* 2004; 54:8–29.

Rugo HS. Cancer. In: Tierney LM, McPhee SJ, Papadakis MA, eds. *Current Medical Diagnosis and Treatment.* 43rd ed. New York: McGraw-Hill/Appleton & Lange; 2004:1577–1635.

Schwayder T. Common skin problems in children. *Patient Care.* 2004; July:32–36.

U.S. Preventive Services Task Force. Recommendations and rationale. *Am Fam Physician.* 1996; 69:903–904.

chapter 52

Geriatrics in Primary Care

Examination questions: Unless instructed otherwise, choose the ONE lettered answer or completion that is BEST in each case.

1 A 67-year-old woman with abdominal pain enters the office of a family physician. Which of the following statements regarding the diagnosis of the pain in this patient is true?

(A) A surgical cause is ruled out by lack of fever and leukocytosis.

(B) Acute cholecystitis is likely to present with radiating flank and back pain.

(C) The patient's chances of having ascending cholangitis are greater than those for a younger person.

(D) One can expect appendicitis to be accompanied by a temperature of 100°F (37.7°C).

(E) Elevated alkaline phosphatase levels will not be helpful in diagnosing ascending cholangitis.

2 Which of the following is the most significant difference between "old-old" patients (>75 years) and younger patients in the diagnosis of perforated peptic ulcer?

(A) The >75 group has devastating pain heralding perforation.

(B) Patients older than 75 years are more likely to demonstrate free air under the diaphragm.

(C) Serum amylase is less helpful in the diagnosis of perforation of these patients than it is in patients younger than 75 years.

(D) Symptoms and signs of perforated viscus are more likely to occur without prior symptoms in patients older than 75 years.

(E) Leukocytosis is more likely to be present in the older patient than in the younger one.

3 A 70-year-old man complains of abdominal pain that is steady and building. Abdominal examination reveals a widened abdominal aortic palpable pulsation; otherwise it is remarkable only for vague deep tenderness (i.e., showing no rebound tenderness). Abdominal ultrasound discloses an aneurysm 5 cm in diameter below the origin of the renal arteries. Which of the following is nearly certainly true regarding atherosclerotic risk factors present in this patient?

(A) Dyslipidemia

(B) Smoking

(C) Hypertension

(D) Psychological stress

(E) Diabetes type II

4 An 80-year-old previously well and self-sufficient great-grandfather who lives alone is brought to the family doctor because of newly occurring falls, urinary incontinence, and confusion over the past 4 days. His temperature and blood pressure are normal for him. Which of the following is the least likely cause of this change?

(A) Acute pneumonia

(B) Urinary tract infection

(C) Acute myocardial infarction

(D) Stroke

(E) Alzheimer disease (AD)

5 A 78-year-old white man is brought to his family doctor for confusion. He is visiting his daughter, son-in-law, and their college-age children. His vital signs, including orthostatic pressures, are within normal limits. The patient's confusion had its onset after he had been at the family's home for 2 days. There had been a recent change of medications for the gentleman, who has established diagnoses of diabetes, hypertension, and depression. Although other factors may cause confusion, which of the following medications is the most likely cause of confusion in this patient?

(A) Hydrochlorothiazide/triamterene (Dyazide)

(B) Verapamil

(C) Lisinopril

(D) Amitriptyline

(E) Metformin

6 A 65-year-old man has persistent blood pressure levels averaging 150/78, although his diastolic pressure has never been above 90 mm Hg. Which of the following drugs would have the best chance of controlling the blood pressure as a single medication in reasonable dosages?

(A) Lisinopril (an angiotensin-converting enzyme inhibitor)

(B) Propranolol (a nonselective beta-adrenergic blocker)

(C) Irbesartan (an angiotensin II receptor inhibitor)

(D) Hydrochlorothiazide/triamterene (a combination thiazide diuretic and potassium-saving diuretic)

(E) Terazosin (Hytrin; an alpha-1 receptor blocker)

7 Each of the following cancers occurs with virtually equal or greater incidence (frequency) in the >65 population than in all younger people, except for which one?

(A) Invasive carcinoma of the cervix (uteri)

(B) Prostate carcinoma

(C) Carcinoma of the lung

(D) Colorectal carcinoma

(E) Carcinoma of the breast

8 A family doctor began seeing patients in a nursing home and assumed care of several dozen patients. One 85-year-old female patient sat impassively during the 3 days required for the family doctor to make initial rounds, familiarizing himself with each patient while still pursuing his office practice. While exchanging a joke with the rounding nurse, the patient suddenly laughed out loud. The doctor found that she fed herself, albeit laboriously. Except for the humorous response, her face remained flat and expressionless. The doctor checked the medication list on the woman's chart and discovered that it included 5 mg of diazepam four times per day. This medication was discontinued forthwith. Within 1 to 2 days she became talkative and began exploiting her

keen sense of humor. Which of the following was the diagnosis if this woman's problem was relevant to the described findings?

(A) AD

(B) Parkinson disease

(C) Supranuclear palsy

(D) Depression

(E) Delirium

9 A 75-year-old woman is brought in by her family because of failure to adequately take care of herself alone in her apartment. Problems include errors and neglect in her private financial records; life-threatening errors concerning her kitchen stove; and a decreasing ability to dress herself. The possibility of AD is considered. Each of the following is a criterion to be fulfilled for diagnosis of AD, except for which one?

(A) Disturbance of consciousness

(B) Progressive impairment of memory and at least one other cognitive function (e.g., language)

(C) Onset between 40 and 90 years of age

(D) Dementia documented by examination and confirmed by testing

(E) Absence of another brain disorder or systemic disease that could cause dementia

10 The patient in Question 9 has been diagnosed with AD and the drug donepezil (Aricept) was started. Which of the following is the best summary of the pharmacologic actions of this drug that are beneficial to the patient with AD?

(A) Anticholinergic activity

(B) Beta-adrenergic blockade

(C) Central nervous system stimulation

(D) Antidepressant activity

(E) Cholinergic agonist activity

11 An 81-year-old father of a 47-year-old female patient of a family physician is brought to the doctor because of urinary retention. Recently he made a trip to a local emergency department and had to be catheterized. In culling the list of medications on which the patient has been placed, you note that each of the following may cause urinary retention, except for which one?

(A) Trihexyphenidyl for Parkinsonian rigidity

(B) Amitriptyline for facilitation of sleep

(C) Amlodipine for hypertension

(D) Terazosin (Hytrin) for benign prostatic hyperplasia

(E) Hydrocodone (Vicodin) for severe pain

Examination Answers

1. The answer is C. Her chances of having ascending cholangitis are greater than those for a younger person. This complication of acute cholecystitis is rare before a person reaches the age of 40; half of all patients older than 65 years of age who have cholecystitis suffer complications including ascending cholangitis, perforated gallbladder, emphysematous gallbladder, bile peritonitis, and gallstone ileus. Older patients are less likely to present with radiating flank and back pain than are younger patients. The majority of people with ascending cholangitis manifest elevated alkaline phosphatase levels. Acute surgical abdomen in patients older than 65 years of age is less likely to present with fever or leukocytosis.

2. The answer is D. Symptoms and signs of perforated viscus are more likely to occur without prior symptoms. The first symptom of ulcer disease is more likely to be that of perforated viscus. Leukocytosis is blunted in old-old individuals in situations that, in younger patients, result in white cell elevation. Amylase levels rise after perforation the same in the older group as in younger patients. Older patients are equally likely as younger ones to demonstrate free air under the diaphragm.

3. The answer is B. Smoking is the strongest risk factor for abdominal aortic aneurysm and 90% of patients with abdominal aortic aneurysm are smokers. The U.S. Preventive Services Task Force has advocated aortic aneurysm screening for all men who are between 65 and 75 years of age and have a history of smoking.

4. The answer is E. AD is unlikely in a previously independent octogenarian. AD would not have such a rapid onset. The point of the vignette is that the old-old (>75 years) frequently develop a set of nonspecific symptoms of mental dysfunction in response to any of the conditions mentioned. Other precipitants of such a change include gastrointestinal bleeding, starting a new sedating medication, or simply moving the venue of the patient's living conditions. Virtually all of the conditions not related to AD that are mentioned in this unit are amenable to treatment of the underlying cause, and for variable periods of time the dementia is thus reversible.

5. The answer is D. Amitriptyline, a tricyclic antidepressant, has a marked anticholinergic action. The latter has a tendency to cause confusion in older people. None of the other drugs' literature mentions this effect in the standard package insert data, though dizziness is reported in association with many other medications.

6. The answer is D. Hydrochlorothiazide/triamterene, a combination thiazide diuretic and potassium-saving diuretic (trade name of Dyazide, among others), may be effective for isolated systolic hypertension, the form of hypertension seen most often in elderly people. The pathophysiology of isolated systolic hypertension leans toward that of salt or water retention (volume load increased) as opposed to increased peripheral vascular resistance. The former is associated with lower renin levels for a given salt balance than normal. As the blood pressure tends to be more or less dependent on blood volume, it responds, in a majority of cases, to a simple diuretic. Angiotensin-converting enzyme inhibitors, angiotensin II receptor inhibitors, alpha-1 adrenergic blockers, and beta-blockers each function to relieve increased peripheral resistance, which is not as likely to be a mechanism of hypertension in the elderly population.

7. The answer is A; 27% of cases of invasive carcinoma of the cervix (uteri) occur in women who are older than 65 years of age. In addition, 45% of breast, 73% of colon, 81% of prostate, 50% of lung, and 48% of oral cancers occur in patients older than 65 years of age. Therefore, it behooves family physicians and other primary care doctors to continue and accelerate screening for these cancers so far as practicable as patients grow older. This activity should be limited only by the interaction of the life expectancy of the given cancer when not diagnosed in a timely fashion as measured against the life expectancy of the patient.

8. The answer is D, depression. There are two messages from this true-life experience. First, true sedatives should be used very judiciously in elderly people and for the most part avoided. Second, treating with a sedative any "nervous" or somewhat agitated state in elderly individuals can aggravate or even precipitate depression. The patient did not demonstrate Parkinsonian or supranuclear palsylike symptoms except for the facial flatness. AD was ruled out by the patient's rapid intellectual recovery when she stopped taking the diazepam. Delirium is acute organic brain syndrome, whose symptoms she did not manifest.

9. The answer is A. Disturbance of consciousness is the one criterion among those listed that does not fit AD. In addition, supporting evidence (but lacking specificity) includes loss of motor skills, family history of AD, and cerebral atrophy on a computed tomography scan. The latter, however, is found frequently in ages even as young as the 70s while the subject may continue to function and grow intellectually. That said, all reversible causes of dementia must be ruled out. In addition to those conditions discussed in Question 4, these conditions include chronic anemia, hypothyroidism, vitamin deficiencies, electrolyte imbalance, disease related to acquired immunodeficiency syndrome and human immunodeficiency virus, congestive heart failure, and seizure disorders.

10. The answer is E. Cholinergic agonist activity is the effect that has been found to convey a limited benefit for AD. This activity has been effected through cholinesterase inhibition in donepezil and tacrine. Tacrine has not worked out well because of a high incidence of gastrointestinal symptoms – particularly gastroesophageal reflux, nausea, and vomiting (28%), as well as diarrhea (14%). Anticholinergic activity aggravates the pathophysiology of AD, as witnessed by the aggravation of confusion in AD patients and precipitation of confusion in other old-old

people by the use of such anticholinergic drugs. Examples of the latter are trihexyphenidyl (Artane) and benztropine (Cogentin), medications that are used to treat rigidity in Parkinson disease.

11. The answer is D. Terazosin (Hytrin), when used to combat benign prostatic hyperplasia or as an antihypertensive, may cause urinary incontinence, especially in women. Each of the other choices has anticholinergic activity as a significant part of their pharmacologic effectiveness or as a significant side effect. Thus, urinary retention is a logical sequela. Each of the choices has legitimate applications in the aged population but must be utilized prudently. Other drugs with anticholinergic side effects include vincristine (anticancer drug); all the other calcium channel blockers; all antihistamines; thioridazine (antipsychotic drug) and many other antipsychotic agents; and opiates, including hydrocodone, benztropine, and many others.

References

Dickman R. Care of the elderly. In: Rakel RE, ed. *Textbook of Family Practice*. 6th ed. Philadelphia: WB Saunders; 2002:88–130.

Johnston B, Harper GM, Landefeld S. Geriatric medicine. In: Tierney LM, McPhee SJ, Papadakis MA, eds. *Current Medical Diagnosis and Treatment*. 45th ed. New York: McGraw-Hill/Appleton & Lange; 2006:49–66.

Lyon C, Clark DC. Diagnosis of acute abdominal pain in older patients. *Am Fam Physician*. 2006; 74:1537–1544.

chapter 53

Hematology in Primary Care

1 The newborn has a relative polycythemia with a hemoglobin range of 16.5 to 21.5 g/dL that declines to levels whose range is roughly 10 to 16 g/dL before slowly correcting to a more narrow range in the pre-teen years. At what age does the infant's hemoglobin range reach the nadir?

(A) 15 to 30 days

(B) 1 to 2 months

(C) 3 to 5 months

(D) 6 to 11 months

(E) 4 to 7 years

2 Which of the following is true regarding iron-deficiency anemia?

(A) Mean cell volume (MCV) is higher than normal.

(B) Mean cell hemoglobin is elevated.

(C) Variability of red blood cell distribution width (RDW; range of red blood cell diameter) is increased.

(D) The ratio between the red blood cell count in millions and the hemoglobin is increased.

(E) Serum ferritin is elevated.

3 A 24-year-old woman has been suffering from prolonged and frequent menses (i.e., menometrorrhagia) for 7 months. She now complains of light-headedness when she stands erect from sitting. She weighs 120 lb (54.4 kg) at a height of 5 ft, 4 in. (1.63 m). Her blood pressure sitting is 110/80 with a regular heart rate at 80 beats per minute, and she exhibits the following readings upon standing erect: Immediately the blood pressure falls to 105/70; at 15 seconds after standing, 100/70; 30 seconds, 95/60 with a heart rate of 120 beats per minute; 45 seconds, 100/60; 60 seconds, 105/70. Her blood hemoglobin

level is 10 g/dL. Which of the following laboratory test results are most likely those of this patient?

(A) Serum iron level of 100 µg/dL, total iron-binding capacity (TIBC) of 300 µg/dL

(B) Serum iron level of 200 µg/dL, TIBC of 300µg/dL

(C) Serum iron level of 40 µg/dL, TIBC of 120 µg/dL

(D) Serum iron level of 40 µg/dL, TIBC of 400 µg/dL

(E) Serum ferritin level of 200 ng/mL

4 A 55-year-old white man has complained of impotence and arthralgia for several months. He complains of morning stiffness involving both proximal and distal interphalangeal (PIP and DIP) joints. His hemoglobin is 17 g/dL and routine chemistries show mild (≤50%) elevations of alanine aminotransferase and aspartate aminotransferase levels. Which of the following test results is most likely to represent this patient?

(A) Serum iron level of 100 µg/dL, TIBC of 300 µg/dL

(B) Serum iron level of 200 µg/dL, TIBC of 300 µg/dL

(C) Serum iron level of 40 µg/dL, TIBC level of 120 µg/dL

(D) Serum iron level of 40 µg/dL, TIBC level of 400 µg/dL

(E) Serum ferritin level of 200 ng/mL

5 An 83-year-old woman who has had late-onset rheumatoid arthritis for the past 10 years arrives for a routine periodic examination. She has had negative stool examinations for occult blood and has had no gastrointestinal symptoms. Her complete blood count showed anemia of chronic disease. Which of the following findings is compatible with that diagnosis?

(A) Decreased mean red cell hemoglobin content

(B) Increased mean red cell volume

(C) Serum iron level of 20 µg/dL, TIBC of 60 µg/dL

(D) Increased reticulocyte count

(E) Serum ferritin level of 1,000 ng/mL

6 Each of the following conditions is characterized by microcytosis and increased RDW variability, except for which one?

(A) Iron deficiency

(B) Lead poisoning

(C) Beta thalassemia

(D) Red cell fragmentation

(E) Renal insufficiency

7 A 55-year-old man enters the health care system in the office of a family doctor, complaining of problems of maintaining balance. His complete blood cell (CBC) count shows a hemoglobin of 6 g/dL (14 to 16) and an MCV of 110 fL (80 to 96). The neutrophil count is $2,500 \times 10^6$/L (3,000 to 5,800) and the platelet count is 100,000/mm^3 (150,000 to 300,000). The man takes no medications. He has also complained of lessening of his appetite and some diarrhea. Which of the following most likely explains his symptoms?

(A) Aplastic anemia

(B) Malnutrition

(C) Malaborption syndrome

(D) Blood dyscrasia

(E) Pernicious anemia

8 Regarding the patient in Question 7, for which of the following is he at increased risk?

(A) Peptic ulcer of the stomach

(B) Carcinoma of the stomach

(C) Carcinoma of the pancreas

(D) Colorectal cancer

(E) Prostate cancer

9 Which of the following is the best specific treatment for the patient in Questions 7 and 8?

(A) Folic acid 1 mg daily by mouth

(B) Vitamin B$_{12}$ 1 mg daily by mouth as maintenance therapy

(C) Vitamin B$_{12}$ 1 mg daily by intramuscular injection (IM) for maintenance therapy

(D) Vitamin B$_{12}$ 1 mg daily IM for 8 weeks followed by monthly dosing as maintenance therapy

(E) Vitamin B$_{12}$ 1,000 mg IM monthly as maintenance therapy

10 A 55-year-old overweight, smoking professional man with poorly controlled hypertension begins to complain of fatigue and anorexia. He decides to revisit his family doctor 6 months after he was originally scheduled. His medications are verapamil 80 mg three times per day and lisinopril 5 mg twice daily. However, the patient admits he often refilled his prescription late, and his medications lapsed an unknown numbers of weeks ago (after several telephoned refills well after the first missed scheduled follow-up visit, the doctor refused to refill further without a revisit). His blood pressure is 160/105. His serum creatinine level is 3.5 mg/dL (0.6 to 1.2) and his blood urea nitrogen (BUN) level is 85 mg/dL (11 to 23). His hemoglobin level is 10 g/dL (14 to 16) and hematocrit is 30; MCV is 85 fL (80 to 96) and mean red cell hemoglobin concentration is 32 g/dL (34 to 36). Urine urobilinogen is within normal limits and serum bilirubin is normal. A review of history finds no symptoms of gastrointestinal bleeding. The man's last renal function studies 1.5 years ago were within normal limits. Which of the following accounts for this patient's anemia?

(A) Blood loss

(B) Iron deficiency

(C) Nutritional folic acid deficiency

(D) Hemolysis

(E) Suppression of erythropoietin

11 A 34-year-old woman has had four bouts of deep vein thrombosis, one of which resulted in pulmonary embolism. None was associated with trauma or occurred after a surgical procedure. A thorough evaluation for occult malignancy has turned up none. There is therefore a strong possibility of an inherited coagulopathy. Which of the following is the most likely cause?

(A) Protein C deficiency

(B) Resistance to protein C activation

(C) Deficiency of protein S

(D) Antithrombin III deficiency

(E) Prothrombin nucleotide mutation

12 A 45-year-old man suffered a pulmonary embolus during his second bout of deep vein thrombosis. During the therapeutic phase, it was noted that heparinization was not quite successful in bringing the partial thromboplastin time into the therapeutic range and that anticoagulation was not achieved until the fifth day through normal oral warfarin anticoagulation. Which of the following was the cause of the hypercoagulability?

(A) Protein C deficiency

(B) Resistance to protein C activation

(C) Deficiency of protein S

(D) Antithrombin III deficiency

(E) Prothrombin nucleotide mutation

13 A 45-year-old man of Greek descent reports to his primary care physician with complaint of fatigue. Examination of the skin reveals telangiectasias about the face and upper chest. His weight is 195 lb (88 kg) at a height of 5 ft, 6 in. (1.68 m). Neurological review and examination are grossly normal, including position sense and stability with heels together standing and eyes closed and acral sensation. Routine laboratory studies show a BUN level of 10 mg/dL, a creatinine level of 0.8, an alanine aminotransferase level of 110 U/L (1 to 45), and an aspartate aminotransferase level of 76 U/L (1 to 36). The hemoglobin level is 10 g/dL. Hematocrit is 29, MCV is 120 fL (80 to 96), and the mean corpuscular hemoglobin concentration is 34 g/dL (32 to 26). Which of the following accounts for this patient's hematologic findings?

(A) Pernicious anemia

(B) Iron-deficiency anemia

(C) Hemolytic anemia

(D) Folic acid deficiency

(E) Beta thalassemia

14 A 16-year-old male African American patient has been seriously ill all his life with sickle cell disease. He displays sickled red cells with hemoglobin SS and generally runs a hemoglobin level of 8 g/dL. Each of the following is a potential cause of crisis in this patient, except for which one?

(A) Splenic sequestration

(B) Vaso-occlusive events

(C) Acute chest syndrome

(D) Hemolytic crisis

(E) Infarctions caused by polycythemic crises

15 A 45-year-old busy male attorney complains of headaches and generalized pruritus. He flew into this eastern American city from Denver, Colorado to attend a high-level legal conference. He smokes 1 pack of cigarettes per day. He denies recent upper respiratory tract infection, foci of specific pain, and urinary and gastrointestinal symptoms. On examination he manifests a blood pressure of 160/105, a temperature of 98.6°F, a ruddy complexion, and splenomegaly and hepatomegaly. Blood gases are not immediately available. His CBC showed the hemoglobin level to be 18 g/dL, the white blood cell count to be 14,000, and the platelet count to be 700,000. Red blood cells are normochromic and normocytic. The BUN level is 18 mg/dL and the creatinine level is 1.1 mg/dL. Urinalysis is within normal limits with a specific gravity of 1.015. Which of the following is the diagnosis?

(A) Polycythemia vera

(B) Secondary polycythemia from altitude accommodation

(C) Secondary polycythemia caused by chronic obstructive pulmonary disease

(D) Spurious polycythemia from dehydration caused by air travel

(E) Secondary polycythemia compensating for carboxyhemoglobin in a heavy smoker

16 A 65-year-old woman complains of pain in the back and chest with localized tenderness at the spine of T8 and ribcage pain with tenderness at the right seventh rib. The patient appears to be quite pale and admits to fatigue. These symptoms have come on gradually over a period of several weeks, with the back pain becoming the reason for consulting the physician. A dip urinalysis shows proteinuria. Screening CBC reveals a normochromic, normocytic anemia with 8 g/dL of hemoglobin and marked rouleau formation with normal platelets and white cell counts and morphology. Serum chemistry results include calcium elevation to 12.2 mg/dL with normal alkaline phosphatase. Plain x-rays show a fracture of the right seventh rib and compression of the eighth vertebra. Of the following, which is the most likely diagnosis?

(A) Alcoholism

(B) Metastatic carcinoma

(C) Multiple myeloma

(D) Waldenström macroglobulinemia

(E) Severe osteoporosis

17 A 26-year-old man has noted painless swelling in the left side of his neck. Further, he has noted afternoon chills and night sweats for several weeks. He has stopped smoking because inhaling tobacco smoke makes him ill. Although he seldom drinks alcohol, during the past week he took a glass of wine and only then noted pain in the swelling about the neck. Examination is unremarkable except for the neck, which exhibits a firm irregular mass measuring approximately 3 cm × 5 cm located in the left anterior cervical region. The CBC and laboratory chemical battery are within normal limits. Which of the following is the most likely significant cause of these symptoms?

(A) Hodgkin disease

(B) Sialoadenitis

(C) Viral respiratory tract infection

(D) Streptococcal pharyngitis

(E) Carotid artery aneurysm

Examination Answers

1. The answer is B; 1 to 2 months is the low point of hemoglobin and the level at which it remains until the child reaches about the age of 8 years. In a comparison of the analogous hematocrit level, the months of 3 to 11 reveal a relative hypochromia (hemoglobin-to-hematocrit ratio of <1:3). This begins to be corrected after the growth rate slows markedly after the child's first birthday. If we assume these data apply to the population at large and all socioeconomic groups, then the reason for the lag in correction to the teen levels is quite likely due to iron deficiency, which reflects the rapid growth in the first year that outruns the dietary iron. The latter reveals that too often the hemoglobin of the growing infant is still not checked frequently enough or that iron-fortified formula is not being prescribed as a routine in the majority of well baby care practice. Either is acceptable, as some practitioners prefer to forego iron-fortified formula because of frequent gastrointestinal side effects, usually hard stools. In lieu of fortified formula, hemoglobin should be checked by about 9 months; in many cases, iron should be prescribed separately when needed.

2. The answer is C. Variability of red cell width (range of RDW) is increased in iron deficiency. MCV is lower than normal in iron deficiency (i.e., the anemia is microcytic). Mean cell hemoglobin is lower than normal (i.e., hypochromic). The ratio between the red cell count in millions and the hemoglobin is lower than normal, which is another indication of hypochromia. The serum ferritin level is low, reflecting low total body iron stores, a condition that exists before the hemoglobin begins to fall in iron deficiency.

3. The answer is D. A serum iron level of 40 μg/dL and a TIBC of 400 μg/dL would be an expected relationship between serum iron and TIBC, given the probability of iron-deficiency anemia in a woman with prolonged menometrorrhagia. A serum iron level of 100 μg/dL and a TIBC of 300 μg/dL (Choice A) represents virtually the median normal values for iron and TIBC and the ratio of 1:3 is expected (i.e., the transferrin saturation of 33% is the median point of normal). In iron deficiency, as the serum iron falls, the iron-binding capacity rises in a homeostatic response. A serum ferritin level of 200 ng/mL, an indirect measure of total body iron, represents 2 g, where normal is 1 to 4 g of total body iron. In iron

deficiency, the total body iron level will have fallen to well less than 1 g by the time the serum iron level begins to fall.

4. The answer is B, serum iron level of 200 μg/dL and TIBC of 300 μg/dL. The transferrin saturation (serum iron/TIBC) is 67%, although normally it is about 33%. Elevated transferrin saturation is found in hemochromatosis. This tendency to overabsorb iron is inherited in a Mendellian dominant mode, whereby, by the age of 50, men may become symptomatic with arthritis similar to rheumatoid arthritis, except that the DIP as well as the PIP joints are involved. In rheumatoid arthritis, metacarpophalangeal joints and PIP joints but not the DIP joints are involved. Impotence may be the presenting complaint and hepatocellular liver disease may lead to cirrhosis and ultimately hepatocellular carcinoma. The ferritin level rises throughout life, whereas the elevated transferrin saturation is present virtually from infancy. A ferritin level of 1,000, analogous to 10 g of total body iron, leads to iron deposition in literally the whole body and its organs, causing liver and heart disease most critically. Heterozygotic individuals may also absorb excess iron if they use medicinal iron or vitamin C and if they imbibe alcohol excessively. Females, as a result of their physiological monthly blood loss, are not likely to become symptomatic until the age of 60 years.

5. The answer is C, serum iron level of 20 μg/dL and TIBC of 60 μg/dL. Note that the serum iron level (normal is 100 μg/dL) and the TIBC (250 to 410 μg/dL) are each decreased by the same proportions so that the transferrin saturation remains at about 33%. This is seen most often in aged individuals but may occur as well in younger people who are chronically ill. Mean cell hemoglobin and MCV should be normal. Ferritin level should also be normal, reflecting normal iron stores. The ferritin example given is abnormally high, in the range of hemochromatosis. The reticulocyte count increases in recovery from reversible anemias, such as iron deficiency, and in other conditions calling for increased erythropoiesis, such as hemolytic anemias.

6. The answer is E. Renal insufficiency is not associated with a microcytic anemia and in fact is characterized by a normocytic, normochromic anemia brought about by failure of erythropoiesis. Iron deficiency, as previously discussed, manifests hypochromic, microcytic anemia with increased RDW. The other conditions show microcytosis and increased RDW but are normochromic.

7. The answer is E. Pernicious anemia manifests a macrocytic peripheral picture and may reach strikingly low hemoglobins. Further, late in the course, one finds a neutropenia with hypersegmented cells and thrombocytopenia. The proximate cause is vitamin B_{12} (cobalamin) deficiency, which in pernicious anemia comes about as the result of a lack of intrinsic factor, needed for dietary B_{12} absorption. Cobalamin is also a cofactor in the conversion of folate to its active form; thus, folic acid therapy may go a long way in redressing the macrocytic anemia in pernicious anemia. Cobalamin deficiency may occur in dietary deficiency and malabsorption (e.g., in sprue) but these two conditions are comparatively rare. The red cell aberrations are identical in the three diseases. Marrow aplasia, which may be expressed as aplastic anemia or as pure red cell aplasia, is characterized by normochromic, normocytic red cells. The neurologic complications of pernicious anemia are peripheral neuropathy (stocking–glove hypesthesia) followed later by posterior column degeneration, which accounts for balance problems (subacute combined degeneration). Atrophic gastritis is a heralding condition and is associated with other gastrointestinal symptoms. Differentiation from blood dyscrasias and the other macrocytic anemias in the absence of neurologic complications is achieved by the finding of an abnormally low B_{12} level. Differentiation from nutritional B_{12} deficiency is effected by the finding of elevated methymalonic acid, the product of the metabolic arrest in the development of cobalamin.

8. The answer is B. Carcinoma of the stomach is a significant risk for patients with pernicious anemia. Preceding the failure of B_{12} production in the gastric mucosa, it has undergone atrophic change on an autoimmune basis. Atrophic gastritis is subject to carcinoma. Pernicious anemia is an autoimmune disorder and is associated with other autoimmune diseases, such as thyroiditis, Graves disease, and vitiligo.

9. The answer is D. Vitamin B_{12} 1 mg daily IM for 8 weeks followed by monthly dosing as maintenance therapy is the regimen for pernicious anemia with neurologic complications. Treatment of pernicious anemia must be parenteral, as the intrinsic factor produced in the stomach needed for absorption of cobalamin is by definition lacking. Eight weeks of more intense therapy is needed for expedient alleviation of the subacute combined degeneration. At that time, maintenance treatment for prevention of recurrence anemia is just 1 mg monthly IM. Folic acid treatment

reverses the anemia but not the neurologic complications. In the not too distant past, many practitioners were giving monthly doses of intramuscular cobalamin (B_{12}) ten times the maintenance dosage (i.e., 1,000 mg) for pernicious anemia, often for a symptom, such as fatigue. Similarly, iron had been prescribed without specific diagnosis of the anemia or often without any findings whatever except for the symptom of fatigue.

10. The answer is E. Suppression of erythropoietin (EPO) is the proximate cause of anemia in chronic renal failure. Frequently other mechanisms make anemia of renal failure a condition of mixed causation. For example, chronic renal failure is frequently associated with gastrointestinal bleeding and attendant iron deficiency as well as hemolytic mechanisms. However, this patient's anemia is normocytic and normochromic. The patient's lack of elevated urine bilinogen and serum bilirubin levels rules out hemolysis. Folic acid deficiency would produce a macrocytic anemia. Treatment with EPO is the mainstay of management. However, in the frequent presence of low iron stores, many patients with endstage renal disease have had significant blood loss. Insofar as EPO replacement requires iron incorporation in the process of erythropoiesis, iron, often parenteral, should be part of the treatment.

11. The answer is B. Resistance to protein C activation (resistance to anaphase-promoting complex activation) is the cause of 50% of cases of venous thrombosis not accounted for by another explicable cause. This abnormality is a mutation in Leiden factor V and thus produces a functional deficiency of protein C, which normally works in part by inactivating Leiden factor V. Protein C otherwise prevents hypercoagulability by inactivating coagulation factors V and VIII. Inherited deficiency of protein C accounts for 5% of otherwise unexplained deep vein thrombosis. Protein S functions with and depends on vitamin K as an endogenous anticoagulant factor. Inherited deficiency of protein S is a less common form of constitutional hypercoagulability. Prothrombin nucleotide mutation occurs in the prothrombin gene wherein adenine is substituted for guanine at position 20210. The result is excessive levels of prothrombin and hypercoagulabilty, the second most common cause of otherwise unexplained venous thrombosis.

12. The answer is D. Antithrombin III deficiency is associated with a relative resistance to heparin because heparin is a cofactor in the physiologic function of antithrombin III. Thus, heparin needs antithrombin III presence for its effectiveness. In cases in which heparin resistance is encountered, fresh-frozen plasma should be given along with heparin.

13. The answer is D. Folic acid deficiency explains a macrocytic anemia in an alcoholic who displays no signs of posterior column abnormalities or peripheral neuropathy. Alcoholism is nearly certain, given the macrocytic anemia, lower than expected BUN and creatinine levels (insufficient protein intake), mild hepatocellular enzyme elevations with alanine aminotransferase more strikingly so, and the physical stigmata of telangiectasias. (These are the form fruste of spider angiomata.) The discussion of Question 7 covers most of the reasoning for this unit. Pernicious anemia manifests a macrocytosis but with eventual neurologic involvement. Iron deficiency shows a microcytosis and hypochromia; hemolytic anemias manifest increase in urine urbilinogen and elevated unconjugated serum bilirubin levels; beta thalassemia is a hemolytic anemia that happens to manifest microcytosis and normochromia. Both beta and alpha thalassemias tend to occur in Mediterranean ethnic groups. The presentation of the patient as being of Greek descent was a red herring.

14. The answer is E. Infarctions that are due to polycythemic crises do not occur as sequelae of sickle cell disease (SCD). On the contrary, SCD is, of course, a condition of anemia, not polycythemia. The African American infant with SCD is typically well until 6 to 8 months of age while his predominantly fetal hemoglobin is gradually replaced by hemoglobin S (SS), in a homozygous sickle cell sufferer. After that age he may begin suffering from bouts of severe pain caused by splenic red cell sequestration, and he manifests splenomegaly. In addition, the patient often suffers from dactylitis. By the time the infant reaches the age of 2, the spleen has infarcted to the point of atrophy and functional asplenia. Most of the critical events attendant to SCD are directly or indirectly related to sludging of red cells and concomitant vaso-occlusive phenomena. The sludging is based mostly on the central hypovolemia resulting from massive splenic sequestration of red cells. Microinfarctions of various tissues, such as mesentery and bone, are results of sludging. Bone infarctions cause aseptic necrosis of the humorus and femoral heads. There is also an acute chest syndrome that carries a 10% mortality rate and is thought to be based on microvascular pulmonary infarctions, occasionally leading to pulmonary embolism. Unrelated directly to vaso-occlusive disease is the hemolytic crisis that may occur in SCD and, if not recognized, may lead to acute heart failure within a few hours.

15. The answer is A. Polycythemia vera involves increased levels of all the formed blood elements. The only other problem choice that fits that picture would be Choice D, spurious polycythemia caused by dehydration and hemoconcentration. The latter is ruled out by the relatively dilute urine. Secondary polycythemia caused by altitude, chronic lung disease, or smoking should involve only the erythroid elements. Polycythemia vera is a myeloproliferative disorder that is characterized by hypervolemia (hence hypertension), plethora, splenomegaly, and generalized pruritus. There is a significant chance of evolution into myeloid leukemia. Thrombotic disease is a frequent complication caused by the increased viscosity of the blood. Treatment historically has been phlebotomy, and this is still used. Also in the past, more definitive therapy included (radioactive) ^{32}P. Presently hydroxyurea or anagrelide are used for myelosuppression. Low-dose aspirin is employed for prevention of thromboses.

16. The answer is C, multiple myeloma. The most common presentations are complaint of bone pain, pathologic fractures, pallor, and symptoms of fatigue; and laboratory findings of normocytic normochromic anemia and hypercalcemia. Metastatic carcinoma to bone usually is characterized by elevated alkaline phosphatase. Multiple myeloma features lytic but not blastic bone lesions; hence alkaline phosphatase is not elevated and such pathologic fractures will not show on radionuclide bone scan. Plain x-rays may demonstrate the typical lytic "punched out" metastatic lesions. Although proteinuria is not always present, as multiple myeloma proteins are light chain and not often found in the urine, proteinuria may be present early. Waldenström macroglobulinemia does not involve the bones and features heavy chain (hence the term *macroglobulin*) paraprotein. Although osteoporosis results in pathologic fractures, it would not explain the other findings in the vignette. (Occasionally osteoporosis may be the sole skeletal finding in multiple myeloma.) Serum protein electrophoresis readily demonstrates the monoclonal spikes. These occur in the beta or (gamma) globulin region in multiple myeloma, with 60% being immunoglobulin (Ig) G, 25% IgA paraprotein, and 15% light chain only. The spike occurs in the IgM region in Waldenström macroglobulinemia. The latter, because of the large chain protein, is characterized especially by hyperviscosity and problems attendant thereto. Bone marrow examination shows infiltration by plasma cells in multiple myeloma, comprising 5% to 100% of the content; in Waldenström macroglobulinemia, abnormal-appearing plasmacytic lymphocytes are seen in the marrow and in small numbers in the peripheral smear, whereas in multiple myeloma plasma cells are only rarely seen peripherally. One percent of all adults and 3% of people over the age of 70 years have monoclonal gammopathy of unknown significance, most commonly an IgG spike with less than 2.5 g/dL. In 25% of cases this progresses over a period of many years to overt malignancy. Nearly all patients with IgG spikes >3.5 g/dL prove to have multiple myeloma.

17. The answer is A. Hodgkin disease presents as a painless mass, often in the cervical lymph nodes or with constitutional symptoms suggesting low-grade fever. Nearly specific is pain in the lymphoid mass with alcohol ingestion and often intolerance to tobacco.

References

Linker CA. Blood. In: Tierney LM, McPhee SJ, Papadakis MA, eds. *Current Medical Diagnosis and Treatment*. 45th ed. New York: McGraw-Hill/Appleton & Lange; 2006:481–535.

McKnight JT, Eklund EA. Hematology. In: Rakel RE, ed. *Textbook of Family Practice*. 6th ed. Philadelphia: WB Saunders; 2002:1224–1275.

chapter 54

Drug Interactions, Caveats, and Primary Care

Examination questions: Unless instructed otherwise, choose the ONE lettered answer or completion that is BEST in each case.

1 A 34-year-old woman has been diagnosed with type II diabetes, with a 2-hour postprandial blood sugar level of 160 mg/dL. Her glycohemoglobin is 8% of the total. She has had no operations and her health is unremarkable except for her moderate obesity. The family doctor plans to start metformin. Which of the following must be measured before commencing with this plan?

(A) Complete blood cell count

(B) Liver function battery

(C) Lipid screen

(D) Serum creatinine

(E) Chest x-ray

2 Regarding the patient in Question 1, she has been started on metformin 500 mg twice daily. The family doctor considers placing her on an angiotensin-converting enzyme inhibitor (ACEI) in order to maximize preservation of renal function in a diabetic. The patient says that she is attempting to achieve pregnancy. Which of the following is a strict contraindication to this drug?

(A) Chronic renal failure

(B) Chronic obstructive lung disease

(C) Pregnancy in the second trimester

(D) Asthma

(E) Pregnancy in the first trimester

3 A 45-year-old man has been treated for hypertension with clonidine (e.g., Catapres), titrated to 0.2 mg daily. However, he has begun to complain of fatigue, and the primary care doctor makes a decision to change the antihypertensive medication to the beta-1 selective blocking agent, atenolol. Which of the following is the wisest method for making the change?

(A) Start the atenolol as 50 mg daily 2 days before discontinuation of the clonidine

(B) Start atenolol 4 days before the discontinuance of clonidine as 25 mg daily and increase it to 50 mg daily 2 days before the change

(C) Start the atenolol at the maintenance dosage of 50 mg on the day after the last dose of clonidine

(D) Discontinue clonidine and wait 2 days before starting atenolol at a prudent beginning dosage

(E) Taper the clonidine off as the atenolol is started low and accelerates, with the two drugs overlapping in their subtherapeutic levels over a 4-day period

4 A 48-year-old male patient has been treated for hypertension for several months. He weighs 170 lb (77 kg) at a height of 5 ft, 9 in. (1.75 m). A combination of drugs has been worked out for control of his blood pressure. On a routine monthly visit he complains of thirst and polyuria. His 2-hour postprandial blood sugar level is 200 mg/dL. The record shows that his mother and two maternal uncles have type II diabetes. Which of the following actions is the most logical next step?

(A) Start insulin 25 units of 70/30 human N/human R daily

(B) Start glyburide 5 mg twice daily

(C) Start metformin 500 mg twice daily

(D) Review the medication list

(E) Stop all medications, recheck the blood sugar in 2 days, and then add the medications back one every 4 days, while following blood sugars

5 Besides the manifestations of Cushing syndrome, which of the following may be a complication of systemic glucocorticoid administration over several weeks?

(A) Decreased insulin requirements in diabetics

(B) Lymphoproliferative disorder

(C) Atrophic gastritis

(D) Premature closure of epiphyses in growing children

(E) Glaucoma

6 A 24-year-old woman is being counseled for "nervousness." The doctor is contemplating prescribing diazepam (Valium). Each of the following should be caveats (causes to reconsider) in making this decision, except for which one?

(A) Presence of depression

(B) Suspicion of latent depression

(C) Ascertainment that there is no first-trimester pregnancy

(D) Presence of psychosis

(E) Presence of open-angle glaucoma

7 A 33-year-old woman is brought to an emergency department in stupor with a history of attempting suicide with a prescribed benzodiazepine. Which of the following is the specifically indicated drug for this emergency?

(A) Naloxone

(B) Buprenorphine

(C) Flumazenil

(D) Dextroamphetamine

(E) Phenobarbital

8 Trimipramine (Surmontil), a tricyclic antidepressant, has been prescribed for a depressed woman. (She had had an unfavorable experience with sertraline, under the brand name Zoloft; it is a selective serotonin reuptake inhibitor, or SSRI, antidepressant). To which of the following serious side effects must one be alert to if this patient is to be given tolteridine (Detrol, urinary antispasmodic agent) for her recurrent trigonitis that is causing urinary frequency?

(A) Bradycardia

(B) Gastritis

(C) Gastroesophageal reflux disease (GERD)

(D) Hyperpyrexia

(E) Decreased near point of visual focus

9 A 34-year-old male patient is seen by a physician for the first time; he presents himself as depressed and taking tranylcypromine (Parnate) prescribed by a doctor in another city for the past 4 months. The patient expressed doubt, insecurity, and frustration with the current regimen because of the necessity to avoid aged cheeses, wines, and other foods to avoid the risk of serious behavioral and neurological side effects. The adopting physician conducts her own interview and is satisfied that the man is indeed depressed and still in need of completing a 1-year course of medication. The new doctor is considering a change to fluoxetine (Prozac, an SSRI) for the patient's depression. Which of the following is the best technique for effecting the transition from tranylcypromine to fluoxetine?

(A) Continue tranylcypromine and start fluoxetine. Discontinue tranylcypromine after 2 days.

(B) Continue tranylcypromine and start fluoxetine. Discontinue tranylcypromine after 2 weeks.

(C) Discontinue tranylcypromine and start fluoxetine the next day.

(D) Discontinue tranylcypromine; wait 2 weeks before starting fluoxetine.

(E) Discontinue tranylcypromine and wait 4 weeks before starting fluoxetine.

10 A 45-year-old man is being treated for depression with tranylcypromine (Parnate, a monoamine oxidase inhibitor, or MAOI). Which of the following drugs is safe to administer while this patient is taking the MAOI?

(A) Dextroamphetamine

(B) Sertraline

(C) Amitriptyline

(D) Amoxicillin

(E) Dextromethorphan

11 Risperidone (Risperdal), an antipsychotic agent, is contraindicated in which of the following groups of people?

(A) Teenaged patients

(B) Elderly patients

(C) Schizophrenic patients

(D) Patients with pneumonia

(E) Patients with urinary tract infections

12 A 37-year-old male patient with schizophrenia has been treated with pimozide (Orap) with satisfactory control. He now has developed a community-acquired pneumonia. Which of the following antibiotics is contraindicated?

(A) Clarithromycin

(B) Ampicillin

(C) Amoxicillin

(D) Sulfamethoxazole

(E) Doxycycline

13 The high-potency topical glucocorticoid, betamethasone, is indicated for certain inflammatory skin conditions on a temporary basis. Each of the following side effects is known to be caused by prolonged application of this preparation, except for which one?

(A) Cushing syndrome

(B) Adrenocorticotropin suppression

(C) Systemic effects passed through breast milk

(D) Atrophy of the treated area of the skin

(E) Precipitation of diabetes

14 A 26-year-old woman who has a history of epilepsy but was taken off her anticonvulsant medication 5 years ago after 5 years of seizure freedom has now become pregnant and shows signs of developing pre-eclampsia. Initiation of a preventive anticonvulsant is contemplated. Which of the following would be safe for use in pregnancy?

(A) Carbamazepine (e.g., Tegretol)

(B) Phenytoin (e.g., Dilantin)

(C) Valproic acid

(D) Topiramate

(E) Magnesium sulfate

15 If a pregnant woman has been treated for dyslipidemia, which of the following drugs would be safe to continue throughout the period of gestation?

(A) Cholestyramine

(B) Gemfibrozil

(C) Simvastatin

(D) Atorvastatin

(E) Fenofibrate

16 Atorvastatin (Lipton) will have its blood levels increased when given in combination with each of the following, except for which drug?

(A) Ketoconazole

(B) Diltiazem

(C) Gemfibrozil

(D) Grapefruit juice

(E) Beta-adrenergic blocking agents

17 The anticoagulant warfarin interacts with many medications to increase its blood level, risking bleeding complications. Which of the following drugs in combination with warfarin acts to decrease warfarin blood levels?

(A) Dextrophenydate

(B) Rifampin

(C) Amiodarone

(D) Fluconazole

(E) Metronidazole

Examination Answers

1. The answer is D. The serum creatinine level must be checked before metformin is started. Lactic acidosis, albeit rare, has been reported with the usage of metformin in the presence of renal failure. The pharmaceutical guidelines state that metformin should not be prescribed if the serum creatinine level is above 1.5 mg/dL in male patients or 1.4 in female patients. Metformin should be held for 48 hours prior to general anesthesia. The foregoing is emphasized more in diabetics, the very group for whom it is prescribed.

2. The answer is C. Pregnancy in the second or third trimester is a firm contraindication for ACEIs and for angiotensin-converting enzyme receptor blocking agents (e.g., valsartan). These drugs may cause fetal injury or death. Although dry cough may be a side effect of ACEIs (not angiotensin-converting enzyme receptor blocking agents) and this may be a subclinical expression of asthma or reactive airway disease, a history of these conditions is not a contraindication to the use of ACEIs.

3. The answer is D. Discontinue clonidine and wait 2 days before starting atenolol at a prudent beginning dosage. Beta-blockers may exacerbate rebound hypertension following discontinuance of clonidine. Thus, if the beta-blocking agent is present when discontinuance of clonidine is contemplated, then the beta-blocker should be stopped 2 days before the clonidine. If the beta-blocker is to replace clonidine, then it should wait for 2 days after discontinuance of clonidine before being started.

4. The answer is D. Review the medication list. Although this patient is almost certain to become diabetic type II eventually, given the family history and the presence of hypertension, the combination of antihypertensive agents may include hydrochlorothiazide. The thiazide diuretics are said to reduce insulin sensitivity, aggravating the underlying conditions of the metabolic syndrome. In practice it appears that this effect is less a dose-related phenomenon than an individual susceptibility, albeit more likely in patients who have the metabolic syndrome. In such patients the blood may rise dramatically and subside just as dramatically when the hydrochlorothiazide is withdrawn.

5. The answer is E. Glaucoma as a complication of prolonged usage of glucocorticoids is perhaps not appreciated; it is less well known than side effects such as precipitation of diabetes, elevation of blood pressure, Cushing syndrome, aggravation of certain viral infections (varicella, herpes zoster keratitis), and osteoporosis. The other choices have no relationship to glucocorticoids and are true distracters.

6. The answer is E. The presence of open-angle glaucoma is not a contraindication for diazepam. Naturally, such glaucoma must be treated. However, diazepam is contraindicated in acute closed-angle glaucoma. (It may be postulated that the prescription of a sedative might be considered by some practitioners during the markedly painful phase of acute glaucoma; it should not be a benzodiazepine.) All sedatives may aggravate depression. Although one sees sedatives prescribed along with antidepressants by some psychiatrists, some antidepressants potentiate the effects of sedatives. A more imminent pitfall is to overlook latent depression in patients who are acutely anxious or in a panic state. Sedatives are not antipsychotic drugs, though they may be prescribed in adjunct by psychiatrists. Prescription during the first trimester of pregnancy is fraught with risk of fetal abnormality.

7. The answer is C. Flumazenil is a benzodiazepine receptor blocker and is specific for overdose of this family of drugs. Naloxone and buprenorphine are virtually complete and partial opioid antagonists respectively. Phenobarbital, one of the most ancient sedatives, would, of course, aggravate the sedative effects of the benzodiazepine. Dextroamphetamine, though a sympathomimetic medication, is not employed in sedative overdose management. However, dextroamphetamine inhibits gastrointestinal absorption of the sedative phenobarbital.

8. The answer is D. Hyperpyrexia has been reported when a patient on a tricyclic antidepressant is given an anticholinergic medication in addition. The basis of the interaction is the compounding of the anticholinergic effects of the two medications, producing a syndrome of overdose of an anticholinergic drug. Each of the other choices is incorrect as an answer to this question. Each of the "side effects" mentioned as distracters is actually a condition that would be ameliorated by the anticholinergic effects of the medications presented. Thus, this would be tachycardia, not bradycardia; reduction of acid production, salutary for both gastritis and GERD; and increase in near focal distance, concurrent with pupillary mydriasis and paralysis of accommodation.

9. The answer is D. Discontinue tranylcypromine; wait 2 weeks before starting fluoxetine. Under threat of hypertensive crisis, behavioral emergencies, hyperthermia and other problems, these two medications should not be given together and should not overlap in time.

10. The answer is D. Amoxicillin, so far as can be known by standard drug literature, is safe to use in conjunction with tranylcypromine. As an MAOI, tranylcypromine collects a long list of medications with which it should not be given in conjunction. These include all SSRI antidepressants (e.g., sertraline, paroxetine, fluoxetine), sympathomimetic agents (e.g., dextroamphetamine), tricyclic antidepressants (amitriptyline, imipramine), buspirone, bupropion, narcotics (e.g., dextromethorphan, oxycontin), antihypertensives, sedatives, diuretics, antihistamines, and alcohol, as well as the foods listed in the discussion of Question 9. In short, most primary care physicians feel that MAOIs should be prescribed only rarely and when no other drug fits the situation—generally deferring to psychiatrists for such as decision.

11. The answer is B. Elderly patients with dementia should seldom be treated with risperidone. In field studies, elderly individuals were 1.4 to 1.6 times as likely as placebo-taking subjects to die while under treatment. The deaths were most often due to cardiovascular and cerebrovascular events as well as infection. Therefore, if the drug is used in elderly people, those conditions as underlying or symptomatic should be ruled out before deciding in favor of starting the medication. None of the other conditions appears as definite or relative contraindications.

12. The answer is A. Clarithromycin in conjunction with pimozide (and with astimizole, cisapride, and terfenidine) may result in life-threatening ventricular dysrhythmias,

including ventricular tachycardia, ventricular fibrillation, and torsade du pointe. This is assumed to be related to inhibition of metabolism of these drugs by clarithromycin. The phenomenon occurs with erythromycin as well.

13. The answer is C. Systemic effects passed through breast milk have not been shown with topical applications of glucocorticoids on nursing mothers. All of the other effects mentioned, well known in association with oral or injected glucocorticoids, are possible as a result of the topical route.

14. The answer is E. Magnesium sulfate is the only drug among a list of 12 of the most well-known anticonvulsant medications that is known to be safe. The following are listed as posing significant risk to the fetus and are not to be used in pregnancy, especially during the first trimester: carbamazepine, fosphenytoin, phenobarbital, phenytoin, primidone, valproic acid, and lithium. The following show evidence of risk to the fetus and should be used only with caution and after fully informed consent of the prospective mother: clonazepine, ethosuximide, gabapentin, lamotrigigine, tiagabine, and topiramate.

15. The answer is A. Cholestyramine, colesevelam, and colestipol are known to be safe for pregnancy and the fetus. Gemfibrozil, fenofibrate, and especially all HMG-CoA reductase inhibitors place the fetus at risk.

16. The answer is E. Beta-adrenergic blocking agents do not appear on the lengthy list of medications that increase the blood levels of atorvastatin. That list, however, includes not only ketoconazole, diltiazem, gemfibrozil, and grapefruit juice but also bosentan, clarithromycin, cyclosporine, erythromycin, fluconazole, and itraconazole. The presence of fenofibrate with atorvastatin increases the chances of rhabdomyolysis.

17. The answer is B. Rifampin is among the few drugs that interact with warfarin to decrease its blood level, risking hypercoagulability and compromise of the therapeutic goal of the anticoagulant regimen. Other examples are tabulated in Table 54–1. Far longer is the list of drugs

TABLE 54–1 Tabulation of Drugs by Effect on Warfarin Levels or Risk of Hemorrhage

Raise Level	Lower Level or Otherwise Risk Bleeding
Barbiturates	amiodarone dextrophenydate
bosentan	cefamandole
capecitabine	cefmetazole
mercaptopurine	cefoperazone
phenytoin (chronic)	cefotetan
rifampin	chloramphenicol
carbamazepine.	fluconazole
	fluvoxamine
	itraconazole
	ketoconazole
	metronidazole
	phenytoin (acute)
	salicylates (specifically enhance bleeding chances)
	sulfamethoxazole
	ticlopidine
	voriconazole
	zafirlukast

that increase warfarin levels and exaggerate the anticoagulant effect (see Table 54–1).

References

Green GB, Harris IS, Lin GA, et al. *The Washington Manual of Medical Therapeutics.* 31st ed. Philadelphia: Williams & Wilkins; 2004.

Suarez RA, Fleming MF. Abuse of controlled substances. In: Rakel RR, ed. *Textbook of Family Practice.* 6th ed. Philadelphia: WB Saunders; 2002:1539–1547.